AF096876

WILD APOTHECARY

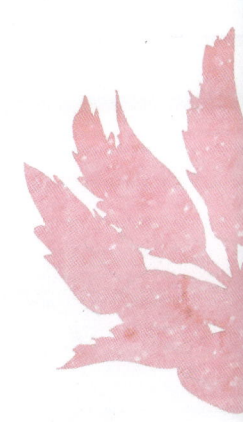

WILD APOTHECARY

Reclaiming Plant Medicine for All

By Amaia Dadachanji
With Claudia Manchanda

AEON

First published 2021 by
Aeon Books Ltd

Copyright © 2021 by Amaia Dadachanji

The right of Amaia Dadachanji to be identified as the author of this work has been asserted in accordance with §§ 77 and 78 of the Copyright Design and Patents Act 1988.

All rights reserved. No part of this publication may be reproduced, stored in a retrieval system, or transmitted, in any form or by any means, electronic, mechanical, photocopying, recording, or otherwise, without the prior written permission of the publisher.

British Library Cataloguing in Publication Data

A C.I.P. for this book is available from the British Library

ISBN-978-1-91280-723-9

Printed in Great Britain

www.aeonbooks.co.uk

With thanks to marbling artists extraordinaire, Luma and Millie, who marbled the galactic backgrounds together and are budding artists themselves and excellent baby herbalists.

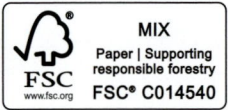
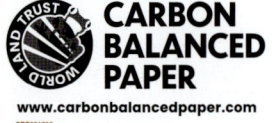

CONTENTS

Acknowledgements and about   vi

A wild welcome   ix

Chapter 1: Wild medicine, plant medicine and us   1

Chapter 2: Life with a wild apothecary   31

Chapter 3: Folk and flora, energetics of wild medicine   61

Chapter 4: Emerging buds: babes and children   73

Chapter 5: Opening buds: youth   117

Chapter 6: From bud to bloom: transitions   143

Chapter 7: Blossom: women   165

Chapter 8: Bloom: men   209

Chapter 9: Plant kin: wisdom of elders   233

Chapter 10: Back to the roots: grief   275

Chapter 11: Radical roots: decolonial reflections   291

The wild journey ahead   331

A few resources   337

Index   345

ACKNOWLEDGEMENTS

Amaia

"For all the baby, growing, and elder herbalists, healers, witches, and folk searching for meaning, understanding, and connection. And, especially, for anyone who didn't fit in, who was a little bit different, who felt on the edges or outside as I did as a light brown girl growing up in a community that didn't see her or her radiating light . . . this book is for you.

I hope this book inspires you to connect with the plants around you, to find a greater sense of yourself within landscape, flora and fauna, elements and spirit. I hope this book encourages you to tend yourself and know your worth.

And I would like to send all my love to my babies, my fire wren and my tiger rose. You have been patient watching Mama write and draw. May this work guide you when you need guidance and grow as you do so you find love, connection, resilience, fun, friends, skills, and plant allies. You know the fairies are there.

Thank you to all you who are already connecting people, plants, communities, elements, and land. To all the herbalists, activists, Land carers, and Indigenous folk who have spread their teachings, shared and cared."

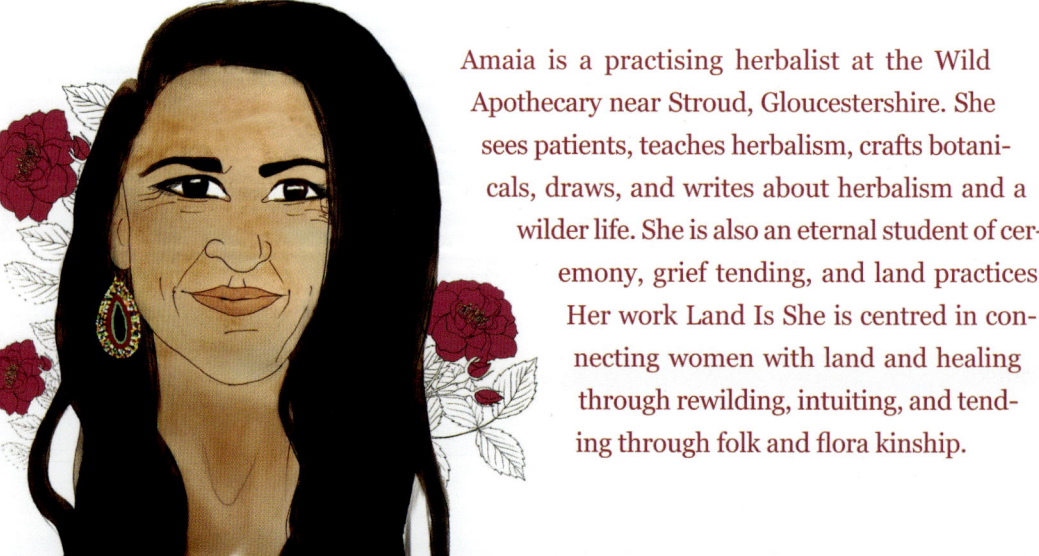

Amaia is a practising herbalist at the Wild Apothecary near Stroud, Gloucestershire. She sees patients, teaches herbalism, crafts botanicals, draws, and writes about herbalism and a wilder life. She is also an eternal student of ceremony, grief tending, and land practices. Her work Land Is She is centred in connecting women with land and healing through rewilding, intuiting, and tending through folk and flora kinship.

& ABOUT

Claudia

"This is dedicated to the memory of Belly Mujinga, (1970-2020) who was not protected. RIP"

Claudia Manchanda is a grandmother, radical herbalist, bioscientist, and lecturer who has a background in social justice activism, community cooking projects and cafes, and campaigns against deaths in custody. She lives in London doing patient advocacy, organising radical herb walks, and teaching integrated cancer care.

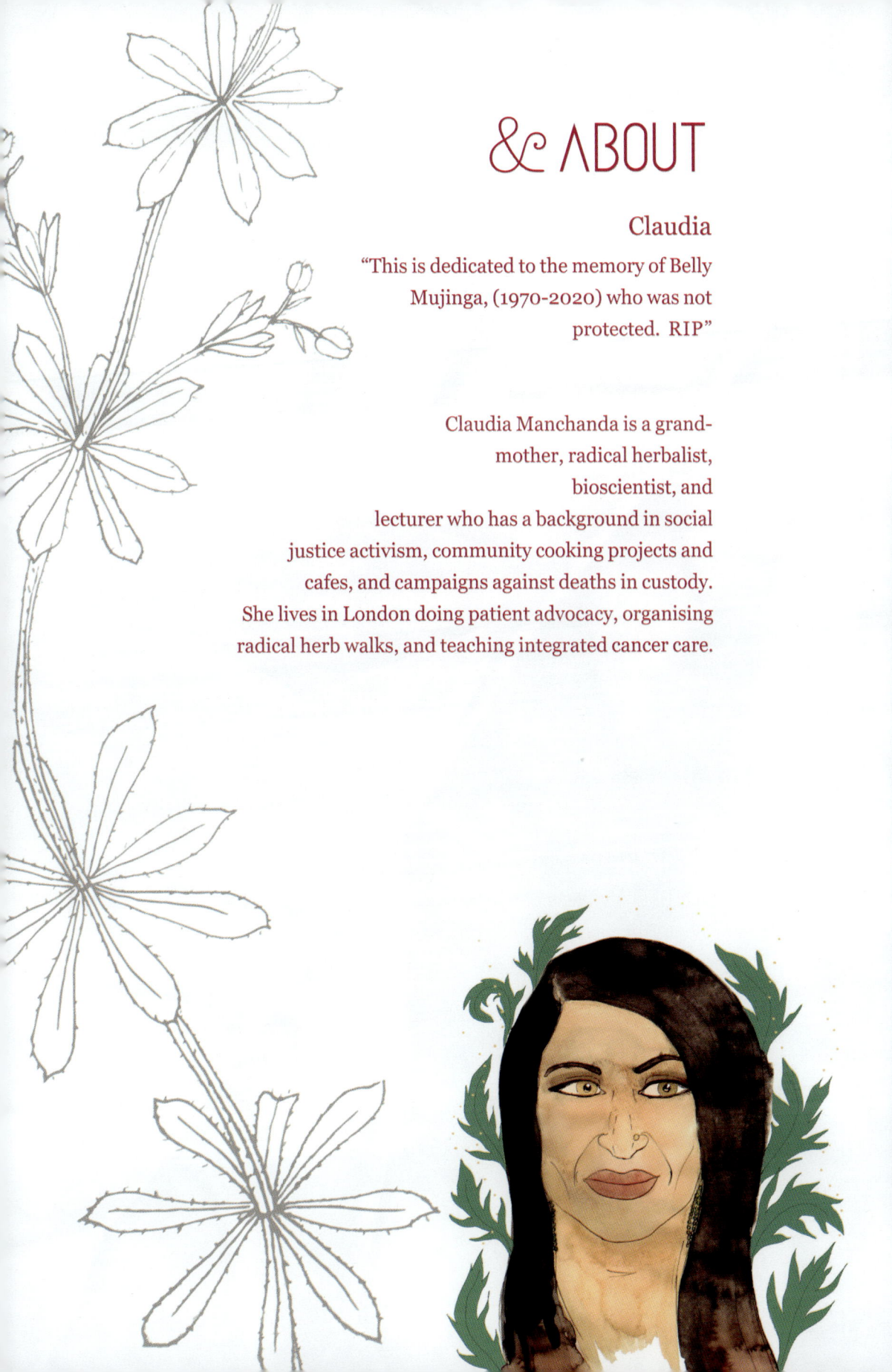

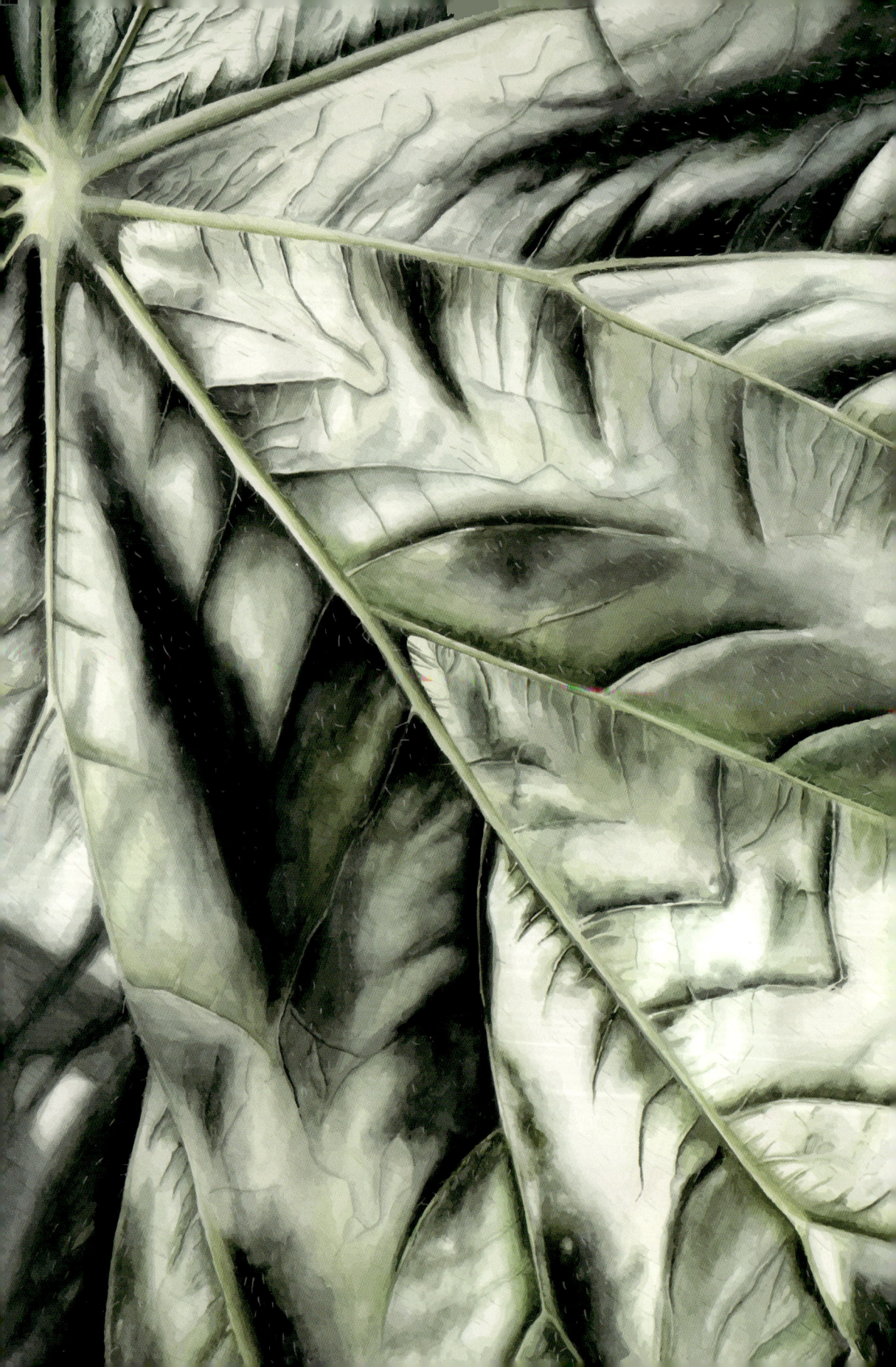

A WILD WELCOME

"What is the heart? A flower opening."

Rumi

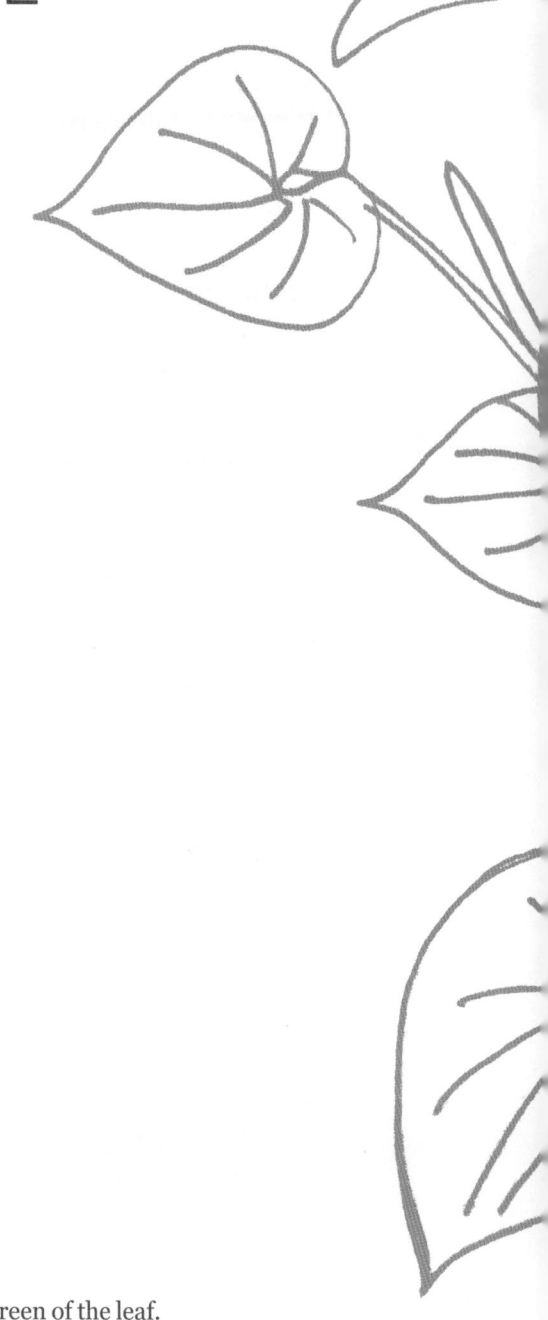

A *Begonia fusca* leaf, studied to enjoy the texture and green of the leaf. Connecting with this little beauty.

Wild | \ 'wī(-ə)ld \
Living in a state of nature and not ordinarily tame or domesticated
Growing or produced without human aid or care
Related to or resembling a corresponding cultivated or domesticated organism
Not inhabited or cultivated
Not amenable to human habitation or cultivation
Going beyond normal or conventional
Indicative of strong passion, desire, or emotion
Characteristic of, appropriate to, or expressive of wilderness, wildlife, or a simple or uncivilized society

Apothecary | \ ə-'pä-thə-ker-ē \
A person who prepared and sold medicines and drugs
"The growing presence of everyday medical practitioners, like apothecaries and druggists, made magic obsolete"
Apothecarius, from Latin apotheca, from Greek apothƒìkƒì ("storehouse")

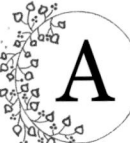

A wild apothecary … have you dreamed of one? I am guessing you have picked up this book because you are attracted to learning more about plant medicine and the relationship between plants and people.

There was a sudden moment in my life when I realised I couldn't do anything else but walk that path. Read on to find out more about wild medicine, people, and connection.

An apothecary has two meanings – it is she, they, or he who knows plants and their medicines, or it is a place in which plant medicines are kept. You could be or have either.

You only need the tiniest apothecary to be an apothecary. You may have peppermint tea in your cupboard or marigold cream in your bathroom. You may well already have an apothecary at home and are looking to expand it.

In these modern times we need to look to the plants to learn more about their uses and our relationship with them and the environment in which they grow.

To be a wild apothecary is a dream of mine, to have a wild apothecary is another.

When I was but a child I would listen. Lie down and listen.

    Hear the rustle of the grasses that lazily shimmered in the late afternoon sunshine.

My squinty eyes making out shapes of oak and ash, beech and birch.

    Slashes of red poppy and yellow hawkweed with splashes of green all around.

I did not know the names of those plants. But.

    I didn't need to then. I was happy to listen and look and just be in nature. A melancholic wistful dreamy child.

I did know some names though.

    There was one I knew well. One I had fallen into many times, gently brushed past many times and avoided many times if I wasn't wearing jeans.

One that stung.

    Yes, I knew stinging nettles. But not as well as I thought. That knowledge came later, and more is still to come.

I knew daisies and dandelions.

    I made daisy chains and learned how to tell the time with dandelion seeds (though perhaps not that well).

I knew oak trees had acorns and I could eat bramble berries.

    I knew that laurel cherries were poisonous but that I could climb to the top of the trees and they would hold me.

I knew that crab apples were worth collecting but were not for eating raw.

    I knew sycamore keys would act as helicopters and I could eat the beech nuts on the way home from school.

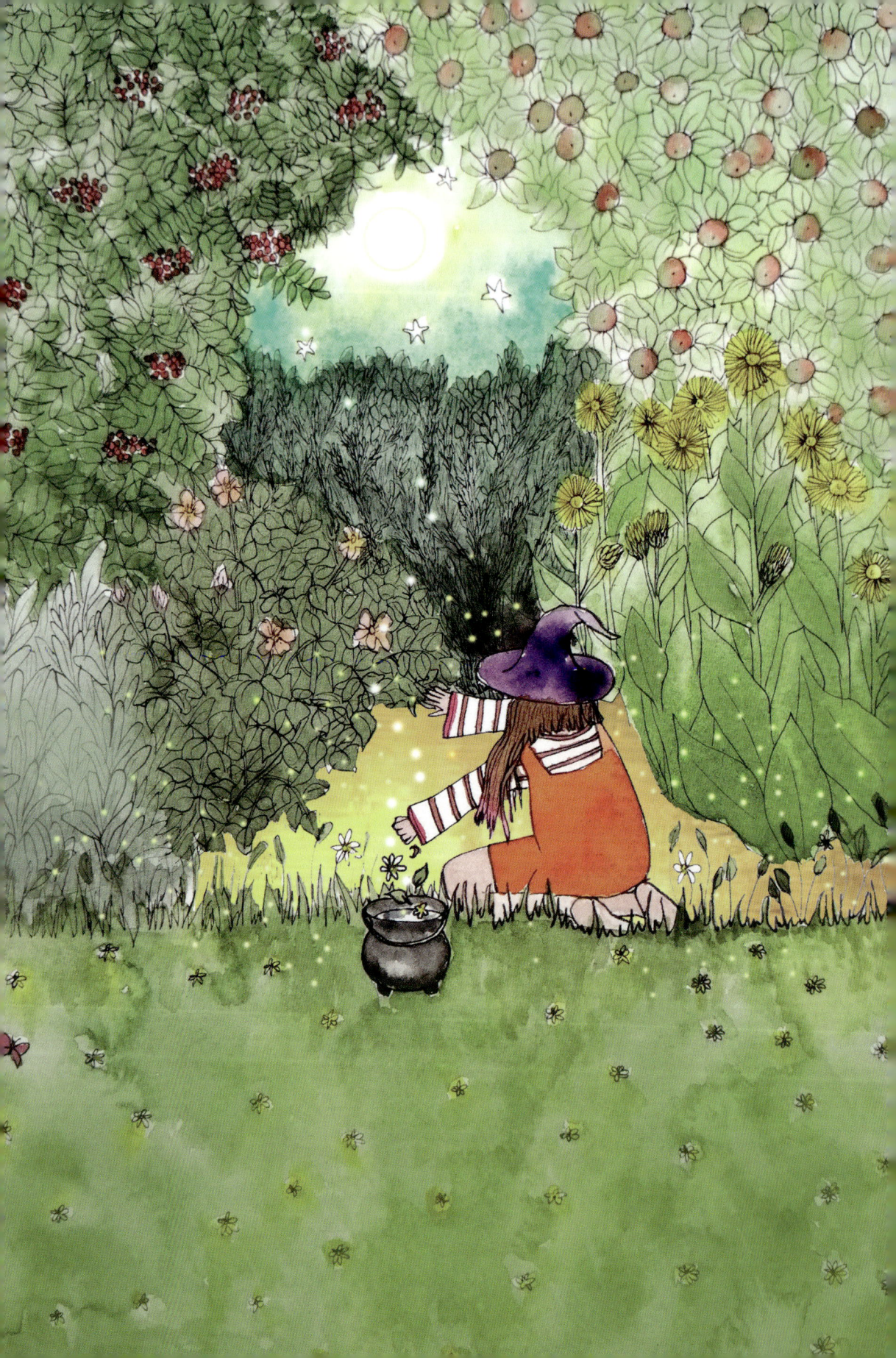

I knew I could suck the white flowers of white deadnettle (though they were just honeydew flowers to me) and taste sweet nectar.

And I wished. I wished, really wished, I would have found little nature spirits at the bottom of those trees and hedges. I wished for the little robins and black crows to come and talk to me. I wished for the foxes to not hide and the hedgehogs to manifest. I contented myself with hedgerow searching. Not sure what for, but searching all the same.

Little hedge witches – children, as a witch to me is genderless, anyone connected to their natural world who sees the magic – are looking under hawthorn hedges and behind foxgloves as we speak, whether for fairies or caterpillars or for what I am not sure, but they are.

I was a child, you were a child, and it is so telling that kids have a natural curious bond with nature – with the plants and trees that surround us. They look to play.

Do you?

Do you remember your first plant connection?

Do you remember the first time you touched a flower, leaf or root?

Do you remember your first fruit, maybe eating a scrumped apple, a wild blackberry or picking a strawberry from the garden or allotment, or cheekily from a local urban farm (I was six years old!)

Or perhaps you remember sitting under a tree, later wondering about how that apple fell directly on Newton's head or hoping the big cones of a pine weren't going to fall on yours.

Perhaps you remember touching objects of wood in your home, or fashioning swords and bows out of sticks.

My little tiger rose finding her magic under the hedgerow. She asks if magic is real and if her spells will work and I tell her of a different kind of magic, one that is nestled right there under that hedge.

Perhaps you remember the incredible scents of bluebells, lilac, or roses.

Maybe you remember the realisation that cucumbers are plants and pineapples grow on top of strange looking shrubs (check them out if you've not seen one!)

If you lived outside the UK, where I grew up, I wonder what the smells of your landscape were, what the colours and feelings were, are. How the different fruits and flowers affected you as a child and how you connected with plants.

I dreamt of finding ways of connecting our wilds with our health. Of walking in the elements and finding medicine to ease our suffering.

I dreamt of slowly becoming more and more knowledgeable about plants and people and the relations we bear or have lost.

I wandered alone trying to listen and be heard.

Sometimes the wind would whisper, sometimes an oak would shiver, sometimes I would find my feet had led me to a tiny plant ally and I would try to learn about that ally as best I could. But . . . often I was consumed in my thoughts of everyday life and they were so loud that listening properly was too difficult.

As I carried on trying to fathom this relationship with nature, *my* relationship with nature, people would sometimes mock me, telling me my connection to nature was false, insincere, or pathetic. Their views perplexed me and made me wonder why and how we, as humans, hurt each other.

Despite their views of me and their hard to hear words, I couldn't help but carry on, and little by little tune into the great wild web of plants and trees and their medicines. Building my own wild apothecary and my own understanding of my landscape.

As I learned to hear and heed my own being, so I learned that my touch upon an apple tree or my stillness by an ash tree are mine to experience and no one else's.

That my own connection cannot be quantified or philosophised, it simply is. It morphs and grows and ebbs and flows but it is what sustains me.

I've grown into a herbalist and through me others will learn, perhaps you will, that they too have deep, superficial, loud, quiet, subtle, beautiful, difficult relations with nature and plants. That they, you, can relate and learn and change and then learn some more. That no one else's experience can dull your own – that we can share and learn and move but we each have our own valid connection.

A WILD WELCOME

In this book I would love for you to find the courage to be your own apothecary, or baby herbalist, or indeed find the time or inclination to connect with nature in whatever way you can.

So thank you for picking up this book – I hope you find words that help you become a wild ally of the plants, or that this book leads you to making your own apothecary. I have travelled down this road and it is a beautiful one that is so vast we can never stop learning.

As I grew further into my herbalist self, I realised what an incredible journey this is. Of course, it doesn't have to be a huge journey for all folks – it may be simply that you would like to make some home remedies for yourself or kith and kin and that would be amazing. It is really important to me that we find wisdom and connection in the smallest of ways as well as in culture-changing systemic ways.

I wanted this book to also illustrate some of the challenges we, myself definitely included, need to rise up to within the world of herbalism. These include a sense of community, dismantling of the modern medicine paradigm and respect for and reconsideration of traditional medicines, the language used in botany and herbalism, cultural appropriation and learning from different cultures, racism and anti-racism, gender and sexual discrimination, and sovereignty. It turns out herbalism isn't immune to oppressive systems and it is up to us to challenge and change and all the while get our hands in the soil and listen.

This book serves to help you connect with nature, landscape, and community. It is a

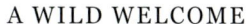

beginner's guide to herbalism and the practical applications of plant medicines in your home or community.

The book moves through the tools and makes of a herbalist, baby herbalists included, and on to the different stages of life from babes to elders and how plant medicines may be incorporated.

Towards the end of the book I have included a small chapter on grief which comes to us all at some point. Following this is a closer examination of the deconstruction of herbal medicine that is needed under the system of colonialisation, patriarchy, and capitalism.

I have invited the wonderful herbalist and sister Claudia Manchanda to write that chapter for us with details of many of the issues that face herbalism as we try to find our way to decolonialise practice.

At the back of the book is a resources guide – people, organisations, books, websites, and more that I or Claudia have found helpful or inspiring.

WEAVING PLANT MEDICINE
THE STRUCTURE OF THIS BOOK

From the page to the wilds and from the wilds to the page again . . . I hope this book will help you with wild harvesting, growing your own herbs, community, and herbal resilience, and of course making medicine and knowing some home remedies for you and your kin.

This book seeks to weave in the magic of the plant world, creating a volume that you can reference if you would like to use wild medicines in your lives.

It is also a companion for those who want to connect to nature more and feel pulled to explore the power of plants and connections with people.

There are so many plant medicines growing in this land and further afield and I want you, the reader, to be able to access some wild medicines that I, and other herbalists, use a lot in clinic.

I would love for you to become a little more empowered as to the best use, or common use, of plant medicine and how to make good remedies. So this book is by no means exhaustive but a prompt as to how and when to use herbs for common conditions.

Each chapter focuses on key herbs and common illnesses relevant to each stage of our lives – beginning with the emerging buds of babes and children and ending with elderhood and grief. At the end of the journey, we move to the realm of herbalism in general as Claudia guides us through the potted history of colonialism and how this affects our practice.

In each section there will be:

>A description of the phase of life and what we may experience
>Common health conditions
>Remedies and blends which are useful for those conditions
>Key plant allies
>Exercises and ceremony which pertain to each phase of life

We will weave in seasons, elements, and energetics, bringing the interconnection of cycles and elemental wonder. I hope we might create a world wild web of herbalistas, radical herbalists, baby herbalists, folk herbalists, medical herbalists, gardening herbalists, foraging folk, medicine makers, wise folk, and wild beauties.

"BIPOC" HEALTH AND HERBALISM

The healthcare system in Britain is not equal for all and health disparities are apparent for marginalised people.

So when thinking of access to health care, treatment of people and the outcomes or even mortality rates among different groups, it is important to be aware that all is not equal.

There is clear and well researched evidence that racialised people have worse experiences or outcomes in our healthcare system at present. Here are but a few of these eventualities, highlighting the need for social justice but also reminding us that each person needs tending and herbal care in their own individual way and based on their experience, taking into consideration genetics, social care, health care, access, their story, dreams, family, support, the list goes on.

Within our national healthcare system a severe lack of support is reported by all ethnic minorities

GALACTIC DANDELION – MOST EXCELLENT "WEED" IN THE WORLD

and in particular people of Pakistani and Bangladeshi origin. "BIPOC" patients are more likely to be given a diagnosis of mental illness than White British people. People of Black Caribbean and African origin or descent are also less likely to access psychiatric care through health services and more likely to access it through the criminal justice system.

Complications in pregnancy and childbirth including pre-eclampsia, as well as dying in childbirth, are vastly higher for Black women. Long-standing illnesses affecting the way we live our lives are most often experienced or reported by Pakistani women and Bangladeshi men. There are many more examples we could list here.

Being acquainted with the prevalence of social, genetic, cultural, and imposed health disparities for racialised people can inform your way of working with plant allies and tending your patients, family, or friends.
In the final chapter, Claudia explores the stories of Black, Indigenous, and People of Colour within herbalism.

ASTROLOGY IN HERBALISM

In the sections on plant allies in each chapter I've included the planet that the plant may be ruled by. I say "may" because there is some discussion about which plant is ruled by which planet.

In all traditional systems of medicine a connection to the astral bodies is significant in terms of diagnosis, cultivation, harvesting and preparation of herbs. Herbs are governed by astral bodies such as planets, the sun, and the moon, and each plant ally mentioned at the end of the chapters has a reference to its astrological affinity. Do find out more about this if it piques your interest.

An example which is commonly used is nettle. Nettle is governed by Mars, the red planet, which is hot and fiery and, thereby, considered masculine. The plants governed by Mars often have spikes or stings for protection and have an association in the body with the colour red. This may be, for example, a red nettle rash or the redness on our skin from the stings, urticaria (a rash which looks like nettle stings), a red face if a plant is heating, red berries, or its action on the blood.

Planets and timing may influence the herbalist to make a remedy with certain plants. You can harvest plants at certain times to increase alignment with planetary forces, according to the astrological charts each month, decade, or even century. Indigenous cultures often harvest this way with a complex knowledge of each plant and its vibration in the world.

A little aside

My name, Dadachanji, most likely means "chief astrologer, with respect" (Dada being chief, chan being moon, and ji, with respect) and while I haven't studied plants and planets in depth, it is something which calls me and there is a wealth of wisdom to be gained. Amazingly, Claudia's name, Manchanda, means "heart of the moon". She has studied planetary forces, alchemy, and medical astrology. I wonder, as I write, whether celestial forces (including the moon) brought us together at our chance meeting a few years ago at the beautiful memorial service for our friend, teacher, and mentor Christopher Hedley.

JOURNALING AND EXERCISES

As well as looking at various ways of approaching health and rewilding with wild medicines at different times of life, we will also explore exercises to help you connect with nature and self.

If you can, get or make yourself a journal just for plant connection in note form, drawing, or prose.

See how it feels to remember your first plant connections or interactions. A simple and yet very telling exercise is to jot down what you remember – any thoughts, feelings, images, colours, family or cultural connections, etc. Get a cuppa and take a little time to connect with that part of yourself. Whenever I think of my first plant experiences, I think of "my" apple tree, sucking dead nettles, and making my feet reach the tops of the "cheese trees" when I was pushed on a swing in the park. See what comes up for you.

When you have a journal, you can write all kinds of observations, from experiences with plants or tastings to medicines that worked well or totally failed (like my rosehip syrup into which I hadn't put enough sugar and bam! – explosion) and to new plants noted on the path to the local shop.

Consider having two books – one journal for writing about your connections with plants, your experience of the exercises we will do, and notes of experiments that you undertake by yourself, kind of like your own recipe book. A second book could be simply for medicine making – with all the notes that will help you in the future.

I am a sucker for a nice notebook so that might just be my own privilege talking. You don't have to spend a pretty penny on a pretty journal – I sometimes staple paper that has only been used on one side to make little notepads. Remember most little pads are made from plants, ink comes from earth . . . we are already connecting.

Plant connections are the beginnings of the herbal journey. Knowing your plants, in some way, is such a good way to get back to health or walk the path of the herbalist – be it as a professional or lay person.

A simple way to get back to your wild self is to spend time communing with and in nature, whether that's your local park, woodlands, the wilds of remote Scotland, a canal path, cracks in the pavement, or a community garden. Of course you can connect and enjoy the green with a plant in a pot or windowsill box.

There are lots of exercises you can do to tune back into plants, natural landscapes, etc. – in each section there will be opportunities to explore how you feel about the season, the elements, and exercises to help you try to connect to the plants around you at those times.

For example, a simple exercise might be:

Rewilding exercise – drawing maps

Take a walk next time you go out, or now if you have the time. Just a short one.

See if you can note down any of the plants you meet in ten minutes. You can do any of the following to get to know your area:

- Note down the plants you know

- Make a map of the plants you know

- Make notes on the plants you don't know – of course you can add them to your map without knowing them – describe them, how they look, how they make you feel (do you like them?)

This is the first of a few exercises in this book encouraging you to get to know your area and the plants that surround you. You could do it of your garden, of the local park, of the woods, of the local plants growing from the cracks in the pavement, etc. and make a map book of plant maps!

If you aren't able to walk, or find going outside challenging or impossible, you can do all of these exercises from your home, even your bed, if you use your senses to feel out to the elements and plants all around the area. You can also ask others to bring you plants and work with them. Adapt any exercise to your own body and ability (movement, senses, emotional needs).

WILDING YOURSELF . . . A LITTLE MORE

This book is a small part of the (re)wilding of ourselves that many of us need. It may be the result of privilege that we need to rewild ourselves – we have infrastructure, technology, urbanisation, transport, money . . . all things which inevitably take us further and further away from nature. While not everyone living in a city disconnected from nature could be called privileged by any means, privilege is certainly wildlessly abundant.

The need to rewild – or wild – ourselves may also be from our loss of connection and culture, our loss of tradition and understanding of the cycles of our land on which we live.

Getting to know our plants, our landscape, our feelings, our connection . . . The rewilding side of herbalism is so important to herbalists like me who find the biggest joy in life comes from the natural world but it is so often put aside to make money, entertain, fit in . . . we all need to reconnect and rewilding is a way of doing this.

What does rewilding yourself mean to you?

What do the words

      wild

                  ancestors

                                      apothecary

          wild medicines

                                                    roots

    plant allies   natural

                    land

                                      forage

  rewild   resilience

                                                herbalism

bring to you?

What do you see in your mind's eye?

How do they make you feel?

Take a moment to see if any excite you or fill you with hope or dread, anger, or wonder. Just a little time spent feeling out these words might illuminate the path you may be instinctively drawn to. It may be that you find wild a difficult word, unsafe and savage (in French *sauvage* is wild, in Spanish *salvaje* is wild . . .) you may find these words too woo woo or crass. Take some time to consider where you're at with them and just notice.

Rewilding. Not to be confused with the now more commonly used term for rewilding the land. No, I'm talking "rewilding the self". Getting to know yourself and your connection in and to nature. We are, of course, part of nature and not distinct from it but we often think of "us" and "nature" as separate. This may be especially true if we live in towns or cities and spend a great deal of time inside, sitting in cars, buses, or trains, and eating food wrapped in plastic or made for us.

Small steps to honour our natural selves is all it takes to become more in tune with natural cycles, local plants, seasonal flora, and the rhythms that nurture us. One small step might be going outside today or tonight and breathing in the scent of the local plants around you, listening for any birdsong, and touching some soil. Cooking, or growing, your own food or using natural products may be another small step.

Each time you spend a little wild time with plants or elements you become a little more rooted or grounded and connected with the magic of the plant world.

In our view (myself and Claudia), there is no such thing as an expert herbalist, there are many experienced and learned herbalists and we try to learn as we grow. We learn and unlearn, then learn some more and then unlearn again. We have tried to make this book inclusive, inspiring and informative and we are aware that language is constantly evolving as is our understanding. We would welcome constructive criticism.

Lucinda Warner's 'Bioluminescence'

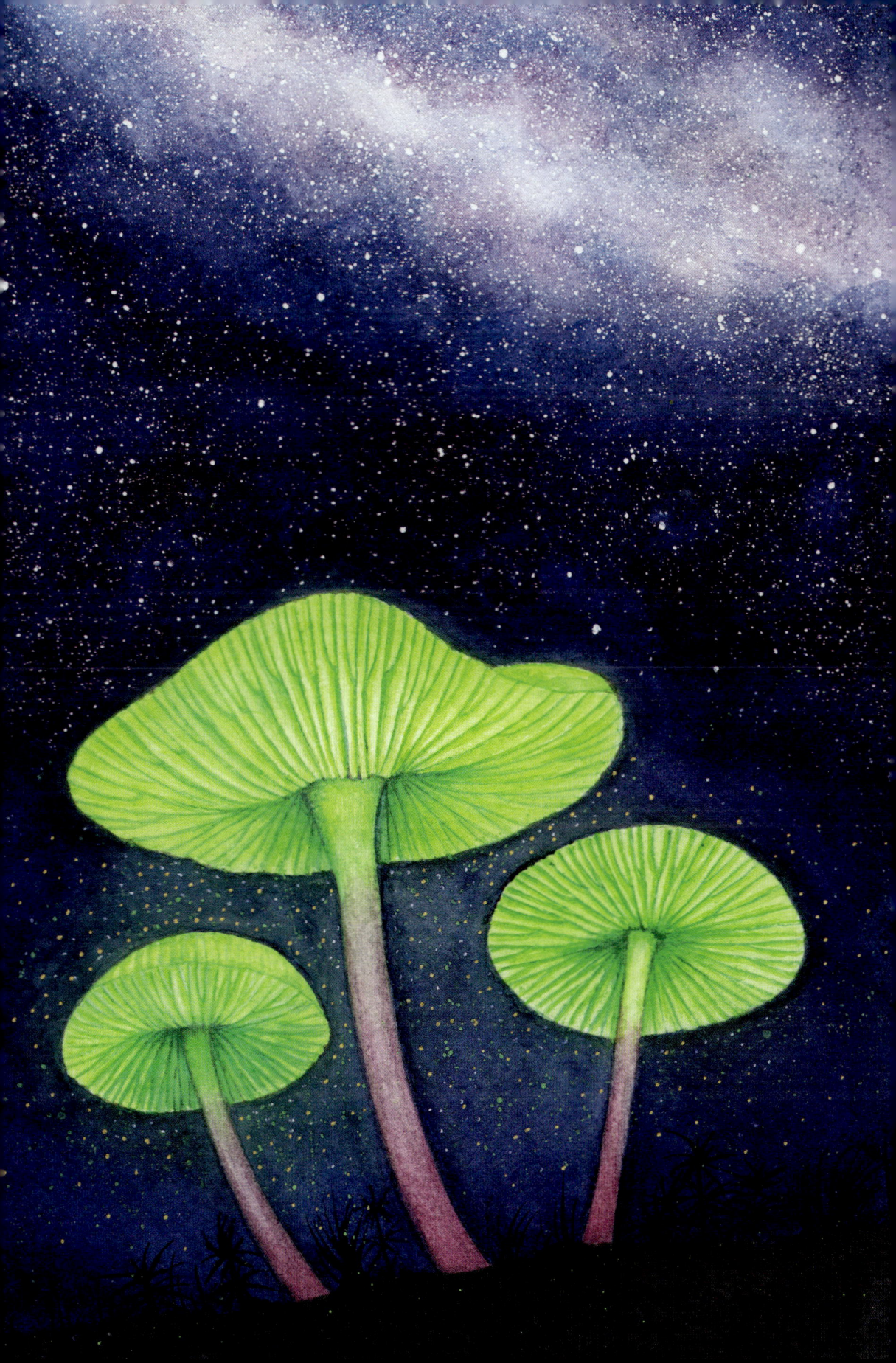

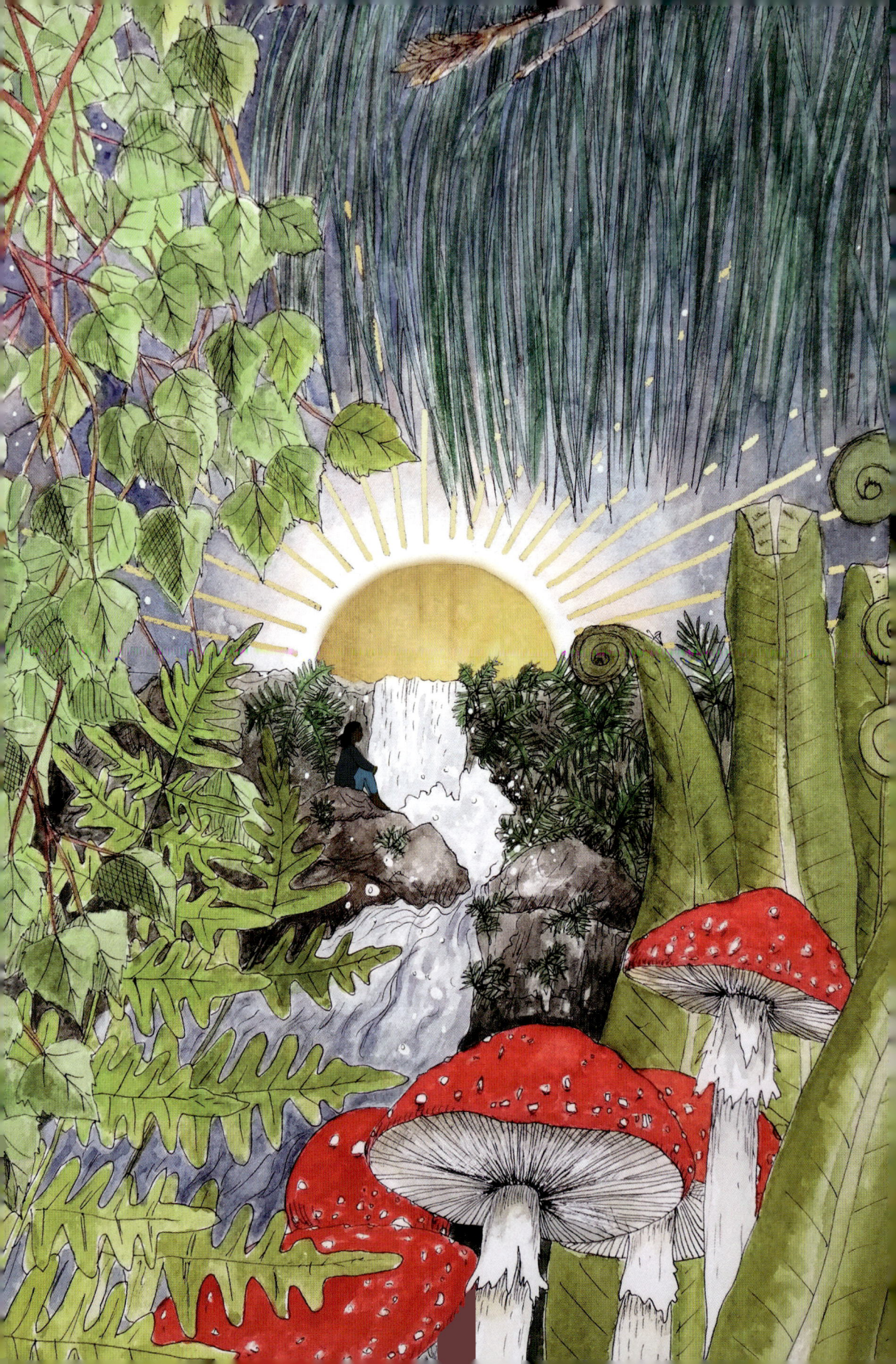

CHAPTER 1

WILD MEDICINE, PLANT MEDICINE AND US

When we lose ourselves midst the trees
When we touch the grace of air on our faces
When we feel the songs of starlight in our blood
We find ourselves back there, wild
Where sometimes we forget, yet always remember.

A womxn alone in nature, being nature. Birch, ferns, fly agaric and pine her plant allies by the water, sun, earth and wind.

Many herbalists, not all, are drawn to herbalism because of the rich connection to the natural world. In terms of herbalism, we can spend a lot of time outside – foraging, harvesting, learning about how and where the plants grow, and why.

Foraging is a big part of being a herbalist. When I was a baby herbalist the term "brown bottle herbalist" was bandied around as a nod to those who used herbal medicines much like orthodox medicine – without the element of nature connection. There is a huge question in herbalism of all kinds (from medical to folk) regarding the structure of the herbal system and the emulation of orthodox medicine which evolved to be elite-medic and white-male centric. We will talk more on this later.

Sometimes we need to be mindful and practise going outside and just get to know the plants in their living spirit so we have an understanding of them, their textures, tastes, and botanical peculiarities, and wonder.

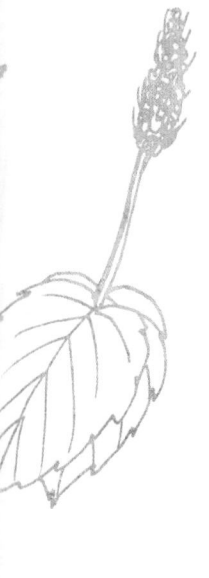

Starting to get to know these traits helps us when we need to know which herb to use, or even to identify a herb in preparations, such as teas and tinctures.

For example if you have two jars of herbs left in your cupboard and you had forgotten to label them and they looked pretty similar but one smelled of mint and the other had little scent, you could probably work out that one was the mint you picked and dried last summer but the other one was the plantain that you were trying as a tea from this summer. Think then of a whole apothecary – unlabelled!

While EVERYTHING should be labelled . . . sometimes we forget to do it and can end up with jars of unlabelled herbs.

If we know the tastes, look, and texture we might be able to easily work out what the herbs are, but if we don't we will not be able to and it becomes a waste of plant matter and potentially dangerous.

When you become more practised in the art of tasting you can start to sense the energy of the plant as well, which will inform you about the plant's actions and effects.

Note though that there are usually a few unlabelled packets of dried green matter at the back of the herbalist's cupboard which were to be labelled "later" and never got labelled. Sometimes they go to waste and this is never good, so, the first rule of herbalism, LABEL (and date)!

In order to get the herbs into your apothecary (or cupboard to begin with), you can either buy them in or get them yourself. If you want to harvest your own herbs you can ethically wild craft them or cultivate them. Both methods are good and have different advantages.

Let's look at the two methods of harvesting.

ETHICAL WILD CRAFTING OF HERBS

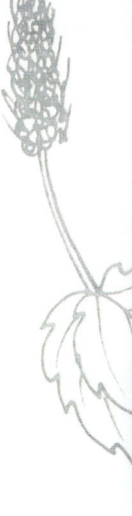

I was reminded recently that it is not simply ethical wild crafting or harvesting that should be ethical. No! It is every single decision we make in our practice (and lives). We as a people choosing to practise herbal medicine in some form need to try to be ethical in all areas. We'll look more at this in the chapter on decolonising herbal medicine.

Wild crafting is another word for foraging; it is the essence and the craft of collecting plants from the wild and then using them for medicine, or food, or similar, perhaps for dyeing or crafting into a basket, for example. It is the craft of harvesting ethically.

The first thing to remember when wild crafting is ethics. If we don't wild craft ethically we begin to destroy the environment around us. When we see a patch of wild medicines, it is too easy to over-gather and decimate the area. If the herbs aren't in abundance we have to leave them. We need to leave plants to seed or spread their rhizomes or continue flowering. We can also find balance: if we pick a few elderberries early we can encourage bigger berries but if we take too many, the birds don't get any and we are not sharing nor caring.

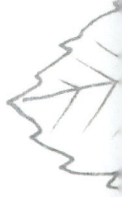

There is so much already that is negatively affecting plants and their habitat, like development and industry, radiation and pollution, etc., we don't need to add to it by ravishing small areas of herbal growth.

When many of us herbalists forage we do so in a manner whereby no one would notice we had been there. For example, a hawthorn tree can be abundant in flower but if it is the only tree in the area, taking only a small amount may be OK. If there are many trees and there are many flowers on those trees, taking a little from each is probably fine. Hawthorns are very common. It may be that you work super locally and in your locality there are various plants you can work with. You need to decipher how your picking will affect the population. Have you picked before there are any new seeds, did you uproot the plant? Have you contaminated it with a dirty blade? Have you made a clean cut? Notice how you harvest.

ETHICS OF INTENTION

Another thing to remember is to wild craft with good intention. Whenever we are involved in any process of herbalism, maintaining an intention of healing is really important. From going out to wild craft, to making medicines, to seeing patients, a herbalist has to maintain a level of responsibility and mindfulness.

If you aren't a practising herbalist you can maintain good discipline by creating good intention around your work. If you've had a tough day or have negative thoughts on your mind, take a few moments to steady yourself and breathe out the negative. Breathe in the beauty of the plants you are going to work with. Tiny adjustments like this can make all the difference in a remedy and your connection with plants. Harvesting plants is often a meditation – harvesting tiny berries is a therapeutic process which you can't rush.

APPROACHING THE PLANT

It is all too easy to only find plants you would like, then pick them and make them into good medicine. However, the practice of approaching plants and trees can be deepened, expanded, and refined. Have you ever approached a plant or tree in different ways? There are many ways to approach plants and trees and the great spirits they are.

We'll look at different plants in each chapter. If you are a beginner, you might like to choose one of the plants in the chapter that you feel fits you or the person you would like to practise this with. There will be different practices in each chapter with different approaches for you to try.

There is so much knowledge of plant medicine and communication, lost and found, it is easy to sit uncomfortably with ideas like these if you have not been around such customs, as is usual in the West now. If you keep an open mind and heart, you can try out different ways of communicating with

WILD MEDICINE, PLANT MEDICINE AND US

plants and see where you are happy. Your relationship with plants will change as you transition into different stages of life, and some of you may deeply connect with this kind of custom, some will mildly resonate, and some will find their strengths elsewhere.

As Claudia mentions in the last chapter, many cultures, including here in Britain, leave an offering for the plant they have spent time with. It might be some wheat, a little mead, it may be coins (the Brits like to leave coins in water, – wishing wells – not such a far cry from this), a weaving, a word, a stone, a ribbon (not plastic), some food, seaweed (to give minerals) and more. An offering for an exchange of sorts, even if you aren't "taking" anything per se.

Rewilding exercise – greeting trees and a step towards opening up our senses

Look for a tree you'd like to greet. Stand easy and comfortably, check your body is relaxed, and try to calm your mind from any rushing or distractions.

Starting at a distance from the tree helps. Just simply make a greeting to the tree and feel or listen for any response or anything that comes up within. Take your time. You can also take note of the shape or textures of the tree from that distance.

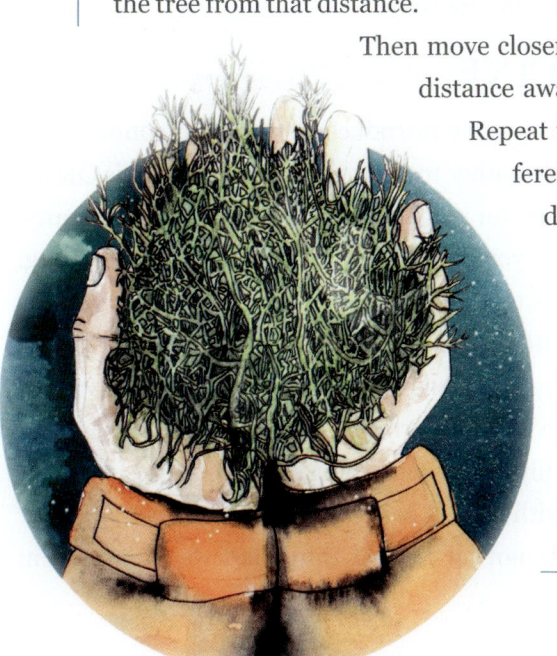

Then move closer to the tree, perhaps roughly at a distance away equal to the height of the tree. Repeat the pattern and also use your different senses to appreciate the tree in different ways.

Go closer as appropriate for you and repeat as desired until you are very close to the tree. Notice how you are feeling and if your thoughts drift. Notice any new or different sensations or words. Some people hear words in the familiar sound of their own voice or language and some hear words in languages they do not understand, while others hear sounds or vibrations. Nothing is wrong as the exercise is about connection and deepening relationship with trees.

I like to feel out my emotional state when I am at different distances.

If you are not comfortable greeting the tree, you can always just notice how you are feeling at different distances from the tree.

When you are ready, after this exercise bid the tree goodbye. It is also a lovely practice to pay your respects – a small bow or a minute spent with your hand touching the tree, or simply looking at the tree sending gratitude from your being or your heart. You can find your way. Then, when ready, slowly move away.

JOURNALING OR SKETCHING

Note in your journal how you feel around trees and about greeting them, or where in nature you feel comfortable. Notice the edges of your comfort and the ease or difficulty you have in communicating with plants. Notice how you do communicate. Write down your own experiences.

GATHERING MEDICINE

Once you feel you have greeted the plant, introduced yourself, or connected in some way, and if you would like to gather medicine, ask the plant if it is OK for you to gather some of its medicines for yourself, your family, your community. Listen for the answer. Sometimes you'll hear it in words, sometimes a feeling. If it doesn't feel good, move on. Listen. The message may be by observation – is the plant alone, abundant, healthy? The natural world and we (remember, we're part of nature) relate through our senses such as sight and touch.

Sometimes I get a feeling when I am gathering that it is just time to stop – if I don't listen to that feeling, I usually fall off something or get scratches or something of that ilk. Listen and go with it. This is a skill I am still developing after twenty years of herbalism. It is not an instant thing and we all attune in different ways but we all have the capacity to listen, observe, feel. We all have the capacity to be in a right relation with our beautiful plant allies.

If this feels totally alien and something you don't want to engage with, see if you can find another way. Always maintain great respect while following an ethical wild crafting protocol.

Once you have met your plants and set your intentions you can now harvest in an ethical way.

Harvest with respect if there is great abundance (nettle, hawthorn, etc.), but even so, only harvest what you need. Waste is not to be encouraged and sometimes a great gathering of one herb may be left at the back of the cupboard. To keep things vibrant, dried herbs are best refreshed every year (this is not a requirement but goes well with vitality in herbalism and seasonal cycles). If you do find you have waste from a previous year, it is a lovely thing to give it back to the earth, rather than throw it away in a bin.

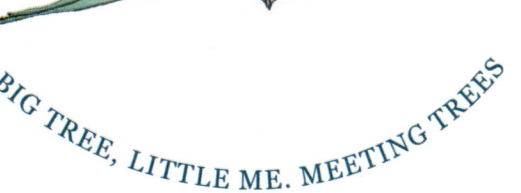

BIG TREE, LITTLE ME. MEETING TREES

Find a suitable place and take your dried herbs as they are or in water if you feel it would be better and gift them back to the earth with gratitude. Gratitude is all about remembering and acknowledging the exchange. You could make an infusion, cooled and appreciated and poured onto the earth, or give the herbs to fire as a smoulder. With intention and blessing. It is key to living well and with nature. Many of us aren't taught to be grateful, we are taught to strive. A simple action like giving unused herbs back to the earth with gratitude can make a difference in how we act and how we develop our herbalism.

A sense of connection to everything is integral to most cultures that are close to the land. Many of us have been forcibly or systematically disconnected from the land, and our understanding of plants, landscapes, and animals is often fragmented. Ethnobotanist Jennie Martin uses the terms "nature literacy" and "dirt time" to describe ways to reconnect and observe nature and our relationships with plants.

Take only what you need when plants are in abundance. If you know you will need lots to make litres of tincture over the year, then plan accordingly; you may need to do different wild crafting sessions in different locations.

If there aren't many plants and you really need the herb, still look elsewhere. It is very tempting to take what you need but we must think of the ecosystem and biodiversity first. If there is a good amount, but not a huge amount, and you need the herb, try asking and listening. Sometimes a plant will lend itself to gathering without you taking too much. Mugwort, for example, will have spikes of flowers on stems that come off the main stem and other major stems, so it is possible to harvest a few spikes off each plant without taking too much from one plant.

Sometimes finding a small patch of medicinal plants is a calling for you to become a guardian of that area.

See if you can connect with local wildflower groups, community gardens, parks, or green spaces and even "landowners", and keep notes about the local flora in your area.

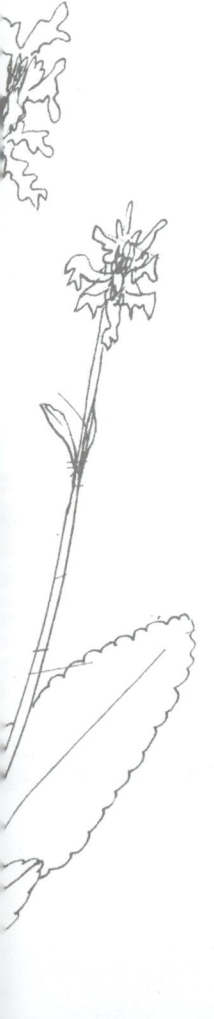

There is a certain patch of wood betony in my locality which is not big enough to harvest much from – enough for an elixir or flower essence but not enough for a litre of tincture or big bag of tea. So I go there to check it and stay a while with it and learn from it. It is a place I sometimes ask my patients to visit and sit a while to think things through or just the opposite, stop thinking and start listening. The patch is a gift but not one to take much from in terms of medicine making. Likewise on the commons near me, there are tiny scatterings of eyebright. Not enough at all to take from but beautiful to see and learn from.

HARVESTING

To harvest cleanly, it is good to take scissors, a small knife, or secateurs. It is lovely to harvest with one's fingers and when picking berries, for example, fingers can seem the best way but with some plants, despite our best efforts, using our fingers leads to more damage to the plant than intended – stems rip awkwardly or smaller plants are uprooted. It is good to cut cleanly to take what you need and no more. If you are picking more than one kind of plant, clean your blade well so you don't contaminate. Forks are really handy too, especially for berries like elder and juniper.

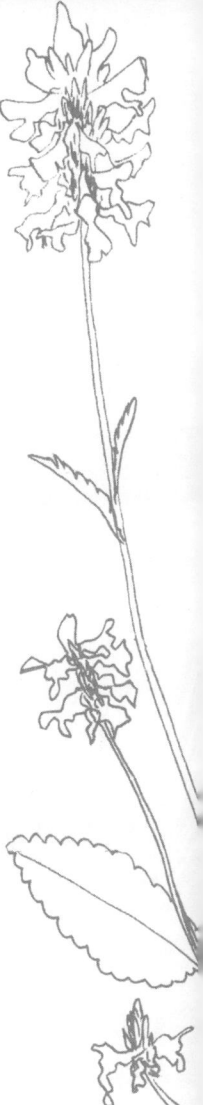

A basket, cloth bag, or paper bag are good receptacles to take with you to put your harvest into. Try to keep plants you collect in their different bags as it can take longer to separate them when you're processing them than it did to harvest them!

If you are picking berries, little boxes can be useful to stop heavy loads becoming squashed and juice leaking everywhere. A juice stained basket is no bad thing really but in terms of caring for our plants and belongings, it is a good idea to work out what works for you in terms of harvesting with ethics and quality in mind.

I don't harvest anything by a main road or sprayed field. This can be problematic because sometimes we don't know that an area is sprayed or built over landfill or rubbish. We have to assess as best we can.

Some of us will only have access to wild medicines in the middle of cities or near major roads or sprayed farms so try to choose well – up paths or along canals or edges or on quieter roadsides. In the UK we are lucky that there are many green areas in towns and cities but not so lucky that the vast majority of land in England is not open to the public.

It is essential that people know where herbs are coming from and how they are harvested. For example, I wouldn't want to buy a batch of wild garlic that was wild crafted by a company that did not know whether its foraging employees stripped areas bare, or picked from busy roadsides or those sprayed fields! Also consider the conditions and fair wages of employees in different areas (especially if your herbs are coming from somewhere you don't know well).

I want my medicines to be as clean and fresh as they can be. It's not always perfect but keeping this in mind means most of your medicine is likely to be better quality, and this kind of practice heightens your own awareness of ecology and environment.

Tips

Generally avoid plants that are at the height onto which dogs like to wee. Dog wee is no medicine. If it is an area where dogs frequently go, think about the height of the plant you are picking. For example there are huge swathes of nettles in a popular walking location near me so I generally wear jeans and boots and wade into the middle of the patch to pick nettles. The odd dog bounds in but rarely stops to wee!

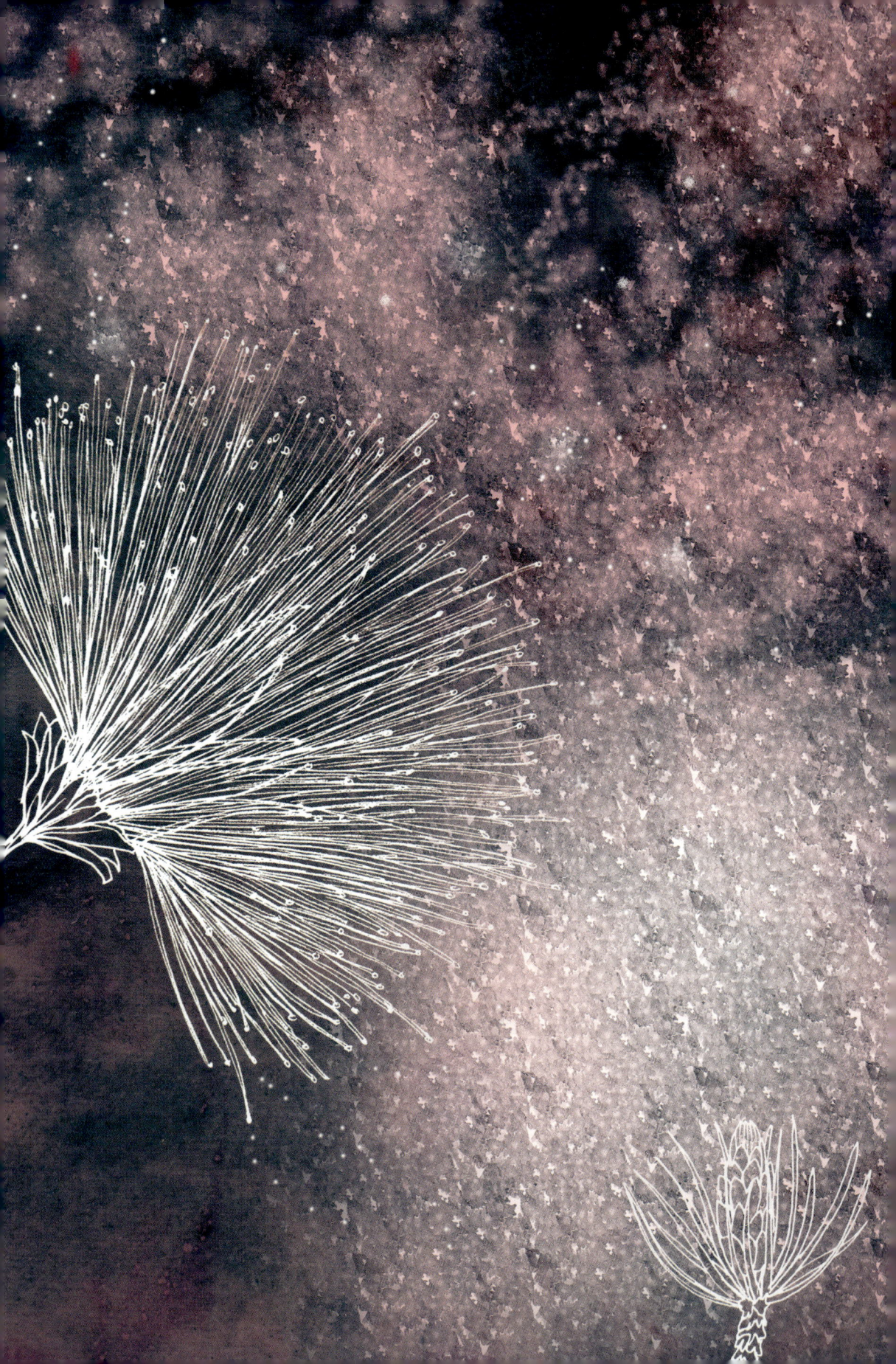

Flowers are best picked on dry days when they have fully enjoyed being open. It is OK to pick flowers on cooler days or cloudy days and even OK after the rain but the optimum is dry sunny days. If you are wanting natural yeasts on flowers for champagne making, for example, sunny days are needed.

If you do pick on rainy days, just pat dry the plants before making them into a tincture or drying them out properly as tea. This will mean you still get to harvest herbs but aren't reliant on good weather, which is a must in some countries!

Make sure you know your plants. If you don't then have a look at the endangered plants in your area and make sure you aren't picking anything on that list. You can also take a small (or big) plant identification book to help you make sure you have the plants you think you have in front of you.

In an age of social media and fast uploading of medicine-making pictures, it is surprisingly common to see misidentified plants being used and described. I have seen people using umbels such as hogweed instead of elderflower to make elderflower champagne (best not to try that). Martin's "dirt time" is just this – spending time observing the characteristics of a plant in real life and not on screen. Plant identification apps can be incorrect and therefore potentially dangerous – especially if ingesting as herbal medicine.

When you start getting to know your local area and keep an eye out for plants, suddenly you start to tune in. When you are interested in something, you suddenly start seeing it everywhere, or reading about it or having conversations about it; well, the same is true for foraging or herbalism. You start to see your plant allies everywhere. As I look out of my window now I see birch, cedar, pine, daisy, lavender, self-heal, and dandelion. Over in the neighbour's garden I see nettle seeds I'd like to go and harvest soon. These skills will develop as you practise over the years and through the seasons.

CULTIVATION OF HERBS
GROW YOUR OWN

It is great to be able to grow herbs – in pots, beds, or around the garden (or ask your neighbours!). The advantages of growing your own include more biodiversity, quality assurance, accessibility, and fun. If you have no outdoor space, inside is good too. If you have a tiny space, think about asking others if you can grow in their outside space, or a community space.

Exploding pollen – pine and albizia

When herbalists help folk design herb gardens, we often choose plants which are suited to health needs, soils, light, and microclimates. A family with small children might like to grow chamomiles and marigolds in big quantities while an older couple or individual with, say, asthmatic issues or frequent colds might choose a lung tonic garden including thymes, sages, echinaceas, hyssops, and elecampane.

The beautiful thing about home grown is that you can easily access the plants, observing them as they grow and change and come back again (or not) in subsequent years. You can take the time to draw them, taste them, understand their needs and in so doing, connect the plants in different ways. You can also manage the way you grow them – using organic soil or planting in gardens that have not been sprayed. You can pick them at optimal times and have quality assurance of their good health.

A lovely thing to do is think about what kind of herbs you want and how they will be presented in your growing space. Reading up a bit about companion planting and which herbs like which conditions (shade, soil type, etc.) will also help the herbs to flourish. If you have a new herb garden or herbs in pots, you need to have time to water them so it does take a level of commitment even for small scale growers. In larger patches you have to have the time to weed and check and water as well sometimes. In community growing spaces you will likely get many tips on growing, tending, and also often a share of the bounty.

These small (or sometimes endless) pockets of time with the plants can be very beneficial for both the growing space and for you. A little quiet time checking the plants are growing well is time when you can release old thoughts, dream up new ideas, breathe deeply, or set intentions. It is also a time when you can channel good energy into your plant medicines.

It has been shown in numerous studies (some done at home, some done in schools, and some in research institutions) that good words help the health of the plants, and we know good words help us too. Time growing can be extremely therapeutic.

Things to think about when cultivating your own herb garden include learning a little about the botany of the plants you have. For example, I once bought a packet of German chamomile seeds, I planted them and harvested them without paying too much attention as they were from a reputable supplier. When I dried and tasted them, I thought they might be Roman chamomile as they were very bitter. I decided to make a tincture from them anyhow as I like Roman chamomile and the colour of the tincture turned out to be much more indicative of Roman rather than German chamomile. After that I realised they certainly were Roman because of their perennial nature, growing back the next year.

I also once bought a wood betony plant from a local herb nursery. As it grew bigger, it became clear that it was in fact figwort and not betony at all!

A great way to grow more plants is to get together with others. Community gardens and shared allotments can really help inspire you, especially if the slugs are rampant . . . the input of others takes away the pressure of doing everything by yourself. Some gardens have different people looking after different plants; some have different people bringing different seeds, cuttings, plants, knowledge; so your own gardening knowledge grows. There are community gardens all around now and many active gardening groups if you seek them out. You'll soon start to see spaces where you could grow a garden – derelict spaces or rooftops. Even little areas of soil amid the asphalt can be tiny gardens that are simply for the pleasure of growing flowers or attracting bees. Walls are great for growing plants up! You'll start to notice (if you don't already). You don't have to have your own growing space. Claudia grows tomatoes up the drainpipes outside her flat; she even has fly agaric on her doorstep when it snows.

Getting to know a little botany is so useful. In fact it can be very important. There are many plants which look similar and if you don't know exactly what you are looking for, you could be picking or growing poisonous plants and then end up with something very different from elderflower fritters, as we saw before.

BOTANY

Getting to know your plants is so worthwhile. Oh so worthwhile! All those little plants you see in the cracks of the pavement or the towering trees above you may be medicinal, edible, or useful to you and your family. You can build relationships with plants you know and through identification you can build up a picture of what is around you and what needs your community or land may have.

It is one thing to know the names of common plants and have some idea of what they look like and another to really get to know your plants – their shapes, their characteristics, their colours, their variations, and their peculiarities. By observing them and drawing them and generally noticing them, you get to build a picture of them in your head or heart, you start to know them at a glance.

Getting a basic book on botany or wild plant identification is a great idea to tap into the structure of trees and plants and to start to recognise different families or traits (see the Resources section).

Basic botany can help you identify your local wild medicines and help you differentiate between similar plants. To help with that, here is just a taste of some very common plant families and their traits.

By looking at plants, ecology, and botany we begin to think about why plants are called what they are called, how they grow, why they are growing in a given location, and various traits of the plant.

Rewilding exercise

Draw three sketches of the nearest "weeds" to you. Those little plants that pop out of the wall or grow along the edges of the paths. See them, draw them, or draw parts of them and label them. Notice the weeds daily, or often – see how they grow, where they move, how they change.

By studying them a little you'll be taking into your consciousness the botanical aspects of plants. This is a beautiful way to begin to see and understand botany.

For example, if you see a flower with five petals and lots of stamens, you'll notice that other flowers on different plants also have the same pattern. Often these flowers are on plants in the same family. A flower with five petals and many stamens could be dog rose, blackberry, apple and hawthorn, all rose family or rosaceae plants.

UNDERSTANDING BOTANICAL LANGUAGE

When we're considering plants and how to identify them, we're taking into account all the elements that make that plant. The divisions that botanists give each plant are through a process of taxonomy which is basically the science of defining and naming groups based on the biological characteristics. Things often get changed about: for example, rosemary was a *Rosmarinus* and now it is a *Salvia*.

The first level of division in taxonomy is the "kingdom" – that's fairly simple: animal, plant, or mineral.

Within the plant kingdom the next layer of identification is the "division", for example dandelion is in the magnoliophyte division, which is a flowering plant.

Next we have a "class" of that division which in the case of dandelion is the magnoliopsida, a dicot plant.

We then have the "order" which is the asterales in this case and then the "family" of the asteraceae (composite family).

Next is the "genus" of dandelion – *Taraxacum* (these always have capital letters).

Coupled with the genus is the "species" – this one is (*Taraxacum*) *officinale* (this is always italics if we're being correct).

Lastly there is the common name which, in this case, is dandelion.

1. Kingdom – plant
2. Division/Phylum – *Magnoliophyta* (flowering plant)
3. Class – *Magnoliopsida* (dicot)
4. Order – *Asterales*
5. Family – *Asteraceae*
6. Genus – *Taraxacum*
7. Species – *Taraxacum officinale*
8. Common name – dandelion

By knowing what these words mean we can start to understand what kind of a plant is in front of us when we go out for a forage. We can easily learn to see if it's a monocotyledon or dicotyledon for example, or if it's likely to be in the mint family with square stems or the rose family because it's got five petals and many stamens.

Let's have a look at that now as there are a few really common families with pretty broadly shared characteristics.

PLANT FAMILIES

Really common plant families with many medicinal gems include:

    Roseaceae family which is the rose family
    Lamiaceae family which is the mint family
    Asteraceae family which is the daisy family (formally compositae family)
    Apiaceae family which is the celery/ (formally umbelliferaceae family)

Rose family

The rose family bears many common wild medicinals in the UK. If you think about blackberry, apple, rose, and hawthorn and you think of the flowers (check them out if you're not familiar with them), you'll notice they have five petals and many stamens and are really quite similar looking.

There are usually five stamens or more, often in clusters of five. The fruit from the flowers can vary but they are often astringent. Think of rose hips and sloe berries – they are very different but can both be quite drying (especially the sloes: if you haven't bitten into the blackthorn fruit, identify it properly and then bite into the fruit; note in your journal what happens to your face!) The cause of that astringency is usually tannins in the rose family which pucker and tighten mucous membranes.

Mint family

The obvious botanical traits are square stems and opposite leaves. Mints are also often aromatic.

Think about the smell of mint – it can be overpowering and that strong scent is due to the volatile oils. In some of the mint family herbs, including peppermint, spearmint, and apple mint, menthol is a commonly seen volatile oil.

Lots of our common household herbs, especially in the UK, are mints – lavender, basil, thyme, sage, and rosemary. The flowers in this family are quite distinct: they have five sepals which are fused together and five petals which are fused together and they are generally irregular in shape with two petals pointing up and three pointing down. This shape will become fairly familiar to you as you get to know your plants. Unlike the rose family with its many stamens the mint family plants generally have four stamens inside the petals, two of which are longer than the other two.

Daisy family

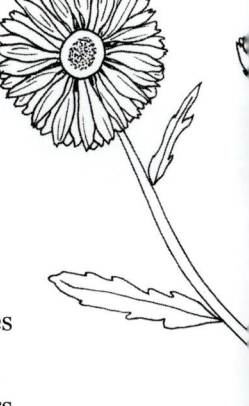

The compositae or asteraceae family is a big one and includes a great variety of plants from the lovely little daisy to the big heads of sunflowers. These plants are distinctive for their flowers which have composite parts.

Each tiny flower in a composite head has a disc flower and ray flowers. Each disc has five petals and five stamens. What we commonly think of as the petals are in fact the ray flowers and on a daisy, for example, the two types are fused together.

Beneath the flowers are green bracts, which look like sepals. Multiple layers of these bracts are pretty common and an obvious example of that is an artichoke flower which has all the spiky multiple layers of these green bracts making the distinct artichoke shape.

There are 19,000 species of composite plants! Common ones that we can grow easily include marigold, chamomile, and milk thistle. These plants all have a mild bitterness or cleansing property.

Celery family

This family, which is called apiaceae, is made up of many incredibly medicinal plants. However, there are lots of plants in this family which are highly poisonous. In fact some of the most poisonous plants in the UK are in this family, such as water dropwort. Go and look that up if you are not familiar with it! It is very worth getting to know the poisonous plants that grow all around you because they can easily be mistaken for something you think is a medicinal.

The classic characteristic of the apiaceae family are the umbels. It used to be called the umbelliferae family and this is due to the tiny clusters of flowers which in turn cluster together on separate little stems forming a flower head which resembles a little umbrella. The stems are often hollow and there are around 3000 species of umbels. Commonly used medicinal plants in this family include wild carrot, fennel, celery seed, cumin, dill, parsley: these are all aromatic and often have an affinity with the urinary system, can irritate in high doses (possibly not fennel), and can cleanse the palate.

The key here is to get to know your plants. If you know them by looking at them and by being able to identify various traits you will inevitably get to know your local area better. With this in mind you'll know how to identify wild plants, and therefore wild medicines if you get to know which plants are useful medicinally.

This is a resilience skill and really helpful in rewilding of the self. This is because you will know what is around you as you identify plants. Knowing what is around means you can identify local edibles, medicinals, poisonous herbs, or those that you could use in some way in your life. For example, you could distinguish willows and begin to harvest and replant willow whips for basket making or you could identify nettles (which is pretty easy) in order to make food, medicine, or material.

NOMENCLATURE – WHAT'S IN A NAME?

So what is in a name? Nomenclature is the naming of plants and the most interesting thing about this is what the name tells you about the plant. If we think about dandelion again, the French name *pis-en-lit* means "wet the bed" and this is because dandelion leaves are a diuretic and make you wee. I love this name because it's fun, and descriptive, but the Brits' name for it, dandelion, is also very telling as the leaves are deeply toothed, reminiscent of a lion's tooth. This word comes from the French *dent de lion* meaning lion's tooth.

Nomenclature can give you an insight into what the plant was used for in different times. For example, meadowsweet was called bridewort or meadwort – wort meaning leaf – so bride's leaf or mead leaf. Indeed the herb was most likely strewn or put into garlands at weddings (bridewort) and meadowsweet was the key ingredient in the sweet mead drink. Claudia will expand on the history of taxonomy later in the book.

A little nod to bridewort . . . I recall a really special day some years ago. It was the wedding of a fellow herbalist and it was July. Meadowsweet was in flower all around so we picked it with its beautiful creamy spray of sweet scented flowers and put it on the tables. She indeed had bridewort for her wedding.

> ### Rewilding exercise
> See if you can look up five to ten common names of plants, especially medicinals, and find out where the name came from. If you have access to those plants, have a look at them in their habitat and see if the name makes any sense.

HERBARIUM

A good way to get to know the local flora and your own changing or emerging herb garden is to make a mini herbarium.

her·bar·i·um
(hûr-bâr'ē-əm, ûr-)
n.pl. her·bar·i·ums or her·bar·i·a (-ə-ē)

1. A collection of dried plants mounted, labelled, and systematically arranged (for use in scientific study)
2. A place or institution where such a collection is kept

You need:

>A flower press (or some very heavy books)
>Some good absorbent paper
>Some newspaper, or similar absorbent paper

I like to make my own plant press with old bits of wood, a drill, and some nuts and bolts. You need to be able to apply a little pressure to what is being pressed (screwing down or layering books!).

If you press the plants you find and keep them together in a volume of sorts, labelled, you start to see what kind of plant allies are growing in your area or your garden. It's a lovely thing to do as they keep well and look beautiful. Drawings are also great and can be added around your pressing or on different pages with different parts of the plant.

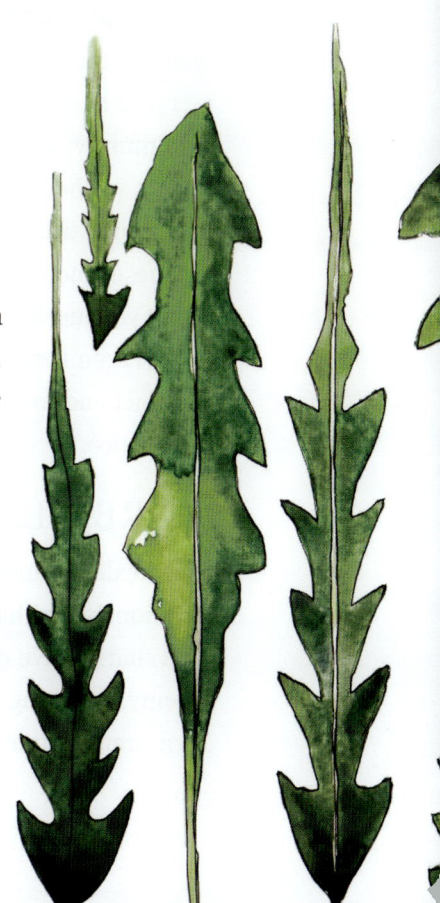

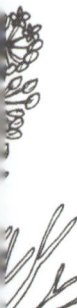

> ### Rewilding exercise
>
> A lovely exercise for all, including kids, is to do simple tiny pressings in a little sketch book. On each little page with a pressed flower or small plant, just add a few things you know about the plants - some constituents, some actions, and your experiences. A little bound book is a beautiful addition to your library and easy to make and carry around.
>
> It's also lovely to frame your favourite pressings and have them around, reminding you of the traits or personality or medicinal actions of the plants.

DRAWING

If you don't think you can draw (but are able), try to drop that notion now! It doesn't matter if it's not botanically accurate or even identifiable (and I bet you can make it so), the act of drawing will provide information you might not notice without such time spent looking and working out how the plant is formed. It's an invaluable experience and doesn't even have to be a botanical rendition, it can be an expression of how you feel around the plant, the colours you see, the negative shapes you see around the plant, etc.

I love herbariums because you can bring in all kinds of additions from your community: ask others to make pressings of the wild or cultivated medicinal plants in their garden or on their walks and you can start to map out what medicinals are growing where.

These kinds of activities may seem daunting if you haven't done them before but if you just have a go, you'll see how easy and what fun it is, with all kinds of unforeseen benefits and experiences. There is a lot of help out there (on the internet and in books, etc.) on how to do pressings if you need some technical assistance.

HERB/PLANT SOVEREIGNTY

The healing journey with plants is often about reclaiming your own sovereign relationship with plants and delving into connection, understanding, learning, and sharing. We can be our own healer or own best friend, or at times our own enemy. By taking up the mantle of herbalist or plantsperson we begin to engage in a practice that is as ancient as the hills (well, almost) and become much more connected to our wild medicine and healing journey and or our wild landscape and environment. Knowing about the plants growing around you can be so rewarding and can be done in so many different ways. I like talking to people – friends, family, neighbours, people on the bus, etc. – about their favourite plants or trees. Such conversations can shed some understanding on a hugely varied subject and then, if you're lucky, you get the gems that are sometimes called old wives' tales (more on that later).

Woah.

Some of those tales! Folk had so much knowledge. I would like to encourage you to ask your granny or your friend's grandpa, or your granddaughter's elder teacher or any elder you know if they used any herbals or grew certain plants for a specific reason. Or for any top tips on making balms, teas, remedies for pain or cuts and scrapes, period pain, childbirth recovery, coughs and colds, getting to sleep, feeling good, and more. Lost knowledge is lost power.

Growing your own herbs and herbal sovereignty means you know the plants and where they've been growing, what they've had sprayed on them (hopefully nothing except garlic spray or similar!) and how they've managed to grow in certain locations.

In Stroud we're doing a project called Herbal Rebellion: Stroud Community Medicine Garden. It is a community-wide project that encourages many people to come together and create a community apothecary. Folk range from those with land to those with space for a plant pot or two and those who aren't growing anything but like to harvest elderflowers in June or rosehips in autumn. We make medicines together on certain days and by doing that create a small apothecary for those involved. In the future we will also be able to sell our wares at the local farmer's market.

The rebel side of this comes into play as a stand against the system which encourages capitalist gain rather than community spirit, but it is not really rebellion at all, it is so, so natural and sadly being forgotten. Stroud is a town of activism and alternative lifestyle (amongst other walks of life) and many here seek community, inclusion, and sharing. Part of this is about becoming resilient, and we will need wild medicines

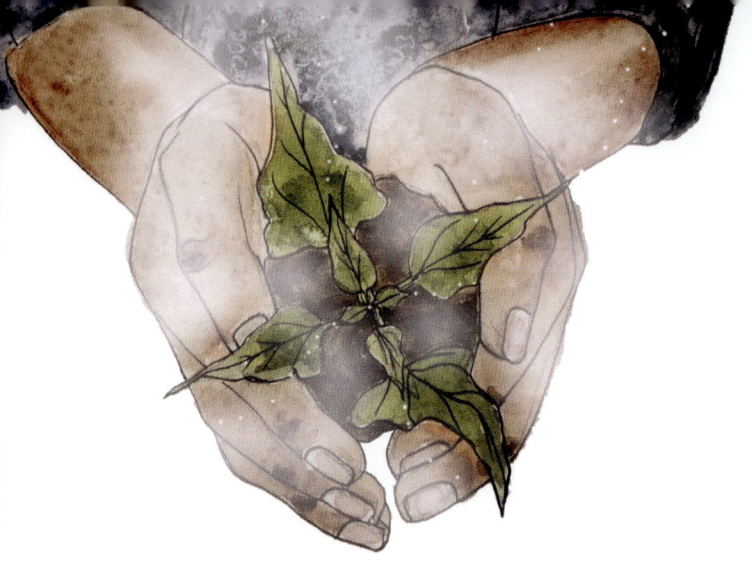

and the knowledge to cultivate them more and more as the climate affects us and we realise we can't consume as we have become accustomed.

You might well fall in love with a community apothecary or herbal rebellion. It is all part of deep adaptation to change and herbal sovereignty.

If you would like a community garden and can't find one – start one! Even if it's tiny. You can always grow. Social cohesion naturally happens when plants and people grow together.

PLANT INITIATION

There are many ways to become more familiar with plants. Plant initiations are one of those ways. If you walk the path to deep interconnectedness with plants, this is a beautiful way to do it.

A plant initiation usually means spending time with a plant of choice. Let's take nettle. If I want to become aware of nettle and the powers nettle may have in healing, I may create an initiation.

Initiations are something that have been all but lost in modern society, except perhaps in some dubious elite university rituals. They were often long lasting (sometimes up to a year or more, for example) and were about passing into a new phase of life. Often fasting would be required before the initiation begun, or at least a restricted diet. Certain times of the year would be chosen to elicit a new growth within the participant.

In terms of plant initiations, a fast is often called for before beginning the work. Some kind of settling into a new paradigm or mindset is needed for this work. Often one plant is chosen and worked with for a few consecutive days.

The work with the plant is intended to go deeper into our beings than just simply a cerebral understanding of the plant.

Our diet and the time taken with the plant all contribute to a different kind of understanding of that plant. We may feel a bonding with the plant that we had not experienced before, a deeply personal relationship to that plant that will carry on resonating far beyond the initiation.

It may be that we receive gifts of understanding, healing, or action through initiation with a certain plant. Different plants will bring about different experiences for different people. Often there is some kind of similarity in understanding when the same plant is used for initiation with more than one person. It is quite amazing when you experience that.

The plant preparation used will have been prepared in ceremony and with intention, likely by an elder or more experienced plantsperson. The time spent in ceremony with the plant allows for breathwork, meditation, dreaming, journeying and connection.

TASTINGS

Tastings are mini-initiations. They can be done without the ceremony and time needed for deeper work but are the start of a relationship with the plant. They are usually done with an infusion of a single plant but sometimes using elixirs, tinctures and teas, or chewing the plant itself.

Time is given for mindful relaxation and emptying of the mind. A connective exercise like a guided meditation or breathwork might be done first. Then, when ready and often in a group, we smell the herbal infusion. Each person notices what they smell, where they experience that in their body, and how they feel. That is then shared. Whether the plants are aromatic, earthy, grassy, sweet, pungent, floral, for example, are noted.

Then a small tasting is done and the same process is repeated. Often we use a picture of the outline of a body (in my classes we try hard not to use the same typical white male outline) and someone leading the tasting will note what people say. These are collated and so often they bear the same patterns. I like to utilise and connect with the old ways of learning but also then reference my herbal books to see what is being said about a plant and see if it tallies with my own understanding and experience – and if not, why not. For example, if I was taking a herb with anthraquinones (a bitter element), why am I sweating? Is it the hot tea, is it my body and something I need to think about, is it something commonly experienced with that herb, or is it that I've isolated a compound in my mind and expected a cooling response?

Tastings are useful on a personal note too as sometimes you react very strongly positive or negative and you learn about your relationship to the plant. For instance, you might adore marigold flowers but their taste is just too astringent and bitter for you. Or you might love willow trees but find the medicine too cooling for your constitution. It is all for learning and deepening our understanding of plants and how their medicines work.

Example tea tasting: ginger (fresh ginger tea)

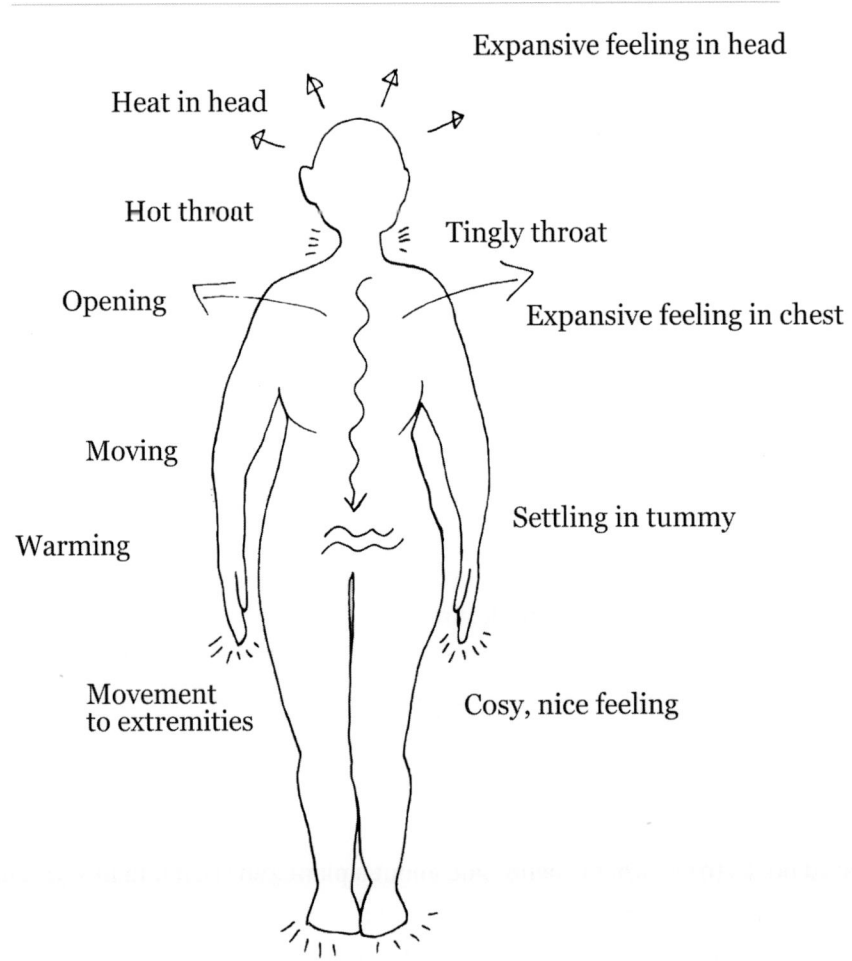

Possible tastes and feelings in the mouth:

Astringent – drying, puckering.

Demulcent – round, soft, full, soothing.

Bitter – move downwards or feel consolidating, cooling, and there are warming bitters too.

Saponin – sweet, soapy.

Mineral and salt – salty.

Resin – sticky, bitter, pungent, waxy, oily, aromatic, hard.

Aromatic – warming and directional.

If you drink a chamomile or mint tea, just see if you can discern the tastes themselves. Or when you try new teas or herbs see if you can notice the tastes and feelings in your mouth or body which may help identify both the plant and some of the constituents.

NATURAL CYCLES

Cycles are an intrinsic part of life. They are everywhere. Our sleep cycle, the seasonal cycle, my menstrual cycle, your breath, their digestion, the water cycle, and so on. Cycles range from tiny bodily cycles at a cellular level to worldwide elemental phenomena. There are even political cycles which come around again and again as the centuries pass. There are cultures that saw/see the world in millennia-long cycles – the Mayans, Aztecs, and many more cultures had or have a deep understanding of cycles.

In herbalism the most obvious cycles for the growth of plants and seeds are the cycles of seasonal patterns of the year, from spring through to winter and to spring again and the plant life cycle within these seasons, depending on the plant – tropical plants will have different cycles than temperate plants.

When we are learning about herbalism, whether as an apprentice, a student in academia, or a wilder student self-taught through experience in nature, try to notice all the cycles and patterns of action and replenishment such as dark and light, of cold and hot. Through understanding cycles, we tune in a little more and get a little closer to plant wisdom. It is an innate need of humans to follow and tune in with cycles.

> ### Rewilding exercise
>
> Think of as many cycles as you can in the natural world and in our bodies. For example:
>
> > Seasons
> >
> > Water cycle
> >
> > ATP cycle
> >
> > Cell cycle
> >
> > Hormonal cycles
> >
> > Seven year cycles
> >
> > Sleep cycles
> >
> > Astrological cycles
> >
> > Menstrual cycle, etc, etc.
>
> Keep space for when you learn new ones.
>
> Think about what these cycles need and the interconnected web of life that sustains all cycles.
>
> Warning: it can get a bit mind blowing.

CEREMONY

My teacher, the dear and late Christopher Hedley, always used to say there wasn't enough ceremony in herbalism or indeed in modern life. He would make little ceremonies for the faeries, or for the roots or shoots. He would create new ones as needed and if he was by a tree that needed introduction, he would embody ceremony, bringing tiny acts of connection with reverence and spirited quiet joy to each encounter. It was a way of connecting with the wild, a way of connecting with the cycles.

Ceremony has morphed in the Western world as it became more secular. However, it is not totally gone, we do hold on to daily rituals and ceremony, unacknowledged: tea at 11, flowers picked freshly, prayer, mantras, walks, lighting a candle, tiny rituals and repetitions we make in our daily lives. Ceremony practised by pagans, druids, and witches is very much pushed to the edges of society whereas mainstream religious ceremony is normalised. Ceremony can really help us.

We do still see some use of ceremony in modern life, marking births, weddings, or deaths, and some religious transitions such as the Thread ceremony for Zoroastrian folk or Confirmation for Catholic folk. These are usually big events in the life of the participant.

We also see the marking of some pagan festivals with Samhain (Halloween) at a similar time to el Dia de los Muertos (the Day of the Dead) and harvest festivals all over the world. Even Christmas is the festival of light and is at a similar time of year to other festivals of light (Chanukah, Diwali, etc.) in the northern hemisphere.

Ceremony doesn't have to be elaborate; even tiny ceremonies can become part of your connection with the wild, or with plants.

You might mark your foraging with a cyclical ceremony, such as every new moon giving thanks for your bounty and blessings from the plants that have made you an apothecary.

You may choose to use natural objects like feathers and sticks and stones you have found near the plants to make a little offering or earth temple.

A WORD ON NATURE'S GEMS

For a long time I thought crystals were the perfect object. Natural, beautiful, of the earth, great for adults and children as gifts, natural wonders from the tooth fairy.

However, so many crystals are ripped from the earth. Children are sent into mines which are created through explosions. We've all heard of blood diamonds, but in fact many crystals have sad beginnings. They were once part of the magic of our earth and while they hold much power, if they are harvested unethically, they don't serve the purpose we often use them for – to attune to a higher vibration or to feel the power and resonance of the earth.

There are natural objects around which are plentiful, beautiful, and worthy. I've seen many mandalas made in offering to the earth or spirit using shop-bought flowers because they truly look beautiful, but I would suggest trying to avoid that which has been sprayed or grown in flower farms on the other side of the world where workers are paid little, the flowers wrapped in plastic and sent thousands of miles to be sold in supermarkets, and then become part of a practice of earth tending or rewilding, most often in good intention. It doesn't quite add up. We have incredible flora all around, even in the most urban wall or pavement crack.

In some ways if you are connecting with the earth, then connecting with your surroundings makes the most sense. Bringing gratitude into the environment you are in through play, manifestation of beauty, and quiet earth-dreaming holds much power and is something I find very rewarding and rewilding.

There are also ceremonies you can do with plants to help move energy – burning plant wands (smouldering) and resins is a practice that is found all over the world. Local plants are used, without the need of white sage, palo santo, or frankincense unless local to you. The ethics of harvesting for commercial sale is dubious due to a variety of circumstances including development, endangered status, or fad culture. This is explored more in the book's final chapter on "Radical Roots: Decolonial Reflections". Burning local herbs to cleanse an area or oneself is traditional practice worldwide and usually done in ceremony.

Ecuadorian curandera (healer) Rocío Alarcón teaches "Limpia" ceremony with the plants she uses in the mountains of Quito or the jungle of the Amazon. She uses the plants that she is called to and through the wisdom of her ancestors and spirit she brings ceremony forth. She encourages us to use our local plants – the aromatic ones, or medicinal ones. Limpia involves using the plants to "cleanse" the body, mind, and spirit by tapping the body with the plant bundle, with similar effects to burning plant wands or resin. We have the wisdom, and if we have forgotten it, we can reclaim it. Listen. Learn. Communicate. It will come and many of us are so in need of healing and connection.

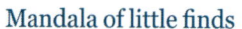

Mandala of little finds

> ### Rewilding exercise
>
> Start with a few natural objects you collect from the ground.
>
> - Arrange them as it feels right to you. It could be a pattern, a scattering, a building – notice what you do.
> - Take a while to stay with what you have created and then either keep it to come back to or disperse into nature once more.
>
> You need not do any more than this. As you create your earth temple consider what your intentions are and be mindful of your own agenda.

Small ceremonies like this can enhance our practice as the mindfulness of doing them creates a different level of humility, service, and awareness.

If you have the skills, working with others to create or learn ceremony is a great idea. In Stroud (and in many other places) folk are coming together to share, care, and create a sisterhood, brotherhood, otherhood, crone connection, kinship, community. Red tents, moon lodges, barefoot walking, and wild dancing are among the many offerings of local folks all seeking to connect us and empower us in some way.

Using ceremony in our lives allows this kind of community. It is there for everyone. We aren't all drawn to it and some of us will be put off participating in ceremony due to the language associated – "sacred", "bliss", "deep" . . . but regardless, we can try to become part of a community rooted in understanding of the nature which surrounds us, with ceremonies that work for us and align us with the wilds as best they can.

A note on living in the city

It is easy to see how someone who lives in the Cotswolds or in Cornwall can simply step out and connect with the natural landscape, with the spirit of Mother Earth. If you are in a city, worry not, it is all there. When I lived in London, I noticed plants all the more. Herb Robert growing out of the vertices between wall and pavement, willow twigs along the canal, bright in their orange glow while everything else is brown and grey. Fleabane along the side of a bit of scrub between home and my neighbour's house. Autumnal sunsets and murmurations of birds are beautiful in the city.

Keep an eye out because there are thousands of plants all around you.

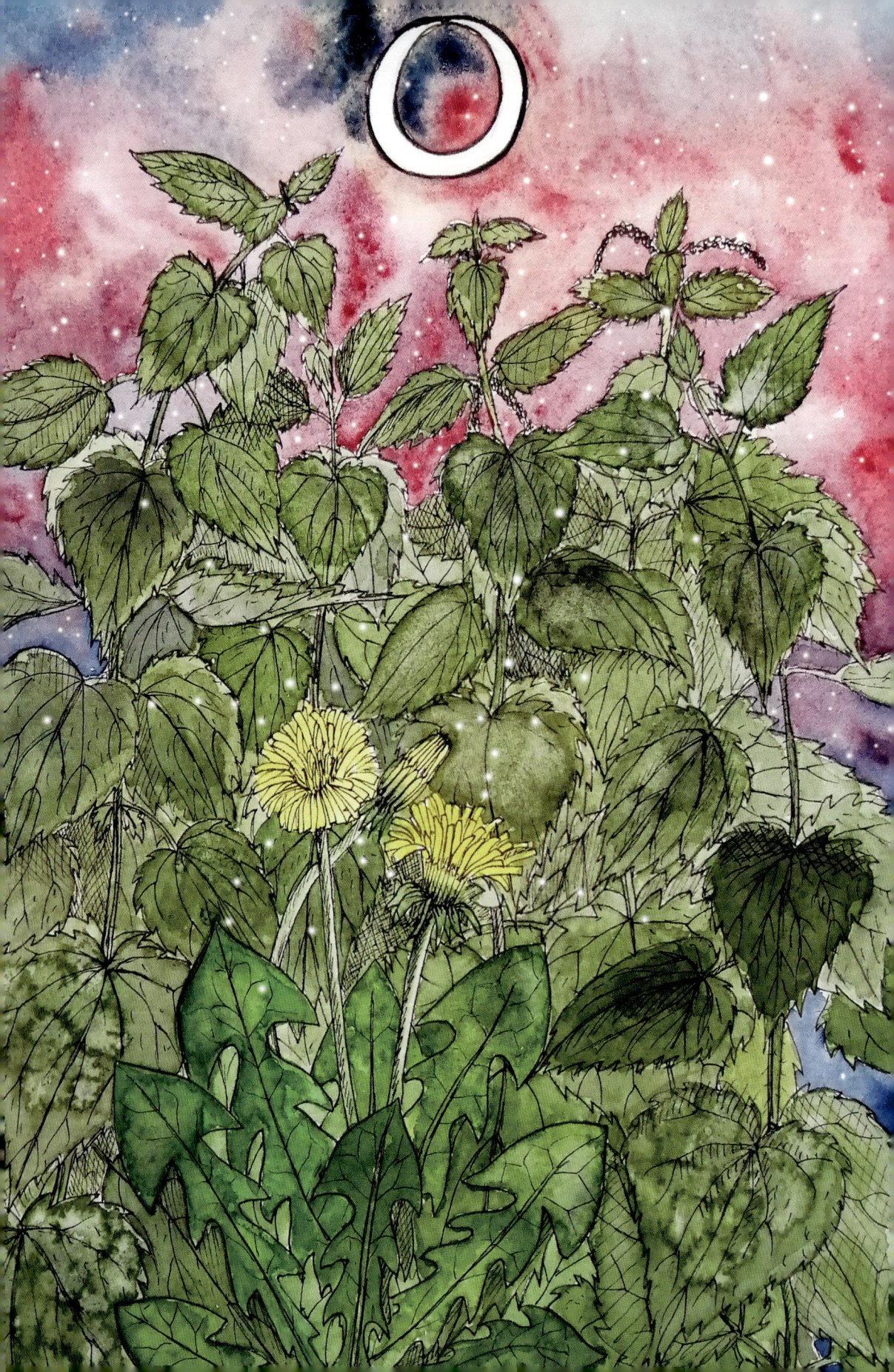

CHAPTER 2

LIFE WITH A WILD APOTHECARY

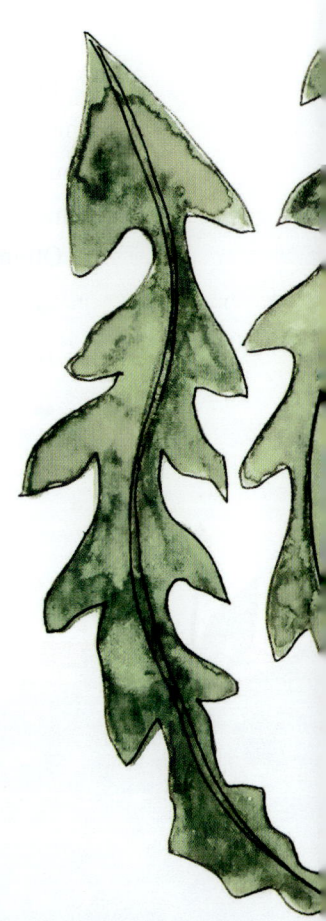

Find your teachers in the voice of the forests
Unplug, you can't ignore this
Wisdom of the voiceless
Remedies are bountiful and surround us
From the garden to the farthest
Prayer made of star dust

From "Medicine" by Rising Appalachia

Nettle and dandelion under the moon

Y ou may find your life is about to be irrevocably changed. A life in connection with plants and landscapes usually means bringing home oodles of plant matter – from roots and twigs to baskets of flowers and fruits, to little bottles of magical (or slightly mysterious if you've forgotten what you've made) liquids, to bags of dried leaves and buds.

Your cupboards may begin to become a haven for all things (forgotten) plant matter. This seems very typical of most herbalists (by no means all – I'm not including everyone!) and is a problem really.

We are in a time which demands we reduce our consumption. Reducing our driving or flying or fossil fuels will never be enough if we don't change the way we, or those of us who make up the culture of mass consumption, live. We simply consume too much and herbalists and foragers aren't immune.

Remember to ethically wild craft, taking only what you need and only if there is an abundance. Is there plenty elsewhere or should we seek cultivated sources? We should also consider whether we will use this exciting plant ally or a more common one such as hawthorn berries instead of bilberries.

Often if we are not sure there are other ways to connect:

❤ Make a flower remedy (or plant remedy) or other energetic medicine that uses very little plant matter (see later in the chapter for recipe).

❤ Meditation with plants.

❤ Initiation – listening and intuiting your needs.

❤ Drawing plants.

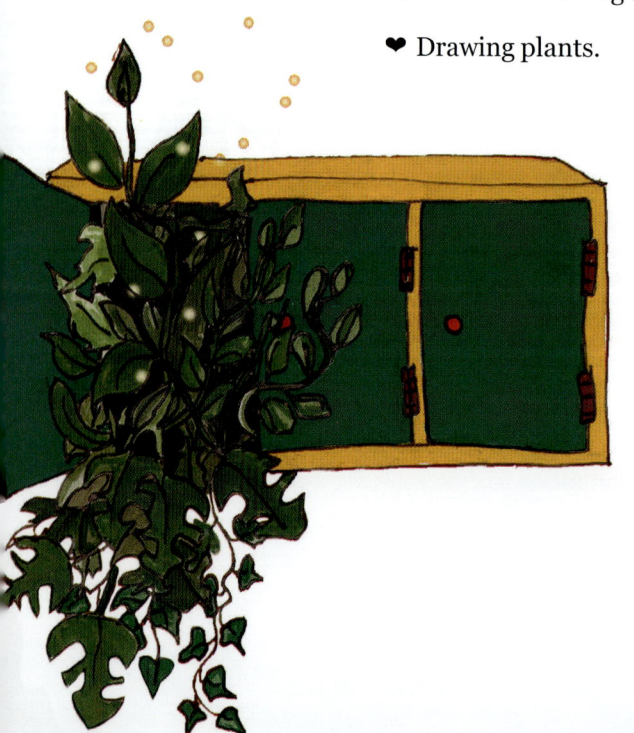

❤ Time with the plant, observing the habitat, what it is growing around, whether it looks healthy, what time of year it is, etc. Get to know the plant and the habitat and how common or uncommon it is.

❤ Observe the growth cycle of that plant and add to your plant maps.

❤ Nibbling leaves, fruits, flower. or roots – plants are living! We connect in when we nibble a leaf as many herbalists do every single day. A sage leaf or a marigold petal is a great start. Claudia's favourite is to nibble on rosemary flowers and leaves or rose and lavender flowers. We know in modern life we have many concerns about nutrient deficiencies; we also have phytonutrient or phytochemical deficiencies around the world as our intake of wild plants is so tiny. Nibbling safe wild edible or medicinal plants can bring our bodies so much benefit.

Dried herbs or syrups have a shorter shelf life than tinctures. Before the year is out if you haven't used up your remedies, find somebody who needs that herb or remedy so it doesn't become clutter at the back of your cupboard and wasted. For tinctures, make sure you use up all of the remedy before beginning new batches of remedies. People will often come to you (or a herbalist) for the remedies you have just prepared. This may be an indication of connection with the seasons or something more mystical.

It is often the case that a remedy you already have could be used instead of another you'd have to buy in. That takes a little knowledge but is worth remembering at any stage of the herbal path. For example, if I wanted ashwagandha for a patient who needed nourishing but I had nettle and oat straw, I might choose the local herbs as long as they worked constitutionally for that patient. I might choose vervain over rose for grief if I've run out of local rose, instead of buying in beautiful organic but foreign rose with all its air miles.

My choice of herb sourcing would be in this order:

1. Local, foraged, or cultivated by me or my kin or kith
2. National or nearby ethical and organic supplies of herbs
3. International organic herbs with ethics in mind
4. Ethical but non-organic herbs from UK, then abroad

It is a bit like your apple choices – do you buy the UK ones that might be a little marked or odd shaped or the organic ones from New Zealand that look perfect? While I hope you say the former, I realise that we are all trying to live within our means and sometimes that means making less ethical choices. But we can try our best.

There are many considerations to be made to really become ethical in your medicine making and relationship with plant medicines, but waste has to be a big consideration. If you do find there are herbs that you just haven't used or piles of unknown wonders, remember to give them back to the earth. Composting them will also allow their nutrient rich return to Mother Earth.

All the remedies in your cupboard should be labelled and dated (first rule, remember). Tinctures and oils should have all the ingredients and ratios on them and whether the plant was fresh or dried. Oils should be kept in a cool dark place.

Herbs you might like to add to the apothecary

Agrimony herb (*Agrimonia eupatoria*)

Alfalfa herb (*Medicago sativa*)

Angelica root (*Angelica archangelica*)

Ashwagandha root (*Withania somnifera*)

Astragalus root (*Astragalus membranaceus*)

Barbary fruit (*Lycium barbarum*)

Barberry bark (*Berberis vulgaris*)

Bearberry (*Arctostaphylos uva-ursi*)

Bilberry fruit (*Vaccinium myrtillis*)

Black cohosh root (*Actaea racemosa* formerly *Cimicifuga racemosa*)

Black horehound herb (*Ballota nigra*)

Black psyllium seed (*Plantago psyllium*)

Black walnut hulls (*Juglans nigra*)

Blackhaw bark (*Viburnum prunifolium*)

Bladderwrack seaweed (*Fucus vesiculosus*)

Blue flag root (*Iris versicolor*)

Boneset herb (*Eupatorium perfoliatum*)

Borage herb (*Borago officinalis*)

Buchu leaf (*Barosma betulina*)

Bugleweed, gypsywort herb (*Lycopus europaeus*)

Burdock root (*Arctium lappa*)

Californian poppy leaves (*Eschscholtzia californica*)

Cardamom seed (*Elettaria cardamomum*)

Catnip (catmint) herb (*Nepeta cataria*)

Cat's claw fruit (*Uncaria tomentosa*)

Cayenne fruit (*Capsicum annum*)

Celery (*Apium graveolens*) seed

Chamomile (German) flowers (*Matricaria recutita*)

Chaste tree berries (*Vitex agnus-castus*)

Chickweed herb (*Stellaria media*)

Chinese (red) sage root (*Salvia miltiorrhiza radix*)

Chinese angelica, dong quai root (*Angelica sinensis*)

(Chinese) ginseng root (*Panax ginseng*)

Cinnamon bark squills (*Cinnamomum zeylanicum*)

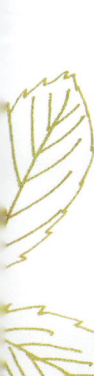

Cleavers herb (*Galium aparine*)

Coltsfoot (*Tussilago farfara*)

Comfrey leaf or root (*Symphytum officinale*)

Coneflower aerial or root (*Echinacea angustifolia, purpurea* or *pallida*)

Coriander seed (*Coriandrum sativum*)

Cornsilk fibre (*Zea mays*)

Couchgrass rhizome (*Agropyron repens*)

Cramp-bark (*Viburnum opulus*)

Damiana leaf (*Turnera diffusa*)

Dandelion leaf or root (*Taraxacum officinalis*)

Devil's claw root (*Harpagophytum procumbens*)

Elder berry and flower (*Sambucus nigra*)

Elecampane root (*Inula helenium*)

Eyebright herb (*Euphrasia officinalis*)

Fennel seed (*Foeniculum vulgare*)

Fenugreek seed (*Trigonella foenum-graecum*)

Feverfew herb (*Tanacetum parthenium*)

Figwort herb (*Scrophularia nodosa*)

Garlic cloves (*Allium sativum*)

Gentian root (*Gentiana lutea*)

Ginger root (*Zingiber officinale*)

Globe artichoke leaves (*Cynara scolymus*)

Goat's rue herb (*Galega officinalis*)

Golden-rod herb (*Solidago virgaurea*)

Goldenseal root (*Hydrastis canadensis*)

Gotu kola herb (*Hydrocotyle asiatica*)

Gravelroot (*Eupatorium purpureum*)

Greater celandine herb (*Chelidonium majus*)

Ground ivy herb (*Glechoma hederacea*)

Hawthorn berry, flowering tops (*Crataegus monoyna*)

Heartsease flowering herb (*Viola tricolor*)

He shou wu (fleeceflower) root (*Polygonum multiflorum*)

Hops strobiles (*Humulus lupulus*)

Horsechestnut (*Aesculus hippocastanum*)

Horsetail herb (*Equisetum arvense*)

Hyssop herb (*Hyssopus officinalis*)

Jamaican dogwood bark (*Piscidia erythrina*)

Juniper berries (*Juniperus communis*)

Lady's mantle herb (*Alchemilla vulgaris*)

Lavender herb, seed (*Lavandula angustifolia*)

Lemon balm herb (*Melissa officinalis*)

Liquorice root (*Glycyrrhiza glabra*)

Lily of the valley leaf (*Convallaria majalis*)

Linden, Lime flowers and bract (*Tilia europea*)

Linseed seed (*Linum usitatissimum*)

Lobelia herb (*Lobelia inflata*)

Maidenhair tree (ginkgo) leaf (*Ginkgo biloba*)

Marigold flowers (*Calendula officinalis*)

Marshmallow root, herb (*Althaea officinalis*)

Meadowsweet herb (*Filipendula ulmaria*)

Milk thistle seed (*Carduus marianus, Silybum marianum*)

Milkvetch root, Huang Qi (*Astragalus membranaceus*)

Motherwort herb (*Leonurus cardiaca*)

Mugwort herb (*Artemisia vulgaris*)

Mullein flowers, herb (*Verbascum thapsus*)

Myrrh resin (*Commiphora molmol*)

Nettle herb, root, seed (*Urtica dioica*)

Oat seeds, straw (*Avena sativa*)

Olive leaf (*Olea europea*)

Oregon grape root (*Berberis aquifolium*)

Osha root (*Ligusticum porteri*)

Pasqueflower herb (*Anemone pulsatilla*)

Passionflower herb (*Passiflora incarnata*)

Pau d'arco bark (*Tabebuia impetiginosa*)

Pellitory of the wall herb (*Parietaria diffusa*)

Peony root (*Paeonia lactiflora*)

Peppermint herb (*Mentha x piperita*)

Plantain leaf, root (*Plantago lanceolata or major*)

Pokeroot root (*Phytolacca decandra*)

Prickly ash (*Zanthoxylum piperitum*)

Raspberry leaf (*Rubus idaeus*)

Red clover flowers (*Trifolium pratense*)

Rehmannia root (*Rehmannia glutinosa*)

Reishi mushroom (*Ganoderma lucidum*)

Rose flowers, petals, buds (*Rosa damascena or gallica*)

Rosemary herb (*Salvia rosmarinus* – formerly known as *Rosmarinus officinalis*)

Roseroot root (*Rhodiola rosea*)

Sage herb (*Salvia officinalis*)

Sarsparilla root (*Smilax ornata*)

Saw palmetto berries (*Serenoa repens*)

Schisandra berries, wu wei zi (*Schisandra chinensis*)

Selfheal herb (*Prunella vulgaris*)

Senna pod (*Cassia angustifolia*)

Shepherd's purse herb (*Capsella bursa-pastoris*)

Siberian ginseng root (Eleuthero) (*Eleutherococcus senticosus*)

Skullcap herb (*Scutellaria lateriflora*)

Spearmint herb (*Mentha spicata*)

St John's wort herb (*Hypericum perforatum*)

LIFE WITH A WILD APOTHECARY

Sweet Annie, qing hao (*Artemisia annua*)

Sweet flag root (*Acorus calamus*)

Sweet violet herb (*Viola odorata*)

Thyme herb (*Thymus vulgaris*)

Tree of life tips (*Thuja occidentalis*)

Turmeric root (*Curcuma longa*)

Valerian root (*Valeriana officinalis*)

Vervain herb (*Verbena officinalis, Verbena hastata*)

White dead nettle herb (*Lamium album*)

White horehound leaf (*Marrubium vulgare*)

White willow bark (*Salix alba*)

Wild cherry bark (*Prunus serotina*)

Wild dog-rose flowers, hips (*Rosa canina*)

Wild indigo root (*Baptisia tinctoria*)

Wild lettuce herb (*Lactuca virosa*)

Wild yam root (*Dioscorea villosa*)

Witch hazel bark (*Hamamelis virginiana*)

Wood betony herb (*Stachys betonica*)

Wormwood herb (*Artemisia absinthium*)

Yarrow herb (*Achillea millefolium*)

Yellow dock root (*Rumex crispus*)

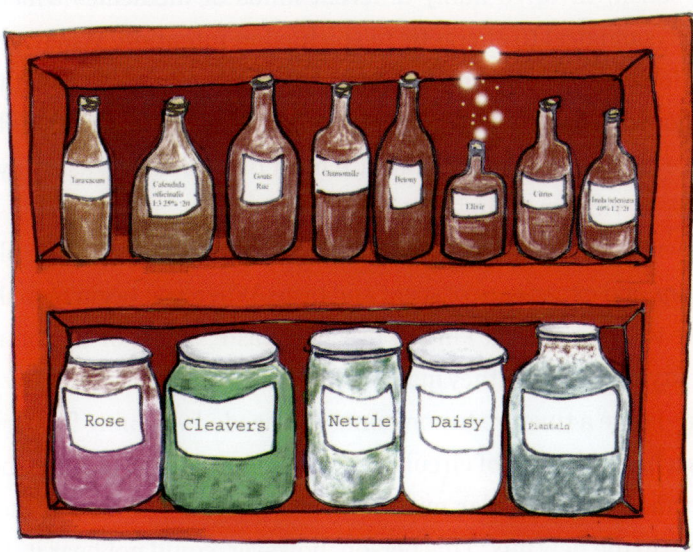

If English is not your first language, or you live in another country, make a list of these herbs in your own language and add any that are commonly used in your culture.

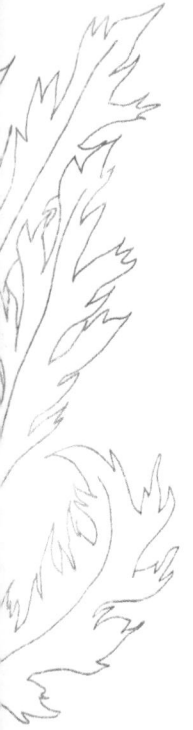

HOW TO CREATE A WILD APOTHECARY

MEDICINE MAKING

What do you think of when you think of herbal remedies? Possibly infusions or little glass bottles with foul tasting liquids. Maybe sweet scented rose oil or even bubbling cauldrons. There are many images that can be conjured with the words "herbal medicine". Many of them from films and books describing the mysterious apothecary or witch selling their wares to the desperate public.

Often films, like The Lord of the Rings for example, portray one flower in high favour. That flower or plant might provide immortality or be an elixir for life or save the life of the protagonist. Sometimes plants are revered and depicted as magical, as in Black Panther where the new king tries to destroy the glowing plants that the shaman needs. It is clear that there is much interest in plants and their power to heal, transform, or hurt; however, it is sometimes in the context of saviour plants rather than grounded wild medicine.

Herbalism involves many different kinds of medicines which range from very physiological to energetic to spiritual in intention. When we make medicines, ideally it is with the intention of doing so in service, with intention to heal, nourish, or help. Even if we are making our living from herbalism, those that are called to use wild plants are most often doing so as a way of life, community, service, or calling.

We wrote a little about tastings before – getting to know the plants through infusions and experience of scent and taste. When you begin to make medicines, be sure to carry on that kind of practice. Taste, smell, or try the remedies you make so you know how they may be experienced (to some extent) by the recipient.

Once I gave a tincture to someone who needed warming for various reasons. It was a beautiful mix of circulatory stimulants and pungent herbs. A previous patient had had a similar mix and loved it and I duly added the 1% cayenne tincture to the new mix. This person, however, could not bear it. It was just too much for them. I hadn't tasted this tincture and considered it enough as I had given it before and it was fine. However, it was fine for a much more choleric person who loved the heat and pungency and the directness of that medicine. If I had tasted it once more, I might have softened the heat knowing that this person was softer and less choleric. So I learned to taste all the tinctures, even those blends I thought I knew really well. (See Chapter 3 for more information on words like "choleric".)

As herbalists we blend, and create and formulate and reformulate many different medicines; as baby herbalists you can too, and just know that you can try again and again until you get remedies that work really well for you and your friends and family.

Developing these skills will also help you in your quality control. If you need to taste an old tea or smell an old oil, you will quickly see if it is comparable to your original blend. You will also be able to assess any herbs you buy in.

I once bought St John's wort when I was a baby herbalist and it was a rusty brown colour. I was surprised as the flowers are yellow and the leaves green and I expected it to be picked at the time of flowering. I shrugged and thought that must be how it dries. The following summer I harvested my own St John's wort which was growing wild in huge swathes. I took only a small amount of herb but when it dried, sure enough it had dried yellow flowers and a few dried green leaves. A few flowers were beginning to turn to seed and there was a little rusty colour to those heads but it was vibrant and green and yellow, not rusty coloured dryness!

I wished, at that time, that I had dried my own, or at least asked one of my teachers what it should look like. Years later a herbalist proclaimed her distaste at the St John's wort dried tea that she had received as it was indeed the same rusty colour. She sent that order back. I should have done too.

Quality is definitely an issue in herbalism and the more you know about how the medicines should be, the better.

So, on to making our own medicines! What will you need to begin making medicines? Let's think about equipment.

HERBALIST TOOLKIT

You most likely have some of these at home, others you can source or you can use similar utensils that work for you. Instead of buying new amber bottles you might ask people to save their coloured glass bottles for you. Clear glass is fine if the medicines are kept out of direct light to stop degradation of the product.

Tools

- Teapots
- Steel pans, bain marie (or water bath of any kind)
- Ovenproof dishes
- Tea strainers
- Wooden spoons
- Funnels (different sizes)
- Sharp knives – moon knives or even meat cleavers are useful for tougher herbs (dried mushrooms, bark, etc.)
- Chopping boards
- Bowls
- Pestle and mortar
- Jelly bag
- Glass jars
- Amber bottles
- Labels
- Notebook
- Scissors
- Whisk
- Clean cotton cloths
- Scales
- Press (eg. apple or wine press)
- Grinder
- Blender
- Food mill (non-electric)
- Juicer (not essential but very useful)

General materials (organic where possible)

- Vegetable oils (or other stable oils)
- Vodka – 40% (or other spirits, each of which will have their own properties; rum for instance has some affinity with the lungs)
- Beeswax
- Cocoa butter, shea butter, etc.
- Honey, sugar
- Spring water (if possible) or filtered water
- Cider vinegar
- Base cream or emulsifying wax
- Essential oils (for external use)
- Vinegars
- Glycerine (vegetable food grade)

MEDICINES WE MAKE

HERBAL TEAS

Herbal teas, or infusions, are great because they are well tolerated, cheap, easy, and often (but by no means always) tasty.

Infusions are great for extracting carbohydrates (gums, mucilage, and more), glycosides (saponins, anthraquinone glycosides, tannins, and flavonoid glycosides), and some salt alkaloids. They are also fairly good at extracting essential oil components of the herbs. That means that if you want certain actions from certain constituents of the plant – perhaps like peppermint oil without taking simply the oil alone, you can use specific methods of extraction to obtain them. In the case of herbal teas it is hot water which acts as the solvent extracting the constituents, and in the case of peppermint tea you will extract some of the essential oils.

It is not just about extraction though. The whole process of making a tea and sitting and tasting and drinking it is very different from the quick swig of the tincture or the application of an external remedy. It may be that someone needs a small ritual or

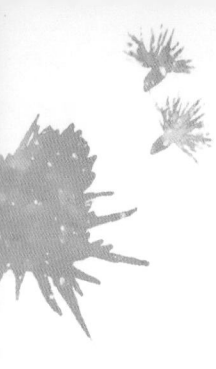

ceremony of tea making as part of the medicine. In some countries tea is highly respected as a way of life with ceremony and community at the heart of tea drinking.

A rough guide to tea making would be:

>5g dried or fresh herb to 1 cup of boiled water
>Infuse 5–10 minutes and then strain and drink

Longer infusions may be done. Often I'll give an overnight infusion of nettles for nourishment, or my Wild Woman tea blend. You make it the night before, leave to infuse overnight, and strain in the morning. It can be sipped during the day and is a deeper remedy. An example of a tea blend I commonly use is:

WILD WOMAN TEA BLEND

Nettle	2 parts
Red raspberry leaf	1 part
Rose	½ part

Brew for 5-10 mins, strain and enjoy

Or for a more nourishing drink, though one that might be too astringent for some, put half an inch (if cut, more if not) of the blend into a 1L jar and fill with boiled water. Cover and leave overnight. Strain the next morning and sup through the day. This is a great tonic.

A variation on this is with demulcent herbs (mucilage-rich ones) over which you can pour the boiling water as above and then leave in the fridge to go slimy overnight or over a day or two. That mucilage is excellent for soothing irritated membranes. Marshmallow, liquorice, or plantain are good.

Decoctions are like infusions but the herbs are decocted actively rather than infused passively. The herbs are simmered for an amount of time – 10 minutes, half an hour, an hour or more, depending on the plant matter.

Decoctions are usually used for harder herbs but can also be used as a deeper remedy with softer herbs. Sometimes the herbs are decocted and then left to steep overnight. Decoction is also used for some preparations that are made into tinctures and which need the water solvent before the alcohol. This is most often roots, bark, and mushrooms.

A good ratio for decoctions is 1oz herb to 1 pint of water. Once measured and added, reduce to ¾ of the volume and either drink or dilute by adding teaspoons of the preparation to a cup of water as it may be very strong.

If you'd like to preserve a decoction you can add alcohol so that the solution is 20% alcohol to 80% decoction, or glycerine can be used if alcohol is not tolerated.

Reduced decoctions can be made for anyone who can't or doesn't want to take alcohol but who also needs stronger (more concentrated) medicine.

How to make a reduced decoction

Make a decoction (as above).

Once strained put the liquid back on a very low heat until you have reduced the liquid to one quarter of the original amount.

If you manage to reduce further (to one twentieth of the original amount) the herb will keep for a long time.

Bottle and label.

You can also reduce a decoction until completely dry, then scrape the powder up and use that as a concentrated powder. Do not use a coated pan if doing this. These are great mixed into honey or kept in airtight jars.

Cold infusions are great for many herbs including cleavers and bitters. So instead of boiling the water for tea, you simply add cold water and allow to steep overnight. Strain in the morning and sup first thing. You can keep it in the fridge for a couple of days and drink each morning before eating.

Hand soaks, foot baths, baths, and douches are other forms of infusions and

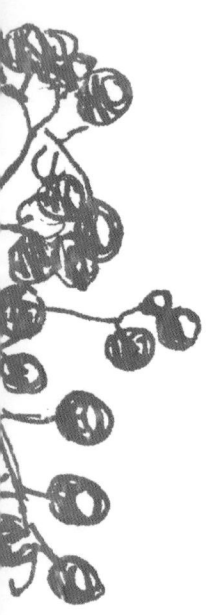

are lovely ways to experience herbal medicine. Baby baths, gargles, eye baths, enemas, can be gentle and effective and were traditionally used much more than they are nowadays.

GARGLES

You can make excellent gargles from infusions and decoctions. You can also add a little tincture to water to make a gargle but for everyday use alcohol is a bit drying on the mouth.

Easy gargles to make are sage and or thyme tea cooled to your liking. Swig a mouthful and swish about the mouth and gargle.

SYRUPS

Syrups are sweet and nourishing, they are a thick sweet soothing liquid that coats the throat. This is excellent for some as it ensures compliancy. Kids love syrups, and they are easy on the throat and suitable for elders. Syrups are particularly useful in lung conditions where phlegm is stuck. The syrup can aid expectoration (expelling phlegm from the lungs) and act as soothing demulcents for the respiratory system.

Sugar, honey, or a concentrated fruit juice may be used to preserve and thicken the infusion of a plant. Glycerine can also be used which is really useful for those who cannot take sugar, for although it is sweet, it is not absorbed in the gut and passes through while delivering the herbs infused in it.

Note: syrups are great for those with a dry constitution and can have a laxative effect.

```
ELDERBERRY SYRUP

1 part fresh ripe black elderberries
2 parts water
1 part honey (raw if possible)
½ cinnamon stick and/or a little ginger root

Gather the fresh berries and make sure no stems remain
- you can use a fork to get them off easily, just use
it as a mini rake and gently prise off the berries.
```

> Place the berries in a saucepan and cover with twice as much water (for 1 cup of berries, use 2 cups of water).
>
> Add cinnamon and ginger to taste, if you like – or similar warming aromatic herbs and spices of your choice.
>
> Place the pan over a medium heat and bring to a simmer.
>
> Simmer gently for around half an hour.
>
> Strain the juice from the cooked elderberries into a glass jar or jug. This makes knowing how much juice you have easier.
>
> Let the juice cool to a warm temperature, then stir in an equal amount of raw honey. Use normal honey or sugar if preferred.
>
> Jar and label. Keep in the fridge.

You can make a decoction or reduced juice – juice your elderberries and then leave over a low heat until ½–¾ of the water evaporates; if enough water is evaporated you don't need to add anything and it will keep very well in the fridge. Sometimes I have made this remedy with elderberry: it is called an elderberry rob – when I paid attention and reduced properly it lasted for years in a small jar. When I was overconfident and took it off the heat as it just thickened, the water content meant it grew mould easily and only last a few weeks.

We usually use this lovely syrup as an anti-viral remedy. One teaspoon 2–3 times a day for an adult, ½ teaspoon 2–3 times daily for child.

There are many elderberry syrup recipes online but getting to know the basics of how much sugar (or other sweetener) you need to preserve is key. Once you have that skill, then you can experiment with syrups. Note down any failures (exploding bottles of syrup, mouldy bottles of syrup, thin syrups, foul-tasting syrups, etc.) and successes so you can draw on that knowledge.

VINEGARS

These are much underused in herbalism. This is probably because people associate vinegar with chips or cleaning. It is a fantastic edible product (when made well) and herbal infused vinegars are very useful and effective. Vinegars, unlike alcoholic tinctures, are well tolerated and can be taken by kids and elders alike with little issue. There are those who won't take vinegars and those who do react so it's not for everyone but generally they are great.

BLACKBERRY VINEGAR

This seasonal vinegar will last for months so if you make it in the autumn, for example, and like to use it a lot, you could make a bigger batch which will last you through the winter.

I prefer using organic and raw apple cider vinegar with the live mother but have a go with different vinegars, or make your own.

Fill a jar with freshly picked blackberries.

If you prefer, you can choose other herbs like rosemary, sage, raspberry leaf, rose and others.

Cover with cider vinegar.

Leave in a cool dark place for 2 weeks and then strain, bottle, and label.

Add a drizzle to salads or a teaspoon in a cup of hot water for a digestive kick first thing in the morning.

To make an oxymel you can simply add honey (very gently heating the honey helps to mix it more evenly). Add a little at a time as you don't want to over-sweeten your vinegar.

If you make a herbal infused vinegar, you can also add honey which turns the vinegar into an oxymel. This may be preferred by many as it is sweet. Vinegars and oxymels promote digestion and are a good base for cooling remedies.

TINCTURES

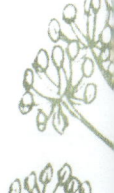

Tinctures are a fast-acting remedy. The alcohol and water base combined is a great solvent for extracting constituents from plants.

They can taste awful and wonderful! By learning about alcohol and its effect at various different strengths, you'll start to see which strength tincture works best with which plant.

The easiest basic tincture is made from fresh plants, and is also known as a "specific" (see below). For the vast majority of very common garden herbs, you can use something similar to vodka in strength (usually around 40% alcohol). To preserve the medicine, a tincture needs a minimum of 20% alcohol.

```
LEMON BALM SPECIFIC TINCTURE
1:3 25%

1 part herb - eg. 100g fresh lemon balm
3 parts vodka - eg. 300ml vodka

Finely (ish) chop the lemon balm: this is because a
greater surface area in contact with the menstruum
will allow easier infusion.

Add to a jar with as little air left as possible, so
choose a jar of an appropriate size for the amount you
are making.

Add the vodka.
```

```
Try to make sure all the herb is covered by the vodka.
If it isn't, push it down or weigh it down with a
ceramic weight or other suitable object. Sometimes I
use a glass or ceramic cup with no handle which sits
under the jar lid keeping all the herbs submerged.

Leave for 2 weeks and shake or mix every day to release
any air pockets.

Strain, bottle, and label.
```

To extract the resins from herbs such as myrrh or marigold a higher percentage of alcohol in the menstruum (liquid) is needed – around 90%. Note that with marigold, you may instead wish to use the flowers for their anti-inflammatory properties, in which case you'd need just 25% alcohol in the menstruum.

Following the recipe above, you will have made beautiful lemon balm fresh plant tincture at a strength of 1:3 25% alcohol.

The water from the leaves will bring the alcohol ratio down, hence the 25%.

The fresh tincture is called an ST (specific tincture).

HYDROSOLS

These are steam distilled remedies which are known as aromatic waters. Water is passed through the still, condensing with volatile oils and more constituents in the liquid captured. They are mostly used for aromatic herbs. The essential oils preserve the hydrosol for around six months to a year depending on the resulting volatile oil content.

A still is worth having to make these remedies, but a home-made version can be absolutely fine.

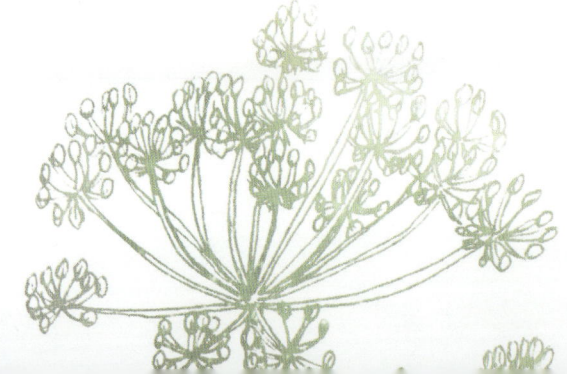

You need a small pot on a trivet that goes inside a larger pan with a lid:

> Pour water into the large pan (not getting any in the littler pot). Add your aromatic herbs to the water all around the small pot – put in as much as you can fit in.
>
> Put the lid on the larger pan upside down so you can put ice cubes in it; the condensation will fall into the small pot.
>
> Heat gently.
>
> Take off the heat when all the water has been used up.
>
> Bottle and label. Store in a cool dark cupboard.

NB. Try to use a small pot that will collect all of the water once condensed.

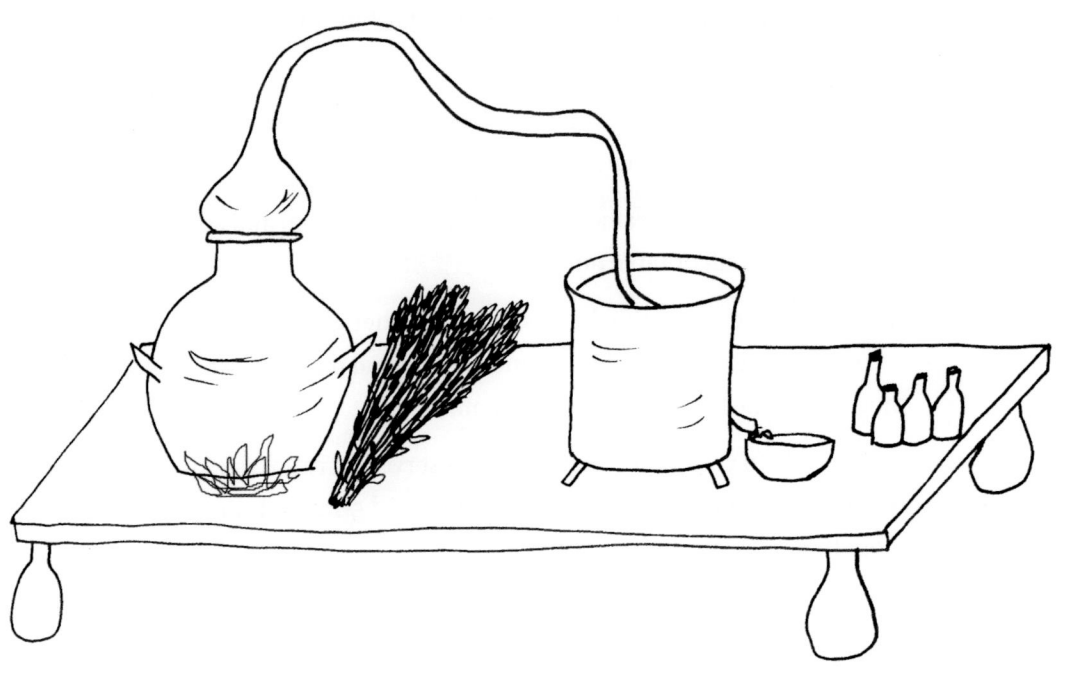

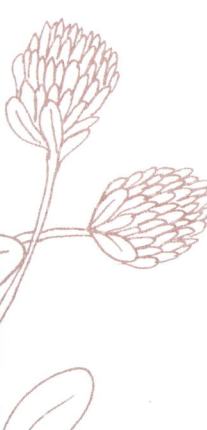

FLOWER REMEDIES

Flower remedies are lovely medicines which work on an energetic level. Flowers are considered to be the highest vibrational frequency of the plant and all that energy is going into the flower remedy on a vibrational level.

Choose which flower remedy you'd like to make. Perhaps one that calls to you at dusk, one that somehow has the wild of the night infused into your connection with it. Or perhaps one that calls to you in full vitality while the sun is hot.

Sit a while with the plant and listen.

Ask if you may take a flower, or a few flowers for your remedy.

If you feel good to proceed then pick the flowers that call to you – the most vital you can find.

Infuse them in a bowl with a little water. I like to use spring water as it is alive but it can feel a little fizzy sometimes due to the bacteria present in this life water. Sometimes I use my filtered water but if you don't have a spring or filter, go ahead and use tap water.

Put your flowers into the water and leave to infuse under the sun or moonlight for 3 hours or all night.

Sometimes I leave my remedy by the plant it was from and sometimes I put it on a windowsill or table outside.

In the morning strain the flowers out and either gift them back to the earth – I often create a little mulch around the original plant, or eat them, or make more medicine from them, or dry them, etc.

Add brandy to your flower remedy to preserve at a ratio of 1:2 parts water to brandy. If you have 50ml of water, you'll need 50ml of brandy as you want more than 20% alcohol to preserve.

Bottle, label, and take drops of it when called to – notice how it affects you when you take it. What happens? It may be exactly what you perceived or it may be entirely different. These are energetic remedies and work in a different way to tinctures or infusions.

Most of the internal preparations listed above eventually mean disregarding the spent plant matter (eg. tea in the pot after drinking). However, if you want to get deeper into the alchemy of plant medicine making you can explore spagyric alchemy where the whole plant, including the spent mark, is processed to include the body, spirit, soul of the plant which is known as the salt, mercury, sulphur.

EXTERNAL REMEDIES

There are many external remedies you can make with infusions and tinctures. The other most common external remedies are oils, creams, liniments, and balms.

INFUSED OILS

Infused oils are a great way to get our plant allies onto our skin and also into the body through transdermal absorption. They are relatively easy to make if you have access to fixed oils like sunflower, olive, or coconut oil. Once ready they store well for around a year or can be added to ointments and creams.

I find the use of oils interesting in an ethical sense. Try to use what is local to you and what is best for the environment. Coconut oil plantations are becoming as common as palm oil plantations and this kind of planting only damages existing biodiversity; olive plantations in great swathes mean that bees struggle. It is all a balancing act but look into your oils of choice and see how ethical they are.

Note it is best to store oils and ointments in darker glass jars or in jars in brown paper bags to prevent light degradation of the ointment. If I don't have dark glass jars, I always keep my ointments in a dark cupboard.

```
RECIPE: COMFREY INFUSED OIL

Pick a good amount of comfrey leaves (root is also
good) and let them dry or leave for a night in a dry
place to allow some moisture loss. Water and oil are
not a great combination: you want your oil to be free
of water.
```

Note: I usually have a full armful of comfrey stems with lots of leaf and I use the leaves themselves and the flowers – with a double infusion this usually makes around 1L of oil or less.

Chop up the leaves. Put half of them aside and add the other half into a bain marie or a water bath. You can also add them to a slow cooker on "warm" setting (anything higher will roast them!).

Cover the leaves with your chosen oil. For herbs like comfrey I use organic olive oil which is a bit heavier; for more aromatic herbs I use lighter oils and prefer organic and local if I can get them.

You should have enough oil to just cover all your leaves. If you have too many leaves or too much oil, try to adjust and always note it down.

Simmer the water in the bottom pan for 2 hours. The oil should be warm but not hot and you should see a difference in the structure of the leaves. Never put the oil on a direct heat source.

Strain and repeat with the other half of the leaves in the same oil. This is called a double infusion.

Bottle and label.

OINTMENTS

Ointments have an oil as their base and are made into balms with the addition of a butter or wax, for example, shea butter or beeswax. They are thicker and heat capturing so are good as rubs and barrier medicine for conditions like chesty coughs or very dry skin conditions. They may not be suitable for hot weepy skin conditions where the heat may become too trapped as oils and ointments act as barriers on the skin.

> **RECIPE: COMFREY OINTMENT**
>
> Use the method above to make your infused oil.
>
> When strained but still hot at the end of the process, add in the beeswax or other hard butter (cocoa, shea, etc.)
>
> Just before adding the beeswax you can also add in essential oils to make a hot (pungent) or aromatic ointment.
>
> If you are using beeswax, a good ratio is 1:6 parts wax to oil.
>
> This can be adapted depending on the wax.
>
> For a muscle rub drops of wintergreen essential oil are great. Try around 5-10 drops for a 30ml pot of ointment.
>
> I like to keep my ointments (balms) in amber glass jars or if they have a great colour, clear glass jars.

CREAMS

Creams are favoured by many. They are light and absorbent and are easily smoothed into the skin. They look appealing and can feel fresh and nourishing. Creams are lighter than ointments so people enjoy them more for daily use.

Creams can be quick and easy to prepare if you have the ingredients going into them ready made. They are also cooler in nature than ointments when applied to the skin. However, they don't keep as well as ointments and don't last as long around the area of skin into which you are rubbing them.

The best uses for creams would be inflammatory skin conditions and skin diseases, cosmetic and nurturing skin/self-care.

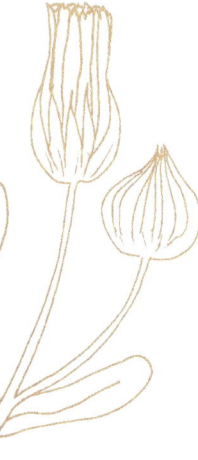

Creams can also be made to suit the skin type of the individual. Folk with dry skin need a little more oil and folk with oilier skin need a little less oil.

Cold folk often enjoy warming creams with a little more oil and appropriate warming herbs, and hot folk on the other hand may suit cooling creams or gels (like aloe vera based gels) or more cooling essential oils.

Here is the first cream recipe I did with my teacher, Christopher Hedley. It is a great cream and easy to make. Have a go at it and then try adding blends of essential oils that you like. It is lovely to be able to whip up your own face cream. If you want it to last a long time you might like to add sufficient essential oils to preserve, a preservative, or keep in the fridge.

```
RECIPE: CHRISTOPHER'S CALENDULA (MARIGOLD) CREAM

4g emulsifying wax

12ml calendula infused oil

32ml calendula concentrated decoction (this is the
water element so water will substitute this, but a
strong infusion or reduced decoction with marigold is
even better!)

Put all the ingredients into a small pan and
heat gently.

Once the wax has melted, stand the pan in cold water
and stir continuously. As it cools, it will
become a cream.

Store in small glass jars and label.

The ratio here is 1:3:8 wax:oil:water.
```

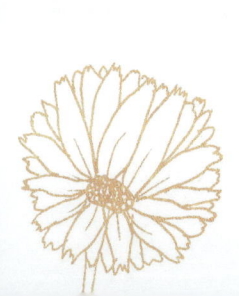
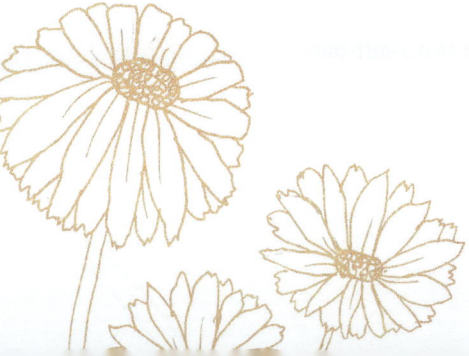

LINIMENTS

These are a useful external preparation used to rub into the skin. They are often a mix of oil and tincture (alcohol), and by rubbing the alcohol into the area the herb is delivered and heat is created which the oil then holds in. This could be useful for cold joints (rheumatism) and could be, for example, a comfrey infused oil mixed with a warming ginger tincture. The two may separate so make sure they are shaken well before rubbing into the area.

You can also add essential oils to a tincture or oil and call it a liniment if you are using it to rub into the skin or muscles to heat or cool. Some people call tiger balm a liniment – it is used to penetrate a joint or muscle with deep heat and contains essential oils like camphor, wintergreen, and menthol in a petroleum jelly base. You could use these oils in a balm such as hot comfrey balm (see p. 242).

Liniments are also considered to be a topical application to soothe skin or muscles so a witch hazel base with some cooling herbs infused in could be classed as a liniment for sunburn. This is a little more simple.

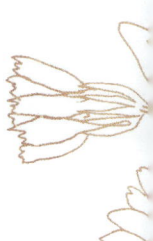

```
HEATING LINIMENT

50ml comfrey infused oil
25ml juniper berry tincture
15ml rosemary tincture
10ml ginger tincture
10 drops wintergreen essential oil

Shake well before applying to aching muscles or pain-
ful joints.

Note if the skin is irritated it may not like alcohol
so use a different base such as aloe gel or witch
hazel.
```

A COOLING LINIMENT

(though this can also be called a lotion!)

Fill a small jar with dried peppermint, lavender, and rose petals. Cover with witch hazel water (this is usually around 85% witch hazel and 15% alcohol) and let infuse for 2 weeks shaking daily. Strain and pour into a bottle – one with a spray top is good as you can simply spray the cooling liniment onto the mild sunburn, for example.

LOTIONS

Lotions really are just liquid remedies which soothe and tone. They are often cooling and I like to include aloe gel which is soothing in itself. I like to mix the aloe gel with a base cream and whichever other herbs I need for the person for whom I am making the lotion. Witch hazel water is another great cooling liquid which can be used alone or mixed with a gel or cream to make a thinner preparation.

COOLING, NOURISHING AND ASTRINGING SKIN TONER

25ml rose hydrosol

25ml fennel hydrosol

25ml frankincense hydrosol (ethical sources only)

25ml rosemary hydrosol

Combine and pour into a spray bottle. Spritz onto skin and gently smoothe across your face.

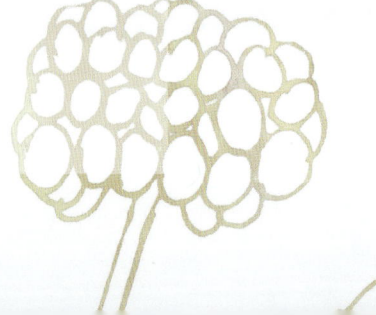

COMPRESSES AND POULTICES

I love compresses and poultices. They are not the easiest of remedies as they can be messy and you need fresh plant to make them but they are so good for us humans – both physiologically and emotionally as they are proper wild medicine.

Compresses are simply crushed up plants applied to the body and wrapped with a thin bandage or cloth if needed. They can be used to disinfect wounds, staunch bleeding, etc.

Poultices are generally used for drawing out of the body – infection, pus, inflammation, etc. We often use demulcent herbs like plantain, chickweed, and comfrey for poultices.

Simply chop up or crush the herbs and mix with a little water, or if wet enough there is no need for extra water. Apply to the skin and wrap in a crepe cloth or strips of muslin. Or if very wet, wrap in thin cloth first and apply to affected area. Leave for a while and take off as needed.

There are many more variations of remedies – sprays, lozenges, powders, percolations, spagyric tinctures, etc.

THE APOTHECARY'S RECORD

It is really good when you are making medicine to record everything you do. Even if it is a remedy you have made before, note down any deviations, such as adding an extra or substitute essential oil or different ratio of waxes. This is because you might fluke an excellent cream and not have noted it down. Have a book solely dedicated to remedies if you can so that you have easy access to your recipes.

You can also expand your range of remedies with body butters, facial oils, shampoo bars, pastes, rubs, powders, etc. A little apothecary's book may just become your best friend one day.

A note about storage

> Keep remedies dry
> Keep remedies out of direct sunlight

Keep remedies away from direct heat sources
Keep remedies labelled

JOURNALING

Note in your journal how it makes you feel to actually make any wild plant medicines.

Did you enjoy it, were you nervous, what parts did you like the most? Did it work? Did you note it down?!

Plan ahead – journal in what kinds of remedies you'd like to make and who for – just yourself or your friends and family? These kinds of thoughts can really help with wild crafting in a busy world – if heart medicine is your draw then think about when you can get out to collect hawthorn or lime blossom, for example. Would you like flowering tops of hawthorn, berries, or both? Do you know where your local hawthorn trees are?

What kinds of remedies are you seeking? Energetic or spiritual remedies to help connect, or remedies with an emotional or physiological effect?

Just journal it out and see what comes.

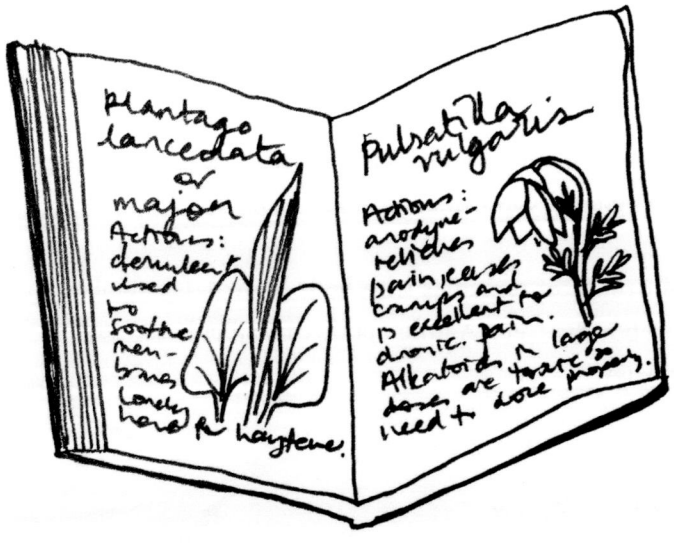

Plant allies wheel of the year

A calendar is helpful too – something for each month of the year is really fun. For example in May you can make hawthorn brandy, in June you can make elderflower fritters, and in July St John's wort oil. If you're completely new and don't have a clue when things come out, use this time to make notes on what you see when and where.

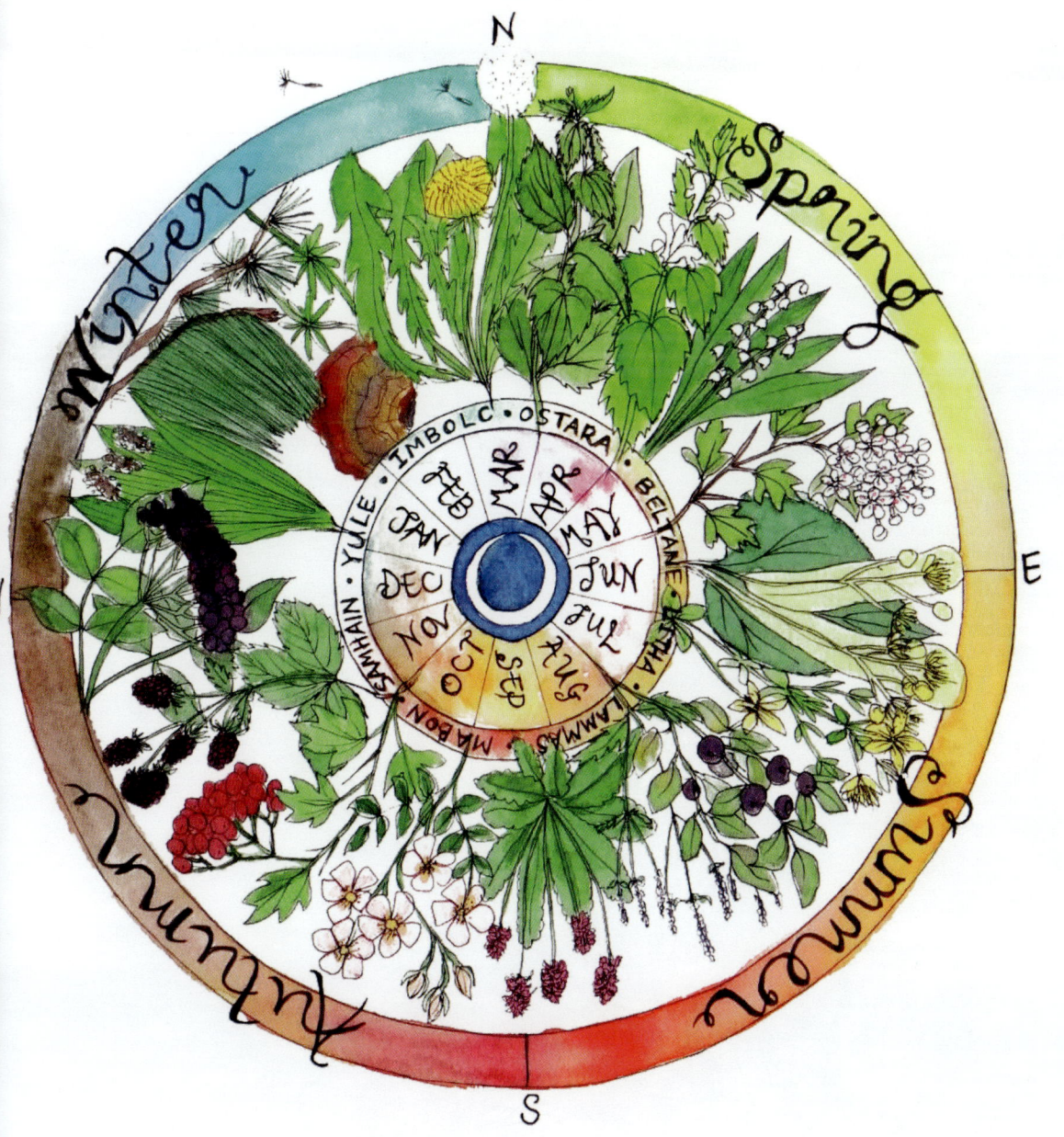

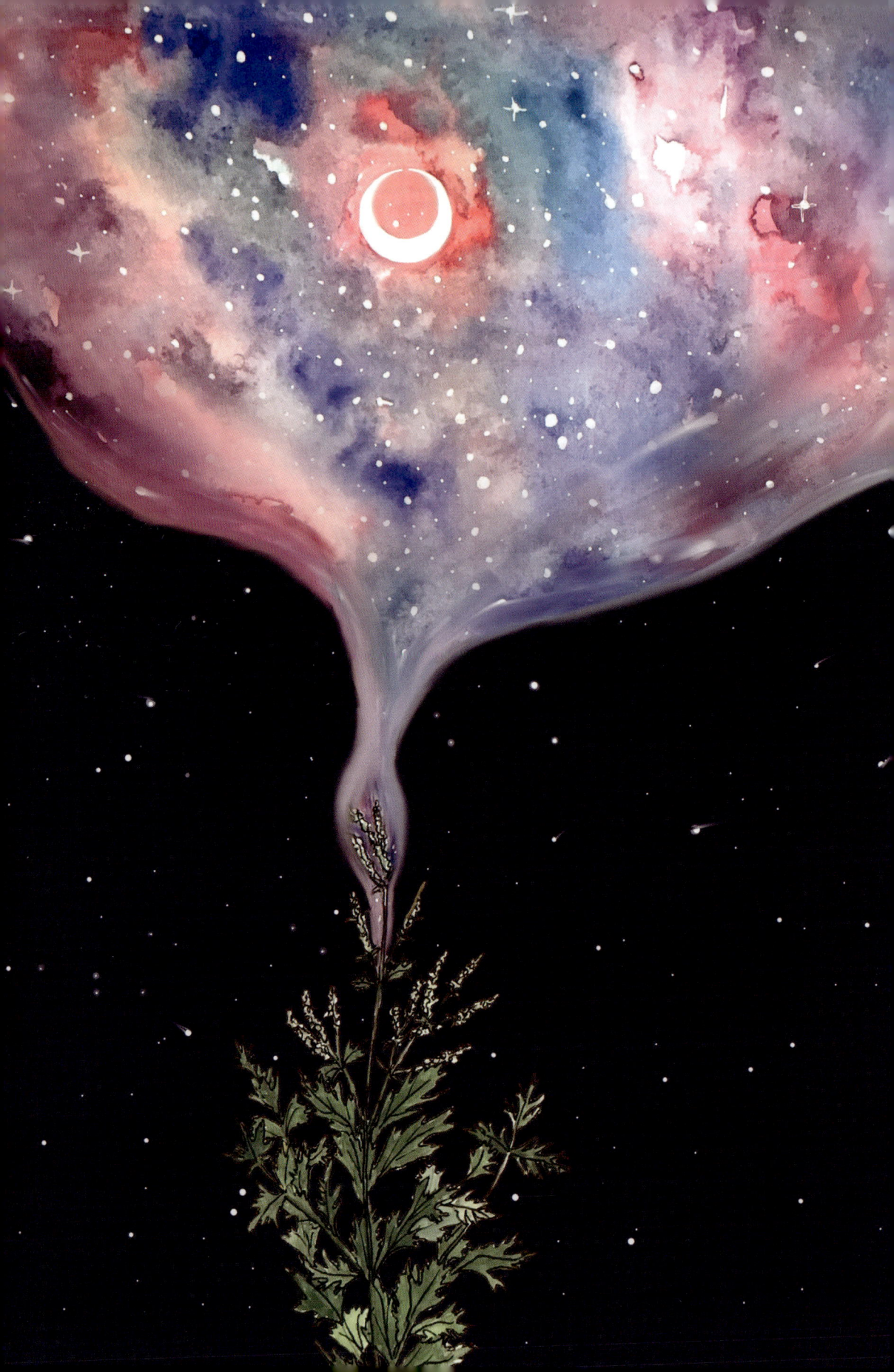

CHAPTER 3

FOLK AND FLORA: ENERGETICS OF WILD MEDICINE

"Of course you love small things, Amaia, you're melancholic"

Rebecca Altman of Wonder Botanica

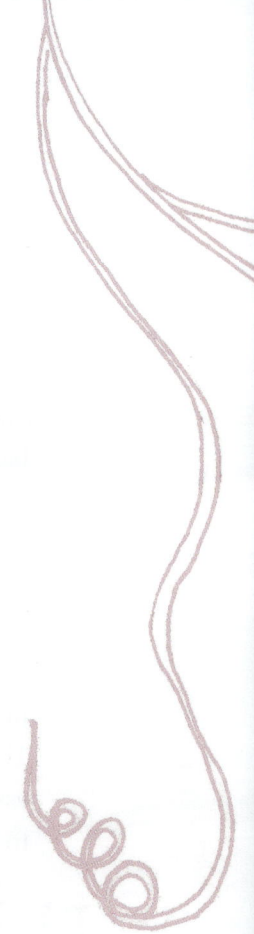

Mugwort dreaming

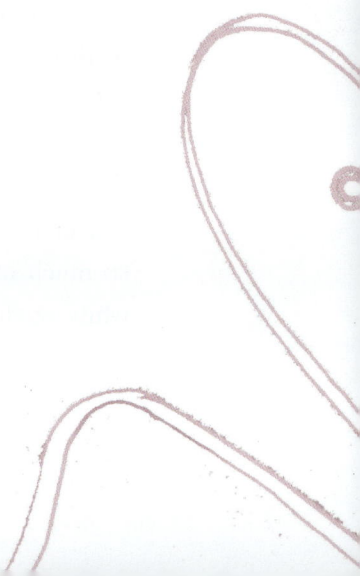

INTRODUCTION TO ENERGETICS OF HERBALISM

We have covered some basics of beginning an apothecary, of how to find and make herbal remedies, and how to reconnect with the earth through herbalism and rewilding. The following chapters will each have a focus on a particular time of life and how to use herbal medicine. We will start with babies and work through to elders and grieving, with conditions and plant medicines to suit. We will look at some gender specific herbalism – gynaecological conditions and male reproductive system medicine to label them in reductive but practical terms. We will also look at transitioning and herbalism in terms of folk being able to access support for their needs.

Before this, however, we'll look just a little at the energetics of herbalism to introduce you to different ways of seeing and understanding plants and people. This will help you to see herbs with different elements of the plant in mind; in essence learning about energetics provides another tool to understanding how to use plants and also helps us interpret what we find in older herbals which can be really useful.

WAYS OF READING THE BODY – THE ENERGETICS AND ELEMENTS

Alongside or in threads through each section, you'll notice words like melancholic, phlegmatic, constitution, and more. These are words that belong to a system of healing.

Around 400 BCE Hippocrates learned his trade in Alexandria, Egypt. He described a system of healing that was based on the philosophy that nature was made up of four elements – earth, air, fire, and water.

Now, it is a strange place from which I write because I was mostly taught by women about the history of herbalism through the work of men. Hippocrates was preceded by Imhotep, a Black man, who was a practising Egyptian medicine man more than 2000 years before Hippocrates. It is very worth noting that so much of our knowledge of the building of orthodox medicine has been white-washed and erased.

In Egypt there were also priestesses, such as Meret and Peseshet who were chief physicians in their time (~2700 BCE), practising medicine for as long as the temples have been standing. The world of medical history is just that. His-story, his White story. This is why decolonising herbal medicine is so vital.

Back to Hippocrates for now. India, Tibet, China and many other countries had their own full health systems such as Ayurveda in India, and the work that Hippocrates focused on was probably the first time that a holistic healthcare system had been recorded in Europe in a medically orthodox sense.

Hippocrates was a philosopher and medic; he thought about the humours of the body. These are the liquid tissues such as blood and phlegm. He also thought about the lifestyle of a person and how much exercise they got, how fresh the air was around them, and how well they slept. He thought food was an essential factor for health and well-being.

In herbalism nowadays these kinds of lifestyle factors are all intrinsic to the health picture of each person. They are of course found in many other systems around the world and weren't only thought about by one White man. Hippocrates' presented healthcare system, however, still largely influences the West in our medicine and his practice of close observation of the patient through the senses, not just the intellect, prevails in any holistic therapy. The senses are the ones you've most likely been familiar with all of your life: taste, touch, sight, smell, and sound. Some also consider nature connection, one's spirit or intuitive instincts too to be a sense.

The four humours made up the body and each humour corresponded to one of the four elements, of which all matter was thought to be composed. Each humour and element corresponds to the four seasons and each also has a stage of life it corresponds to.

Disease was thought to be an imbalance of the humours.

The humours themselves are:

   Blood: air, sanguine, spring, children
   Yellow bile: fire, choleric, summer, youth
   Black bile: earth, melancholic, autumn, adults
   Phlegm: water, phlegmatic, winter, elders

Each humour has its own attributes and when they are in balance the individual is deemed healthy. Often a person has a more dominant humour or two, or displays certain traits when there is imbalance.

Getting to know the humours and how they manifest in the body can be really helpful in assessing and understanding what is going on for someone in terms of health. Just like in Ayurveda where one's balance of doshas (pitta, kapha, vata) affect not only the body but the personality, so too do the humours. Different combinations make up different personality traits, lifestyle choices, and emotional health pictures.

Detailed observation can give hints as to what is going on in someone's health picture. Examples such as a pale face, a red hot cheek, a sweaty layer, a frazzled demeanour or thick luscious hair can point to imbalances, constitution, and health. The way people describe themselves such as, "I just look at food and I put on weight", "I eat like a horse", "Don't mind me, I'm just a worrier", can also be self-describing in terms of constitution.

By reading the body, you begin to understand the physiology, the energetic picture, or emotional state of the patient. These kinds of systems allow for greater understanding of humanity and ill health and are used by herbalists as part of a wider system with modern thought, intuition, grass roots knowledge, and many other factors woven together.

Spiritual practices integral to understanding the body in all its forms (physical, emotional, mental, spiritual, astral), also known as "shamanism", are found throughout the world. They are hugely complex and sophisticated, yet are often belittled (remind you of ceremony?)

When Hippocrates differed from the state in his secular beliefs, he was incarcerated. He did not think that spirit contributed or caused illness. He believed in physiology and paved the way for hundreds of years of orthodox medicine in Europe. This system defined diagnostic practice. This model of health takes us even further from shamanic practices and reduces our understanding of the different layers of life.

Hopefully, most folk appreciate that there are many different ways of working in health and understanding life and illness. If we don't understand how modern medicine came about and what we have because of it, we won't be able to fully understand a holistic system of medicine. In this short introduction, we have noted White-washing, Eurocentrism, male and secular ideals which are now sewn so tightly into medicine that it has been normalised.

The humoral chart

His-story continues with Galen – the next name commonly mentioned when history of herbalism was taught to us. He was another Greek man who took on the work of Hippocrates and he also recorded the uses of plants. The information he meticulously gathered has been worked with by herbalists for hundreds of years. Galen noted down the uses of thousands of plants and is one major source of knowledge. There are other sources of knowledge too, such as shamanic knowledge, physiomedicalism, indigenous knowledge, etc. Much of it wasn't written and ethnobotanists and many others have taken up the mantle of trying to preserve knowledge on paper (or digital files more likely) before it is all but lost.

Each section in this book will have a little bit of humoral medicine and energetic uses of plant medicine, showing you how it can be a useful tool in everyday life working with plants and people.

There are also similar energetic systems into which herbal medicines have been recorded, such as eclectic medicinal distinctions and the defining of classes of plants by, for example, Galen, Culpeper, or modern herbalists. Modern herbalists are a huge mix of women, men, non-binary folk, queer folk, folk of all nationalities, colours, and voices. However, it is still the White male herbalist who has the loudest voice. Things are changing but we each need to take responsibility to make sure all voices are heard.

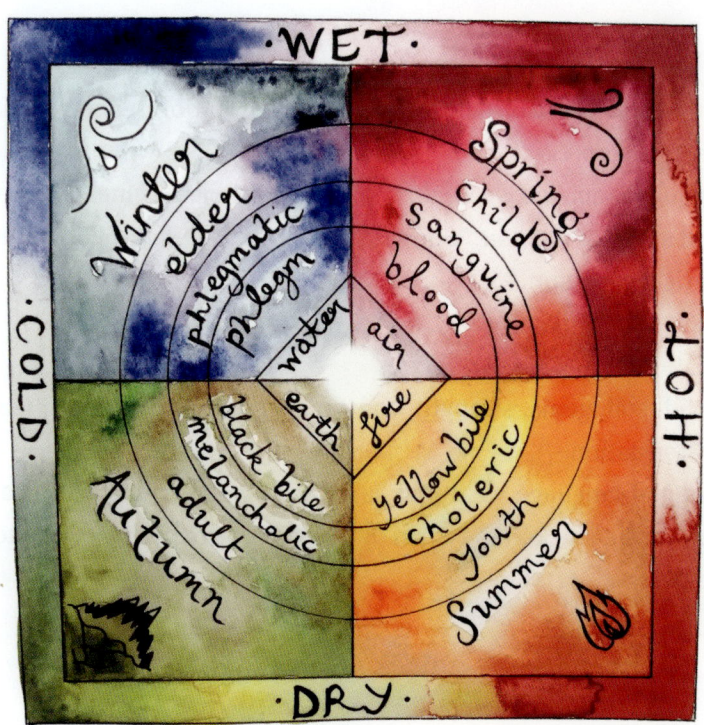

When learning herbs try, if you can, to feel out the qualities or virtues of those herbs – whether they are cooling, heating, drying, moistening, opening, closing, etc. These impressions will give you knowledge you can then cross reference in herbals of old and new, with others in different countries with different systems and with your fellow herbalists' experiences. You'll soon get to know which herbs might suit a hot dry choleric individual and why.

Most chronic illness is born out of an imbalance; in humoral terms, it would be an imbalance usually in the form of a dominant humour in excess. Once brought back into balance, a different state of health may be achieved. It also helps demonstrate why some folk like a certain type of herb or food and others react badly to that same herb or food. Knowledge worth knowing.

For each plant you learn, assess its energetics on yourself – see what it does to you, how it makes you feel.

Elements that affect our temperaments and their nature:

Air (sanguine)

Formless, mobile, drying, dispersive, gentle or wild, feeds fire, thought, ideas, intellect.

In colloquial language we might say, "she was very sanguine about that," meaning optimistic in difficult times.

Fire (choleric)

Form without substance, heat, power, transformation, energy, doing, fast, movement, passion.

In colloquial language we might say, "he's so choleric," meaning he's full of energy and anger or passion. "She's fiery" refers to the same – fierceness could be a choleric disposition.

Earth (melancholic)

Stable, solid, soil, gems, strength, constancy, reliability, support, stuck, nurture, transformation.

In colloquial language we might say, "he just can't shift his melancholy," referring to being stuck in the earth or "they're so earthy," referring to a calm, grounded person.

Water (phlegmatic)

Receptive, flowing, evaporating, condensing, deep, still, powerful, sustaining, turbulent, stagnant, emotive.

In colloquial language we might say, "stiff upper lip" for the stoic nature of phlegmatic folk. "Still waters run deep" – you might not see the depth but phlegmatic folk are deep thinkers and calm (my kids' kindergarten teacher used to say, "be a boring rock in the river" around challenging kids – though this was easier for her as she was phlegmatic and patient).

Herbs are often described with their virtues, or qualities. A basic version of this would include their flavour – bitter, pungent etc. and the temperature. More specific inquiry would illuminate organ specificity, when a herb has an effect on a specific organ, eg. hawthorn for the heart, the direction of effect, energetically or physiologically would also be considered.

Flavours and how they affect the body:

>   Sweet – nourishing, neutral, often demulcent or strengthening
>   Bitter – cooling, downward moving (generally), cleansing
>   Pungent – hot, spicy, dispersive, stimulating
>   Sour – sometimes cooling, heavier
>   Salty – drying, mineralised

Tastes and feelings in the mouth:

>   **Astringents** are drying.
>
>   **Demulcents** are round, soft, full; you can add marshmallow to teas simply to give it a round softness which makes for a better drink.
>
>   **Bitters** move downwards or feel consolidating.
>
>   **Saponins** are sweet.
>
>   **Minerals** and salts are salty.
>
>   **Resins** are sticky, hard.
>
>   **Aromatics** are warming and directional.

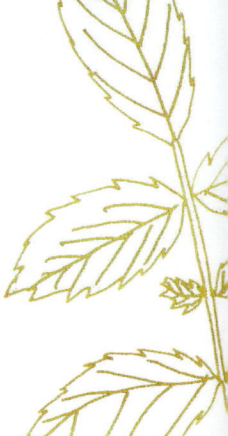

Temperature of herbs as we experience them:

>   Hot
>   Warm
>   Neutral
>   Cooling
>   Cold

Accompanying descriptions might include: drying, damp, tonifying, nutritive, relaxant, stimulant, moving, uplifting.

In each stage of life there will be different amounts of each temperament and we'll introduce each chapter with a little bit more on the time of life, the connected season, element, and temperament.

ACTION	EXAMPLE HERBS
Adaptogens Tonic herbs working to increase the body's resistance to stress via the adrenals	Ashwagandha, Siberian ginseng, liquorice, nettle seed, medicinal mushrooms
Alterative "Cleanses" blood	Burdock, red clover
Anaesthetic/analgesic Produces a partial or complete loss of nervous sensation	Yarrow, cayenne, clove
Anti-allergy (including antihistamine) Reduces symptoms of allergy	Plantain, nettle, eyebright
Anti-infective (including antimicrobial, antiviral, and antiseptic) Helps prevent infection	Echinacea, thyme, St John's wort, elderberry, elderflower, goldenseal, yarrow, sage, garlic
Anti-inflammatory Reduces inflammation – both externally and/or internally	Willow, comfrey, marigold, nettle
Antispasmodic Prevents or eases smooth muscles contractions	Valerian, cramp bark, chamomile

Astringent (including styptic)
Encourage contraction of tissues

Agrimony, witch hazel, rose, green tea

Bitter
Stimulates digestive system including secretions

Gentian, dandelion, vervain

Carminative
Stimulates peristalsis in digestive system

Peppermint, fennel, lemon balm

Cholagogue
Stimulates bile secretion

Dandelion, artichoke leaves

Circulatory stimulant
Excites circulation, increasing blood flow

Ginger, yarrow, rosemary, cayenne

Demulcent
Soothes and protects inflamed tissue

Marshmallow, cornsilk, plantain

Haemostatic
Arrests the flow of blood

Yarrow (note it is also a circulatory stimulant), cayenne, nettle

Hepatic
Tones and strengthens liver and stimulates bile flow

Milk thistle, blessed thistle, artichoke

Lymphatic
Encourages the flow of lymph

Marigold, cleavers, pokeroot

Nervine
Tones and strengthens the nervous system

Oats, skullcap, chamomile

Sedative
Calms the nervous system/excitement

Valerian, hops, wild lettuce

Skeletal muscle relaxant
Relaxes voluntary muscles

Skullcap, wild lettuce

Vulnerary
Aids recovery of tissue from wounds

Marigold, comfrey

So! Let's begin with the sanguine stage of life – babies and children, and then we'll move towards elderhood and beyond.

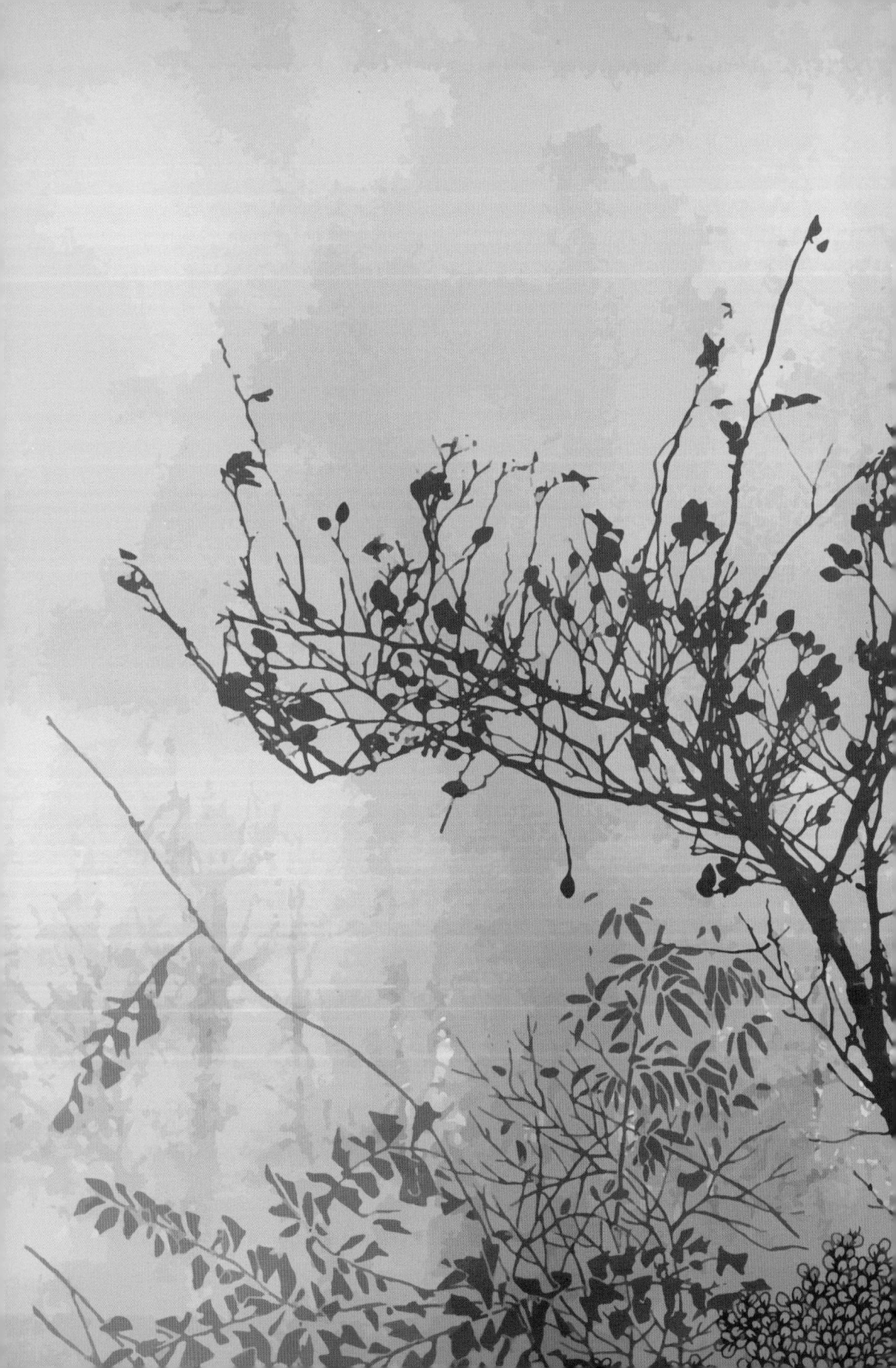

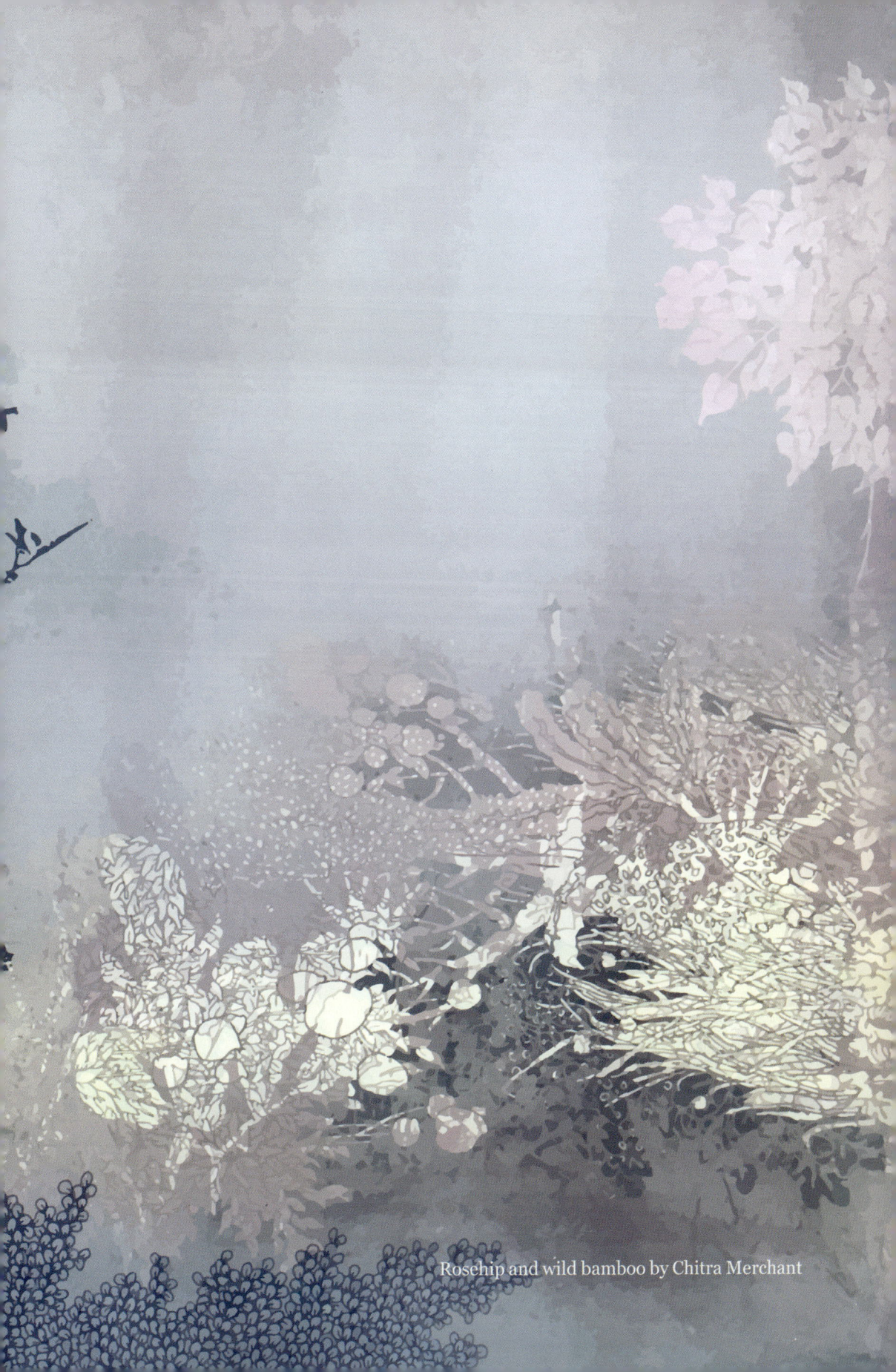
Rosehip and wild bamboo by Chitra Merchant

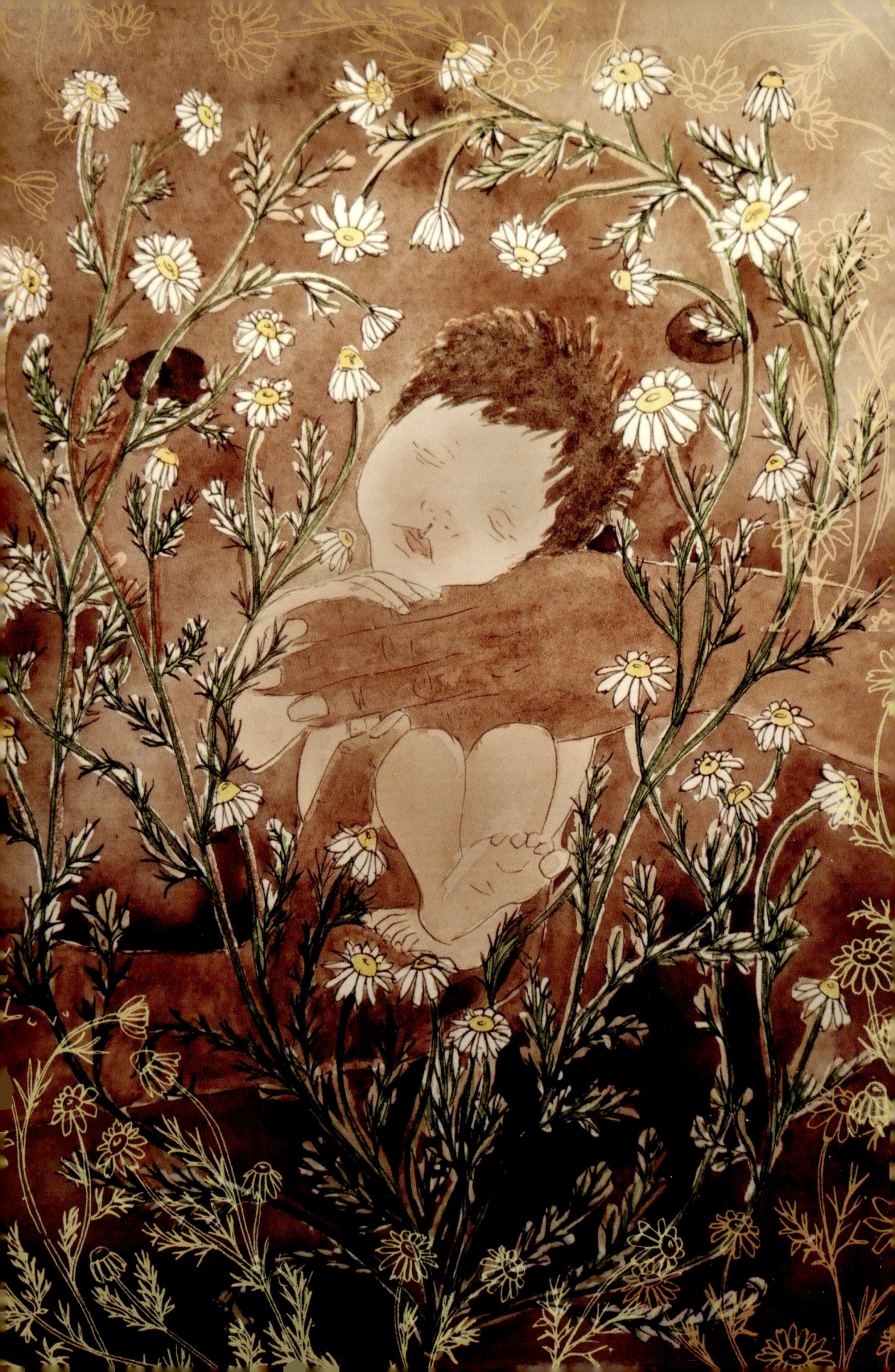

CHAPTER 4

EMERGING BUDS: BABES AND CHILDREN

My eyes are closed
My little body trembles
My knees in the grass. And mud.
The butterfly just out of reach.
The sun warm. Safe.
The water near, a trickle.
The air electric.
Birdsong above. Buzzing below.
Summer in my heart.
I long for the wild of a child.

Father holding baby with chamomile all around

We find the magic that all children know about if we choose to look for it. Rewilding yourself is about that magic. That connection to the divine, the sacred, the natural, the wonder, the big magic. Of course we can be the most beautiful flowers and fruit of adulthood and elder years but keeping that spark of child energy is a beautiful thing. Let's look at babies and children and how wild medicines can help.

ENERGETICS AND ELEMENTS

Kids are the spring of the seasons, fresh, new, blossoming with potential and gorgeousness. They are the buds that open and become the flower. They are the new life force that sustains the old until we part. They are joy and fun, untethered imagination and spirit, if we let them be children.

The sanguine temperament is most active in children and they are in the spring of their lives. Children of course also display other temperaments and grow into any of the four.

The sanguine temperament is associated with air, spring, sweetness; it is seen in folk who have many ideas and projects and can't keep to one task; they are warm and bubbly and, in many ways, childlike.

Sanguine types are revered in our society as they are thinkers, they notice, they socialise, they use intellect, but still feel energising and warm when they enter a room. However, whilst interested in everything you might tell them, they may tire of you and your words just like a child will. They are the least organised of the temperaments and reflect the unsteadiness of air which is in constant flux and movement.

The worst trait of the sanguine person is their disinterest, superficial warmth, or connection and self-importance, but this is normal to see in a child.

Children need support with all these issues, whether they grow to demonstrate a stronger expression of another temperament or not. They need a constant positive model to emulate as they may not listen but mimic or imitate instead. They need nourishing and tender care and for their little selves to be loved, heard, encouraged, and allowed to be.

Ken Robinson, the educationalist says, "We are all born with extraordinary powers of imagination, intelligence, feeling, intuition, spirituality, and of physical and sensory awareness." Children are everything – the buds that bloom hold everything the flowers need, we tend them, water them, feed them, and admire them but they have all the potential, they are extraordinary.

How best can we nourish them and care for them? Keep in mind they are of the spring. That they are the restored life force we are losing as we age, they are not mini versions of us, and do not deserve many of the traits we attribute to them. For example, if children steal a rainbow rubber (mentioning no names) they are not "stealing", they are succumbing to impulse with a simplified view of the action and consequence. We adults attribute theft and stealing and the punishment or admonishment to an adult action and understanding – the consequences are tough for a child. Children are children, their joyful and ever-changing expressions consistent with spring and wonder are a measure to treasure.

However you consider children, they are in need of care and love. When they are sick they need help, when they are hungry they need feeding, when they are curious they need elders.

Our society has done its best to separate us all, keeping children in school from the ages three to eighteen and beyond, in classes of kids who are all the same age. Society keeps adults at work and elders tucked away.

In many ways the system has enabled a loss of the essence of community as we strive to pay our bills. We have lost our togetherness and to get that back we have to seek out community, family, friends, neighbours. Not all of us will want that but if strong community exists, we can dip in and out or be at the centre. Children help elders to remember, elders help children to grow. We are all needed together.

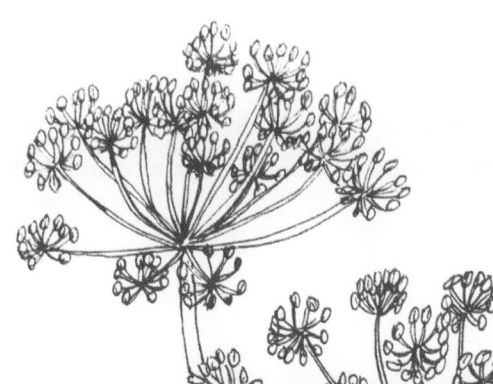

REWILDING EXERCISES

1. Stones and wonder

A simple exercise for children is to get them to turn over rocks and stones and to see what there is underneath. This is such a simple exercise and for young ones may last for hours. For the most sanguine of children, it may just last a little while unless there is a social element to the exercise.

You can let the children do this exercise with no extra help and see what happens, what they naturally experience and enjoy, or you can encourage them to feel the texture of the stones, to compare the hardness, sharpness, weight, look, etc. and also to describe the findings – woodlice (or chucky pigs as they're called here!), squashed grass, mud, cold, wet, faeries, etc.

2. Tracking and listening

Pick a spot for children to tune into the sounds around them – preferably the sounds of nature but if you are in a park or green area near roads also note the man-made sounds.

Make sure the children feel supported and comfortable. Then ask them to close their eyes and tell you or just note to themselves, depending on age, what they hear. Do this for half a minute at first, then build up to a minute and more and just keep noticing. Many of us have lost this skill because we have relatively safe lives and rely heavily on our vision.

Listening! What a skill.

As you practise this exercise, ask the children to point to where the noise is coming from and indicate when a noise, like a bird sound, starts and ends (if appropriate). When they open their eyes you can ask if they can tell where the noises come from.

Let the visuals seep in and see if they can connect the sounds to the visions. For instance, a bird is calling and they need to figure out which tree or post it is calling from.

Allow this skill to develop and see if the children can become more aware in their daily lives of where noise is coming from and what it might mean. If you are in the woods and all is quiet, for example, and birds suddenly start calling, it could be that someone, or an animal, is coming through the woods. This is an exercise of learning the woods, or the land, which is an amazing skill and one that needs practice.

3. Connect with your inner child

Simply remember what your first plant memory is. Is it making a daisy chain or being fed overcooked veggies, nutmeg on semolina, or climbing a tree? Just see if you can remember it. Chat about it to someone if you can or make notes on it – how did it make you feel then? How does it make you feel now?

If you can, remember more plant memories. You might start to see something in them – perhaps you have grown much closer to plants, or perhaps you always loved plants. Perhaps you like flowers but don't have green fingers and now are stepping into your power! Whatever the memories are, they serve to connect us with nature and plants and find ways for us to do that.

CONDITIONS

Let's have a look at some common conditions that affect babies and children. We'll also look at the herbs which can be used when working with kids.

BABIES

Mothers (or primary carers) often have intuitive knowledge of how to tend their babes. There is much empowerment from learning intergenerational and family knowledge of how to tend our bodies and babies.

There is much external pressure from orthodox medicinal practice but there is so much that can be done with an understanding of wild medicines, food, and traditional practice. While by no means exhaustive, here is a taste of some wild medicinal action for ailments of babes.

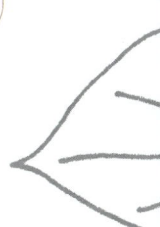
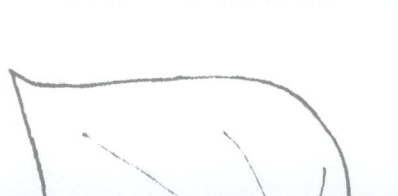
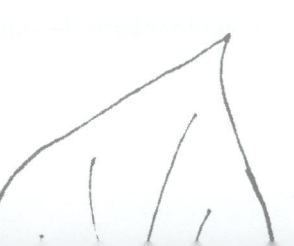

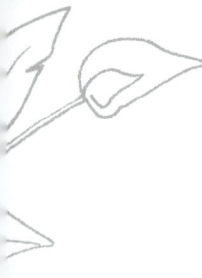

No matter your biological role, the relationship you have with a baby, or children, can be tended, nourished, and assessed. Herbs can be an integral part of your care, as can natural lifestyle or relational tendencies (for example, hand-in-hand parenting, non-violent communication, choice of schooling). So while this section concentrates on mamas as the most common primary carers, it is by no means exclusive.

Colic

Colic is a bit of a vague term. It is the word for when baby is crying with no known cause. It could be that baby needs soothing or is hungry but when soothed or fed baby is still crying. When this happens the term used to describe it in the UK is "colic". It can often be that baby is uncomfortable or there may be something that needs further investigation.

Colic is a common ailment for babies and it may be the case that mothers can tune into what is causing the colic – not always though, so no guilty motherhood feelings if you don't know what's causing the colic. Your baby expressing pain and exhibiting restlessness and crying or being unsettled may cause you to be tense or stressed so both mother (or carer) and baby need addressing.

Checking baby's feeding techniques, hours sleeping, and general well-being is important. Noticing what a breastfeeding mama eats or what the baby is fed if bottle-feeding is also needed. Positive relationship between parents if you are co-parenting is helpful for colic – to soothe the stress that can cause it.

Whatever the cause of the baby's colic, it is likely, in the case of tummy colic, that it is a resulting build-up of gas due to gut bacteria or fermentation in the alimentary canal. Interestingly in some countries babies just don't suffer with colic so it points to the way we are with our babies, be it what food we give them, what stress they experience, or another factor from modern UK living.

Plant allies

Herbs can be given as a tea or via breast milk – lots of carminative herbs are good as they soothe excess wind in the tummy.

Coupling this with baby massage is lovely – lie babies on their back and gently move their legs so their knees bend and a circular motion ensues. You can ask about this at something like MOBS (mothers offering breastfeeding support) or another baby/feeding professional service in your area.

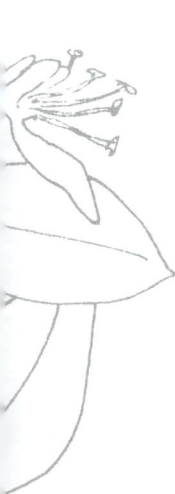

EMERGING BUDS: BABES AND CHILDREN

Rhythmic movement also helps – such as patting the baby as you rock or gently bouncing the babe. You'll learn what helps and be guided intuitively if you can relax enough, but that isn't always easy with limited (sometimes non-existent) sleep and all the other challenges newborn babes gift us with.

Carminatives are generally lovely warming aromatic herbs and include dill, fennel, lemon balm, and chamomile; they disperse gas and settle windy tummies. The latter two mentioned are also nervines so ease an agitated parent or child.

How to get a tea into a baby? Herbal teas can be blended with both breast and other milks in a bottle or they can be added directly to a bottle. Weak teas are good for babies and they can sup as much as they will. You can't easily make a baby drink herbals! Mama can also add to her own diet and some of the herb may reach the baby; sometimes this is enough but not always.

```
TUMMY LOVE TEA

Lemon balm            2 parts
Fennel                2 parts
Chamomile (German)    2 parts
Dill                  1 part
Linden                1 part
Catnip                1 part
```

1 tsp of tea blend infused in a cup of boiled water for 5 mins and strained, given to the baby when cooled to a warm tea – make sure this is NOT hot tea.

This lovely tea will ease both you and babe into gentle calm in body and well-being.

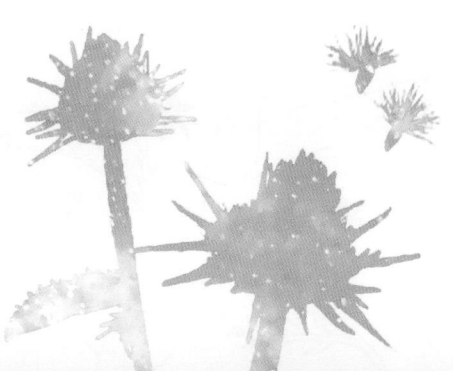

Differences in baby's weight

There can be pressure to maintain a certain weight or your baby may be labelled "failing to thrive" by orthodox standards. First it must be noted that these standards are Eurocentric and don't necessarily apply to babies of different racial heritage. Your baby could indeed be thriving in every way but be on the smaller side or could be bigger and somehow not thriving.

There is a huge amount of pressure pushed onto a mama or parent if she (he, they) feels that they are unable to provide what their baby needs. It can be traumatising for the parents if their baby is not considered to be thriving, or they are considered to be failing at keeping their baby in line with standards.

If your baby isn't meeting the growth he or she might be expected to meet, and you are worried about baby failing to thrive, do check there is nothing amiss in the baby's health. If nothing obvious is found by your GP or chosen professional health carer, you might like to try a little slippery elm while checking dietary issues (yours and the baby's).

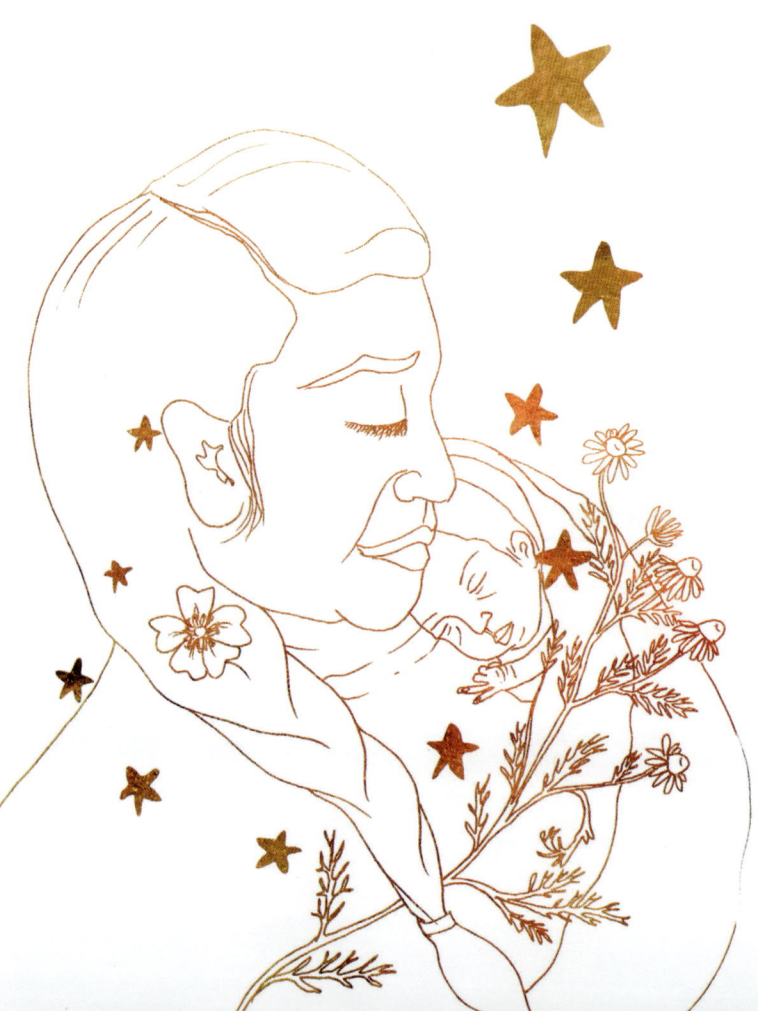

Slippery elm is a lovely herb but must be sourced sustainably. I use it for babies who seem as if they aren't thriving and with persistence and attention nurse babes back to good health.

Sometimes I add nervines to a mix in addition to the slippery elm, like chamomile, and sometimes supporting the mother and her diet has been key – or just being there as a support for the mother so she can follow and trust her intuitive mothering knowledge.

I like to give ¼ tsp of organic and ethically sourced slippery elm powder in water or milk of whichever kind you use a few times a day. The babe must be given fluids to make sure no constipation ensues if you are choosing to use this bulk laxative herb. If in any doubt, see a herbalist who can advise as to what you need.

It may be that a simple tea like chamomile is needed to relieve colic, or any stress that the baby may be feeling. This may be affecting appetite. There may be a variety of reasons why your baby is unhappy so make sure all avenues are explored.

In some cultures, babies are never put down, they are always with mama or someone else, never left alone. Swaddling is also a common practice in traditional tending of a baby. These are beautiful practices. If you are in this position, try out some different care techniques and seek support with this.

Diarrhoea

If your baby suffers with stinky diarrhoea that just doesn't seem healthy, check diet and any other possible conditions that may be causing the upset (consult a herbalist if you don't know what to look for). If nothing is found, you could try slippery elm and chamomile as above (see "Differences in baby's weight"). Ongoing diarrhoea is a red flag and must be checked as it is usually caused by something else which needs addressing.

The most common cause of diarrhoea is rotavirus infection and dehydration. Herbs that pass

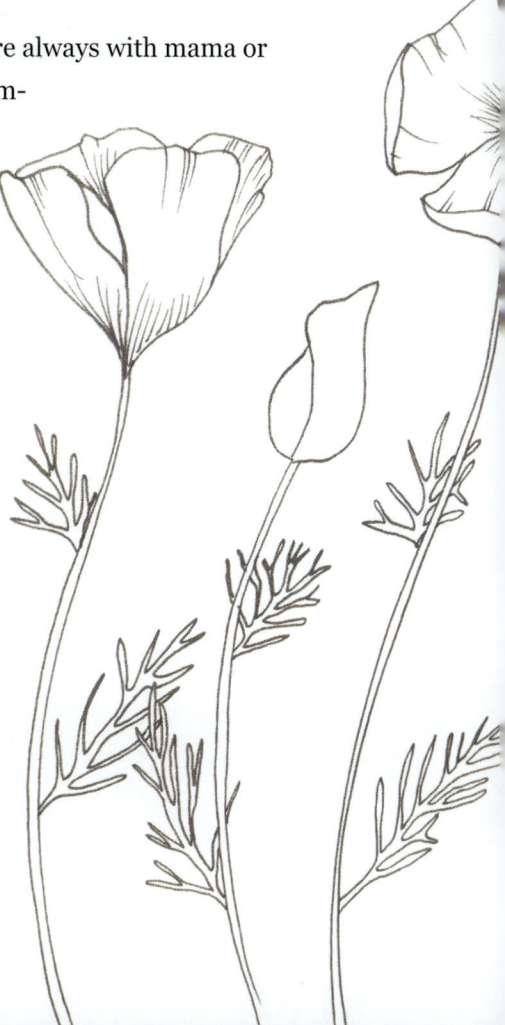

through breast milk can be useful as can settling herbs similar to the Tummy Love Tea.

Nappy rash

If your baby does develop nappy rash, there are various factors to consider. Know though that nappy rash is not a "normal" occurrence but it is so common that it has become normalised. Much like giving dolls to girls and not to boys. But that's another story.

Nappy rash is a redness on a baby's bottom when babies wear nappies. It can be sore and itchy and sobbingly painful or just a bit of uncomfortable swelling around the area. It may be caused by baby's skin reacting to the urine and poo in the nappy, especially if left a long time. It may also be caused by friction, a reaction to washing powder or plastic nappies, and it may be worse when your baby is teething. It may be due to a fungal or bacterial infection or low immunity, or an infection might occur secondary to the rash as an opportunistic infection, for example, thrush.

If you are breastfeeding check your diet for anything the babe is reacting to – for instance if she or he gets a rash when you drink lots of coffee or eat garlic. Check for any sensitivities or intolerances if you are breastfeeding or bottle-feeding.

Whatever the case, it is a great idea to leave the nappies off the skin where possible, bathe your baby's bottom with herbal infusions, and make sure the skin is dry before putting another nappy on. I liked to use chamomile tea and a flannel to clean my babies' bottoms and then when I thought they were fully dry I'd give them a dusting of slippery elm powder. I used this mostly when I thought there was a sign of redness. Nappy rash never really developed and certainly nothing more than a few spots or a little redness that quickly disappeared.

Keeping nappies off a baby's bum is also great, allowing the skin to breathe and heal if needed. If you do this a lot at

EMERGING BUDS: BABES AND CHILDREN

home you may find you know the cues for when your baba will wee or poo, but regardless, it is good to do this for some time each day.

I sometimes use a thick marigold cream which acts like a barrier whilst also being a healing salve to the skin. It is common to find these creams now in health food stores and supermarkets. You can of course make your own as marigold is the easiest herb in the world to grow – just scatter some seeds and they will come up (if this doesn't happen, do try again! Don't be sad!)

Plant allies

Chamomile hydrosol or strong tea is really useful here – it can either be made and sprayed on to the baby's bottom or applied as a wash with a flannel. Both are lovely and gently anti-infective.

Myrrh tincture – very diluted with water as it's a high strength alcohol tincture (90%) – can be helpful if there is infection present but it might sting a little, so sometimes it is best to mix it into a marigold cream and let the skin breathe out of nappies for a while after application. Use up to 1 tsp of tincture in 60ml cream. A dusting of myrrh powder is a good alternative if too strong for baby's skin and it can be mixed with the slippery elm powder.

Chamomile and lavender cream is also very helpful – you can make a cream and add hydrosols or essential oils appropriate to the needs of the child.

St John's wort flowers infused in the oil of your choice is a good oil to gently rub in too, but I like to mix it with aloe gel or chamomile cream and add a few drops of lavender.

If you have none of the above, try a diluted wash of cider vinegar or a herbal infused vinegar (such as rosemary).

You can also bathe the baby in chamomile, oat, and lavender baths. These are strong teas added to the baby bath water – if added to a big bath the teas will be more dilute but worthwhile all the same. Herbal baths infuse through the skin and are very relaxing in aroma. See Chapter 2 for basic recipes.

Teething

Someone once said to me she knew my babies wouldn't have any teething problems. She was right – I'm not sure what made her think that, perhaps their melancholic stoic baby energy or their sanguine smiley faces? Whatever it was, they didn't suffer with teething, their teeth cut through almost unnoticed. Sadly that is not the case for all babies, but it is possible.

The pH of urine changes when babies are teething and ensuing symptoms of teething include nappy rash, dribbling, crying (more than usual), neediness, or a clingy babe wanting to be in your arms more than usual. These symptoms may also be due to other conditions like a cold coming or a childhood illness. It's important to keep an eye open and rule out other possible factors.

From a few days old my babies wore amber teething necklaces. It may well have been these beautiful necklaces that helped, I'll never know for sure, but I think they're great. If you choose to get one, make sure you get one specifically for babies as they have tiny knots between each bead so if they do break, they don't all come off.

Chewing helps – cooled teething rings, cold vegetables such as cucumber in sticks or celery or smooth wooden teethers are good. Dried roots like marshmallow can be great and soothe as they chew on them as best they can.

I like to give teething infusions and settling baths when the babes are uncomfortable.

TEETHING TEA

Catnip	2 parts
Chamomile	2 parts
Lemon balm	2 parts
Rose	1 part
Marigold	1 part

1 tsp of tea blend infused for 5 mins and given to baby in a bottle, or spoon feed – check temperature first. Mamas can also drink this calming, healing tea. Pink roses are lovely for babies.

KIDS

Fever

Your baby might get many high temperatures or few. Babies may get fevers which are high and fast or low and slow. They might carry on as usual with a high temperature or be laid out needing you and sleep. Babies are different just like adults. Normal temperatures for a baby are around 36.4°C and when the baby's temperature rises over 38°C it is considered to be fever and must be monitored.

Fever may be a sign of illnesses like chicken pox, colds, or other infective illnesses, such as the parvovirus, or slapped cheek syndrome, a name which never ceases to surprise me. Fever is not a condition in itself but a reaction when the body is trying to deal with something as part of the immune response. Fever aids the body to combat pathogens by increased immune cell release and uncomfortable heat for the invaders.

Convulsions: high temperatures and frequent fevers could lead to febrile convulsions in some children. It is important to know the level of care that you are confident to give your children. We are frequently told that if our kids have a temperature, Calpol or equivalent is the best remedy. In my experience it hasn't been necessary, except the time when my son had to go to hospital as he was dramatically losing blood.

It turned out that my son has a deficiency we did not know anything about and we are so thankful to the doctors in the NHS kids' acute care unit at Gloucester Royal who diagnosed him, saw him through, and saved his life. However, what also sticks in my mind is the assumption of the medical staff that my son had had any drugs before. No steroids, no antibiotics, and "not even" Calpol. It is so common in our lives that we easily lose the skills to tend the poorly. Knowing your limits as your kid's carer is important so you know when to seek help.

In terms of herbs for fevers, there are lots of things you can do from pepping up the child's immunity in general and thereby preventing the body's need to produce fevers in order to get rid of a pathogen, to working with the fever or illness, to nourishing the child.

Assess the fever – is it high or low and is your child prone to convulsions? Feel out how confident you are and what you know around fevers, illness, recovery, etc.

Be clear that you need to contact a GP or medical help for advice if temperature is high and prolonged. Read around the subject, speak to your healthcare providers, and note when you feel you need more support. Being prepared is a far greater help than not. This is where having a herbal first aid cupboard for children is really useful.

Fevers indicate children need rest first and foremost. As with any illness it is important to nourish children so that they can fight the illness as best they can.

Keeping kids hydrated is really important, and filtered water, broths, and herbal infusions are great here. Note that even if your child has an appetite, it is OK to allow the body to fight the pathogen without too much food burdening the digestive system in the acute stages. Lighter foods – thin soups or porridges – might be enough, or a little fruit. Work with children to find a balance between keeping them comfortable, hydrated, and on the road to wellness. If a baby has a prolonged dry nappy with fever, or fever accompanied with a rash, this warrants a call to a GP.

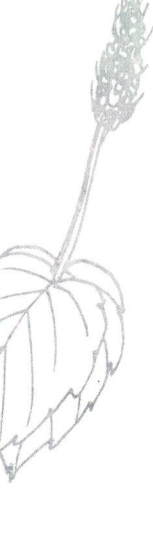

Plant allies

Infusions are key here. You can give teas and make strong teas for baths and washes.

My favourite herb for this is German chamomile as it is so gentle yet effective. In the acute stages of fever yarrow tea, supped or given on teaspoons depending on the age of the child, is an excellent fever herb, helping to break the fever once the body has reached the higher temperature and therefore hopefully killed the pathogen.

Chamomile is great because it's anti-infective and calming. I use chamomile myself when I have a tummy bug and I give it to my children as the first herb to try in illness. Children will need to rest so nervines like chamomile and lavender will be really helpful in aiding them to sleep or just remain calm because sometimes being ill is really boring. I know my (choleric melancholic) son gets agitated when he's ill and just wants to do all the things he normally does, so calming herbs are very beneficial, particularly for sanguine or choleric children.

I like to use the traditional remedy of yarrow, peppermint, and elderflower. This is a tasty tea that your child will probably like and it's cooling while being diaphoretic so will encourage sweating.

If your child won't take this tea try lemon balm, lime flower, lavender, catnip, or thyme infusions until you find one he, she or they will take.

If the child is a bit older, ginger is a great herb for fevers but can feel too hot for some. Remember the sanguine qualities of a child's predominant temperament are hot and moist so some children will not like spicy foods or pungent herbs. However, herbs that encourage blood flow are really beneficial when your child is ill as toxins will be moved out of the body via the blood, through the liver and kidneys.

While peppermint is also really useful, be careful not to give it to very young children because it may be too cooling on the belly. Often gently warming herbs are used in very young children or babies. I like applemint as a slightly gentler mint which tastes lovely in teas.

The great thing about using herbs when your child has a fever is that you will likely prevent other complications. If your child is uncomfortable or feeling pain herbs like meadowsweet can help. Meadowsweet has salicylic acid in it which will act as an analgesic helping to calm the pain; it is also a diaphoretic so will help the sweating and it is anti-inflammatory so an all-round good herb for fevers.

If your child succumbs to fevers often then teas or broths with herbs that nourish the immune system are indicated. Herbal roots such as astragalus, liquorice, or elecampane may be a great addition to your apothecary. Traditionally a root like astragalus is cooked in soups, broths, and stews, and feeding herbs as food is a great way to aid your child's immune system.

I like to give echinacea to older children at the first sign of illness. I often couple it with elderberry or elderflower tincture or tea.

Note – I use fresh (specific) plant tinctures where I can. If you haven't got access to fresh elderberry don't worry – you can make the tincture with dried herbs. Make sure the mixture has a 20% alcohol content to preserve it. With elderberries I might decoct them first as I like to cook them and then make a decocted tincture.

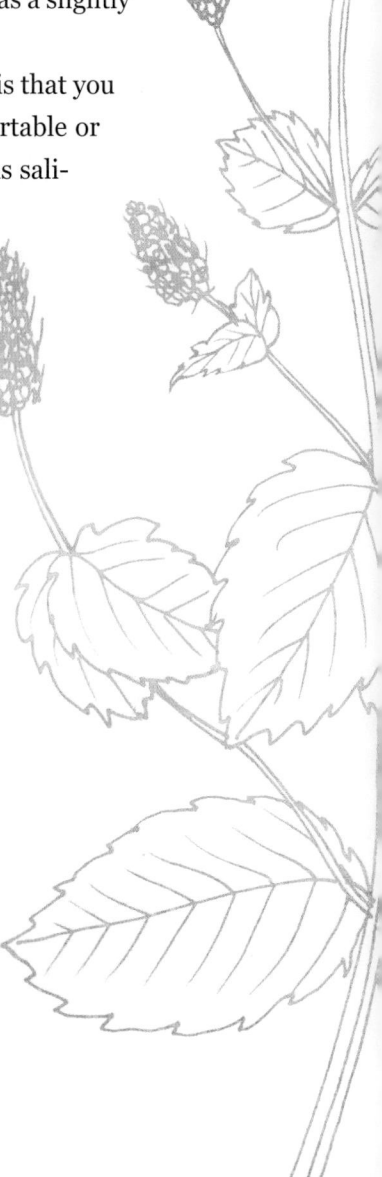

ELDER AND ECHINACEA TINCTURE
(for kids over two years old)

Elderberry ST (specific tincture) 1:2 25%	1 part (eg 25ml)
Elderflower ST 1:3 25%	1 part (eg 25ml)
Echinacea angustifolia root ST 1:3 45%	1 part (eg 25ml)

The dose will depend on the age of the child. Typically, I would give a quarter to half a teaspoon 3-4 times daily when acute infection is present.

FEVER TEA

Elderflower	1 part
Yarrow	1 part
Peppermint	1 part

You can also add herbs like catnip and lavender – experiment and see what you like.

Infuse 1 tsp of the herb blend for 5 mins, strain, cool a little, and give frequently in fever or colds.

If it's not easy to get your kids to take a tincture, you could add a syrup of choice – I like liquorice for colds and lethargy, or rose for soothing and calming. You can also mix with a little honey in a tiny amount of hot water. Or do drop doses in water throughout the day. There are many ways to get the tincture into the child so do experiment.

Chamomile and yarrow bath

Infuse a small handful of each herb for 10 mins in boiled water. Add to really warm (but not hot) baths or sponge onto the child as needed.

Coughs and colds

If your child (or the child you are caring for) is getting lots of coughs and colds then think about how to improve the child's immune system.

There are lots of reasons why a child's immunity might be low. Here are a few examples:

Diet – you might wonder what diet has got to do with your child getting coughs and colds. If your child is reacting to something that is being eaten then the body has to accommodate and use up energy on resolving the issue. For example, if a child is sensitive to dairy and keeps eating it, every single time it's consumed the body has to release adrenaline and then cortisol to cope – this is depleting the adrenals. So your child will have a naturally lower immune function because he or she is constantly having to deal with the dairy though you won't always see this as a child can appear fairly healthy. Keeping an eye on children's stools is a good way to monitor their digestion. Check out the Bristol stool chart which shows what a healthy stool should look like.

Dairy is also a food that increases our bodies' production of phlegm. Children often feel a bit bunged up and tired if they have a sensitivity to dairy, and sometimes even if they aren't sensitive, they will feel more phlegm and tiredness because dairy products are damp cold foods. Wheat may also cause this to happen along with sugar and other stimulants or other inflammatory foods.

Your child might be fussy and refuse to eat greens or coloured vegetables or certain forms of food such as chunky soup or textured meat. When a parent struggles to feed a child healthy food, stress is created and the parent may feel it is easier for everybody if the child eats food that is liked. While a happier dinner time may ensue, sadly the child's immunity may weaken in the long term so a balance has to be found between the child eating foods that nourish and foods that please.

It is not an easy job, feeding kids, and you can only do your best, but preparation and support really help. If you can, prepare a few recipes that the children really like and make tiny changes to them – add in some broccoli or make a smoothie with added kale and spinach, for example. I find the thing that really helps is having the right foods in the home so I can grab them when needed and

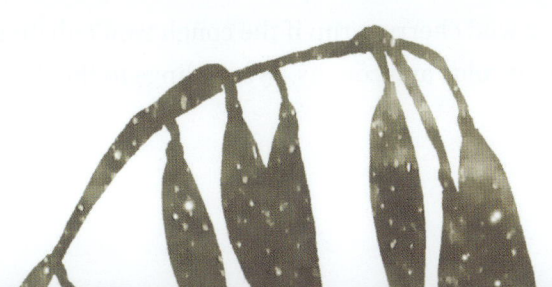

having a set of recipes I use regularly so I know what to do and how. I know some folk are lucky enough to have set up a system where they cook for each other's little family so that they are not cooking every day. Freezing food is also useful – my freezer is usually full of leftovers made for days we're late or days we're tired . . .

Stress can decrease a child's immunity – worry, lack of sleep, anxiety, and anger all take their toll on the body. Encouraging balance, calm, and fun in children's life is important, especially if they are prone to colds and coughs.

Keeping children warm or cool enough is also key. It's healthy to have fresh air in the house and a cool temperature – not too hot or humid or dry. In fact central heating, while keeping a dry atmosphere which is helpful against mould, etc., may irritate the mucous membranes of the throat as the air is too dry. Take a look at your child's environment and assess if you can improve it in any way. Make sure your child is getting enough exercise too in a form that the child finds is fun.

Kids' immunity tip: make sure kids have enough vitamins if they are getting ill easily: vitamin D (sunshine, mushrooms, or fish), selenium (brazil nuts), zinc (shellfish, chickpeas), vitamin C (fresh fruit and veggies).

Plant allies

If your child seems tired or has the first sign of a cough or cold you can prepare syrups or herbal teas, or both.

Yarrow, elder, and peppermint tea is a great one and comes in useful if there's fever but can also be used as an astringent expectorant anti-infective infusion (see "Fevers").

Other herbs to be given as infusions include thyme, liquorice, chamomile, calendula, marshmallow, echinacea, elderflower, and elderberry. Experiment with your child see what he or she likes – some combinations will work and some will be less popular. You can always add some honey or maple syrup to soothe the throat and encourage the child if needed.

If your child will take turmeric which is slightly pungent, a great little remedy is a dollop of turmeric honey either in hot water or milk or just a spoonful of it. Simply mix the dry turmeric powder into honey until a paste.

I like to give wild cherry syrup if the cough won't abate and liquorice and thyme syrup for colds and coughs. Syrup clings to the throat and soothes it.

EMERGING BUDS: BABES AND CHILDREN

You can also gently fry up finely chopped ginger, garlic, and onions in honey or in maple syrup until soft and eat this food as medicine. Pickled ginger, garlic, lemon, or onions also come in handy at this time. These are cheap and easy food-based remedies.

A throat spray can also be of use for kids: they are fun and if you make them tasty compliance is good. I like to use sage, marshmallow, and peppermint tinctures diluted with water and have the children spray the back of their throat frequently throughout the day.

Inhalations are also really useful as they break up phlegm and help expectorate it. Pop your child's head over a steaming bowl of water, making sure it's not too hot to breathe in. You can add one drop of peppermint or lavender oil if you feel the need. Keep a towel over the top of the child's head and bowl to stop the steam escaping.

Kids and adults alike enjoy chest rubs – especially just before bed. A soothing rub with an essential oil-rich ointment can really help a child's chest in the night. It will soak in through the skin and the essential oils will evaporate so the child can breathe them in. You don't want overly strong balms but a good ointment with a few drops of peppermint, cornmint, eucalyptus, thyme essential oils (say 20–30 in total in a 120ml jar). See Chapter 2 for a basic ointment recipe.

Tonsillitis

Tonsils are one of our first lines of defence and we want to do everything we can to keep them. Whipping them out is not such a common practice nowadays and it is well worth seeing a herbalist if your child is experiencing chronic tonsillitis.

Your child may suffer from tonsillitis what seems like all the time or your child may rarely suffer from it but it is good to know how to treat it if this is the case. Tonsillitis can be due to a viral or bacterial infection and often happens when immunity is low (see "Coughs and colds" for how to pep up immunity in your child).

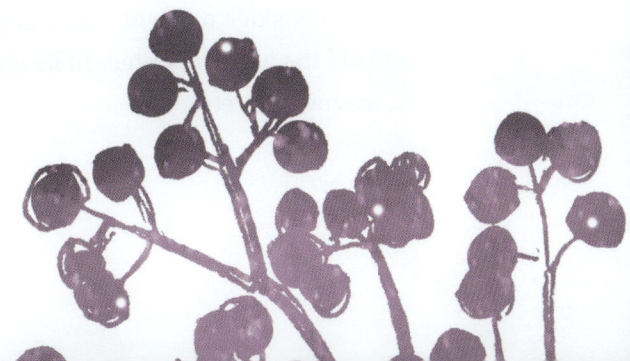

Plant allies

Similar herbal treatment can be given for tonsillitis as for coughs with extra help for soothing the mucosa when the cough is dry or irritating and for spasm; if the coughing gets too much, wild cherry syrup is great for this.

Colds and fever often present together so an extra emphasis on lymphatic drainage and febrifuges is needed. Herbs to encourage the lymph system include marigold, cleavers, and burdock root. Infusions of these herbs can be drunk frequently by children.

Gargles, such as sage, come in handy here because they act directly on the tonsil tissue as the head is thrown back and the infusion or diluted tincture is swashed around the tonsil area.

Yarrow, elderflower, and peppermint tea can be given for fever (see "Fevers").

Astringent herbs such as agrimony and elderflower can also be used to tone the swollen tissue as infusions, syrups, or gargles.

Insomnia and night terrors

Insomnia can be something you see in your child from a very early age. Some babies sleep really well and some babies don't. This is the same with older children.

There may be lots of different reasons that a child does not sleep well and it is really good if you can figure out why your child doesn't sleep well. Reasons for insomnia can include too much stimulation, not enough stimulation, stressful times, emotional disturbances, being too tired, physical issues such as poor digestion or constipation, breathing difficulties, headaches, and other ailments. Conditions that affect the emotional and physical body in our children such as hyperactivity or some neuro-diverse behaviours can also bring about difficulty in relaxing or sleeping.

If you have eliminated any physical ailments that are causing insomnia such as sleep apnoea, discomfort, asthma, or pain, then look to the emotional. Stress, anxiety, fear, agitation, or worry with constant thoughts going around the head can stop a child sleeping.

Also consider nutrient deficiency as certain herbs, vitamins, and minerals will aid the nervous system in its ability to relax – such as B vitamins, vitamin C, magnesium, etc.

A good bedtime routine is encouraged without too much screen stimulation or excitement before bed. Nourishing foods during the day and a good amount of exercise will help good sleep.

Night terrors, or bad dreams that cause children to wake or make them fearful of going to sleep can also be eased with the above considerations and herbs. Talking and body therapies are good here too.

Rewilding exercise: my plant friend

As well as dolls or cuddly toys it is great to have a plant friend next to your child's bed, and in fact next to your bed if it is separate. Plants release oxygen which is excellent when we're sleeping and they're also alive which is a lovely thing for a child with fear. Allow children to choose their plant or choose one which gives out a lot of oxygen and takes in the carbon dioxide such as a parlour palm or aloe vera, and of course get them to name the plant. Children will then know as they're falling asleep that there is a living being who is their friend right next to them.

Encourage children to listen to the plant or to talk to the plant if they would like to. You can also let a child know that plants respond really well to praise and good positive vibes so the child can almost pet the plant. If your plant looks unhealthy learn how to care for it and encourage children to learn about plant care, that plants need their tender loving care.

Exercise: visualisation

Just before bed encourage your child to look at something natural like the plant by the bed, or a stone or the moon or a tree, and to breathe deeply into the lungs.

As the child does this you can do a short guided visualisation that is nourishing for the child. I like to imagine and tell a story of stars lighting up the tree or the plant or the moon and sharing their special magical light which the child can bathe in.

Find your own way of connecting with a child and the story. You might align the visualisation with stories you are telling your children before bed. Become aware of your intuitive voice and allow yourself to be confident that you know what will help your child. If it doesn't work don't be hard on yourself but try again in different ways – you have the power and the intuition. Once you feel your child is relaxed tuck the child in and keep breathing deeply and gently while you hold the space for settling – gentle song is also welcome here.

I only ever managed to remember one verse of one song but ten years later, the kids still like it when I sing it to them before sleep. Some of you may know it:

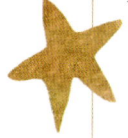

Deep peace of the rolling waves to you
Deep peace of the flowing air to you
Deep peace of the shining stars to you
Deep peace of the quiet earth to you.

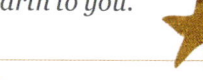

Plant allies

Nervines would be my first port of call for insomnia in children. There are so many ways in which our children can become stressed – difficulties at school, difficulties at home, too much, too little, too fast, too slow, too late . . . about anything.

Thoughts can really affect children and they express it through their physicality. Nervines encourage the nervous system to relax, thereby aiding a child to sleep. Allow your child to choose from herbs with this gentle effect such as lemon balm, lavender, rose, lime flower, and chamomile.

Herbs like passionflower and skullcap can be excellent in relaxing your child enough to sleep. This combination is a lovely one for children and may be given as tincture or tea; it is mildly sedative so will relax the child if there is tension present.

Nervines given during the day are also beneficial. Nourishing nervines like milky oats or oat straw, ashwagandha, and stinging nettle can be really good to calm and nourish during the day in readiness for peaceful sleep.

Traditionally in the UK, warm milky drinks have been given often with a bit of honey before bed. While there are obvious ethical considerations surrounding milk, a warming nourishing calming drink in the evening is a lovely thing for a child and adult.

Ashwagandha powder and maybe a little turmeric in warmed oat milk with a tiny bit of honey or maple syrup in a small cup may be just the ticket, or lavender-infused milk may be something your child likes. Try out your own different nourishing nervine drinks in the evening from the herbs above and just give a little to the child.

You can also make a calming oil to rub on the temples or to put on a handkerchief near the child's head, working in a similar way to a lavender pillow soothing by aroma. I like oils being rubbed in by the children themselves as an act of empowerment or by their parents or someone they love as this is a physical nourishing act.

```
BEDTIME CALM BALM

Make an ointment with calendula infused oil and bees-
wax or shea butter (see Chapter 2 for a basic recipe).

Add a few drops of rose lavender and bergamot essential
oils before the ointment has set. You can ask your
child to colour in a label for it if desired and mas-
sage it into the temples before bed.
```

Wood betony is an excellent herb, particularly for worries whirling around the head. It is also a specific remedy for night terrors which can be very scary and disorienting for the child. An infusion of wood betony and rose is also a great mix for children during the afternoon and evening if they are experiencing night terrors. California poppy (often referred to as Cali poppy) is good for kids with agitation or ants in their pants (variations of attention deficit conditions, frustration, and energy).

```
NIGHT EASE DROPS
(Tincture or glycerite)
Cali poppy      10ml
Wood betony     10ml
Rose            10ml

Take 5 drops before bed in a tiny glass of water.
```

Bed-wetting

Nocturnal enuresis happens for a few different reasons in children. If your child is still young, say under around five years old, he or she may simply not have gained nervous and muscular control of the bladder and hence wet the bed. If, however, children have already gained control and suddenly or unexpectedly start wetting the bed then other causes are possible.

Reasons for wetting the bed include stress and fear or worry and anxiety and these kinds of feelings can be very alienating for a child who wants to belong, and pretty much all children do in their own way. Wetting the bed can be humiliating, especially if you are told off for it or teased about it, and some kids will wet the bed far longer than you expect. Treating it as something that is OK is the best way forward even if it does mean a bit more washing and some disturbed sleep for both you and the child. Reassurance is still needed if it's a very regular occurrence meaning you or the child is not getting enough sleep. This can be hard so if it happens be sure to take soothing nervines and strengthening adaptogens.

Consider dietary factors: sometimes a child may not have enough magnesium or other essential minerals, or may be eating too many sweet things or have an intolerance or sensitivity to dairy. Interestingly, drinking a lot of water just before bed can ease bed-wetting in some children as it seems to calm an irritable bladder, but for most it will make it worse with a wetter bed in the middle of the night. You will be able to assess if there is anything obvious that affects your child in a positive or negative way. These kinds of nutritional imbalances can contribute to bed-wetting and need looking at – if you need professional help with this your local herbalist, naturopath, or nutritionist will be able to provide support and advice.

Good methods of dealing with bed-wetting rest in the way you talk to your children. Reassurance is key. Reminding them that they are normal and have nothing to worry about is essential in whichever way you choose to show them. Children can also wet the bed if they are disturbed in their sleep, or by being too hot, too cold, or restless, so trying to make their environment just right is important too.

Some children will simply grow out of bed-wetting after a while and some will carry on wetting the bed longer. If they are a little bit older and they're getting frustrated that they're wetting the bed, it may be worth working with them through visualisation, meditation, yoga, and exercise. These may be exercises focusing on strong pelvic floor muscles or visualisations in a full night's sleep or calm breathing.

Check for any irritable bladder or infection – this is noticeable if they are urinating frequently or have any pain or burning sensation when passing urine.

Plant allies

A tea of the brilliant St John's wort and the wonderful astringent agrimony can be drunk liberally throughout the day. It is also uplifting for children. You can add various nervines, too, such as chamomile, lemon balm, or lavender for easing anxiety. Nervines similar to the ones mentioned for insomnia can be used to relax the child if stress or worry is present.

If you don't have St John's wort or agrimony to hand a really common herb which is very helpful is herb Robert. This pretty plant can be found all over the place and grows abundantly and easily once settled. An infusion of herb Robert and other astringing herbs may be enough and if you do find this herb growing outside, you'll most likely start seeing it everywhere.

For kids with insomnia or bed-wetting, herbal sleep pillows are lovely, inexpensive, and work well. My daughter makes her own lavender and rose petal pillow (using little old bags she finds and fills).

Chickenpox

Chickenpox is one childhood illness your kids will probably get. At the moment in the UK we do not generally give a vaccination for it, unlike other illnesses such as measles and mumps which are vaccinated against. Not everybody chooses to vaccinate their kids. This is a huge point of contention for many people and respect for each other is still needed.

The Varicella zoster virus is infectious and highly contagious from a couple of days before the spots erupt until the blisters are dry. Children must be kept at home and need rest and gentle nourishment. They may have been incubating the virus for one to three weeks prior to the emergence of spots.

Keep your children well-rested even if they have some energy as chickenpox may be mild and kids like to play whenever they can and so miss out on much-needed rest. Keep kids well hydrated. The immune system can be supported through food such as gentle broths and antioxidant-rich veggies (in soups, gently steamed, etc.) which include vitamin A, beta carotene, and vitamin C.

If the children are a bit older (teenagers) then echinacea and garlic may be useful and if younger (two to twelve years) then infusions of chamomile,

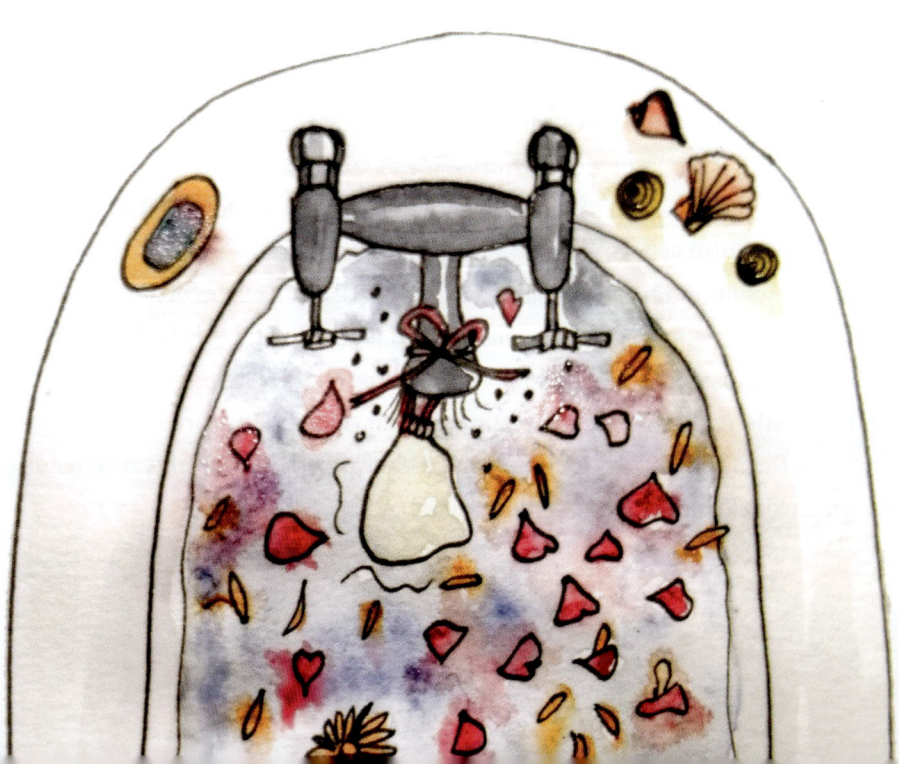

catnip, lime flower, and other nervines can be helpful. If fever is present you may choose to use some diaphoretics alongside nervines (see "Fevers").

If the skin is itching where the spots are, a great herbal remedy is lavender essential oil mixed into aloe vera gel – apply this liberally and frequently. Baths are really good because the water covers the whole body. Lavender essential oil can be added to a bath as can strong chamomile tea or an oat sock (a sock filled with organic oats and tied at the top and left to infuse into the bath water as it runs).

If the child gets vesicles in the mouth then gargles of echinacea tea or tincture, or diluted myrrh tincture can be given. If you don't have these, you can try a concentrated sage tea as a gargle.

```
COOLING GEL

Aloe gel                   60g
St John's wort             5ml
Lavender essential oil     10 drops

Mix together and apply to itchy spots as needed
```

```
ANTI-VIRAL TONIC TINCTURE

Elderberry      2 parts (eg 50ml)
Echinacea       2 parts (eg 50ml)
Olive leaf      2 parts (eg 50ml)
Liquorice       1 part  (eg 25ml)

Dosage is dependent on age/size of the child. Roughly
a quarter to half a teaspoon of the blend 3-4 times
daily in water during acute stage of illness. Glycer-
ites and hydrosols can be used instead of tinctures if
no alcohol is preferred.
```

Measles

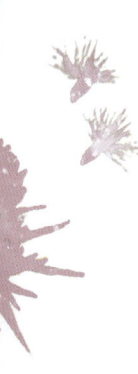

A similar approach to chickenpox should be used for measles, and serious care given if the child is in any way immunocompromised. Make sure vitamin A and beta-carotene levels are good and keep the child in a dark room and well-rested. It is common practice to supplement with vitamin A as soon as you know your child has measles. This should protect the eyes if any vitamin A stores are lost due to the viral load.

More complications arise in measles than chickenpox just after infection when temperatures can rise sharply. Ear infections are a possibility, along with rarer encephalitis.

If you are not confident to care for your child during measles, ask your GP and a herbalist and make informed choices.

```
EAR INFECTION OIL

St John's wort infused oil    1 part
Mullein infused oil           1 part

Ask your child to lie on one side. Apply a few drops of
oil (depending on how big your child is) into the ear
presented to you and let it sit for a few minutes. Ask
the child to turn over and let the oil run out onto a
hankie or similar. Repeat in the other ear and do this
3 times daily. It is very soothing and can stop painful
ears very quickly.
```

Eye wash

Strong chamomile and eyebright tea can be made and strained thoroughly before washing the eyes with it when cool enough. A hot flannel soaked in it is lovely over the eyes if they are irritated.

If you have chamomile teabags in the house, these can be dipped in boiled water and placed over the eyes.

Asthma

Asthma is a serious condition that affects over 1 million children in the UK alone. Over a thousand people die from asthma each year in the UK. This is shocking and must be taken seriously. There are great herbal interventions that can reduce or resolve asthma in many people.

Note: never simply take away an inhaler from a child (or anyone) and replace it with herbs. If your child already has an inhaler, work with herbs and monitor the need for the inhaler. Consult a herbalist for help with asthma in a child.

Symptoms include difficulty breathing, wheezing, panic attacks, and coughing, and can be indicative of other respiratory ailments such as bronchitis or croup. Acute asthma can be seen in asthmatic bronchitis which mainly affects children less than six years old.

In asthma, when the bronchioles are constricted and the child has difficulty breathing, panic can occur, so learning about breathing and calm responding is also really good. Check out yogic breathing or the Buteyko method for more help.

Allergens may bring on an asthma attack and often asthma presents as part of an atopic picture where hay fever or eczema may also present. Pollen, dust, mites, and certain chemicals may affect a child so keep an eye out and a diary if possible.

Children with asthma can also be prone to phlegm, so cutting out dairy and other inflammatory foods may help, and increasing the child's immune system efficacy and vitality is essential.

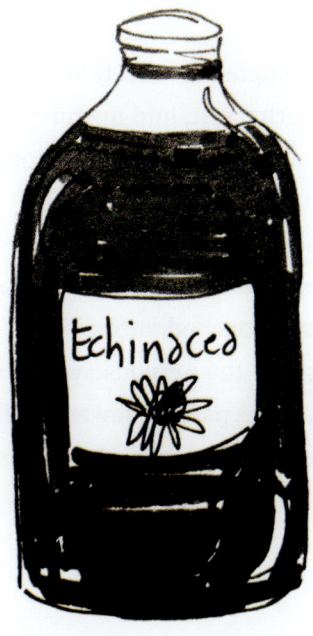

BRONCHEASE TEA FOR KIDS

Liquorice root
Thyme
Peppermint
Applemint
Mullein
Ginkgo

Equal parts of each herb.

Infuse 2 tsps of the tea blend for 10 mins and strain, cool enough for the child to drink. Add honey if desired but the liquorice is quite sweet. Encourage the child to breathe slowly and deeply between sips.

Plant allies

Use the herbs and food protocol suggested in the section on "Fevers" to help immunity.

To aid with expectoration, regular steam inhalations are beneficial, as is good gentle exercise such as yoga or fast walking, along with expectorant herbs. These include elecampane, thyme, and hyssop. Teas, tinctures, and syrups may be used for this.

Deal with any colds, coughs, or infectious respiratory conditions as these aggravate asthma; use herbs, rest, and nurture. Anti-infectives include garlic, echinacea, elderberry and elder flower, thyme, liquorice, catnip, yarrow, and hyssop.

A herbalist might choose to use bronchodilators that are a bit stronger than common home remedies. These include lobelia, jimsonweed, or ephedra which are all restricted but great bronchodilators.

Support the adrenals and the nervous system with gentle adaptogens like liquorice and nervines such as passionflower and lime flower.

Ginkgo may also be given as an infusion or drops and has been shown to help asthma and is also packed full of antioxidants.

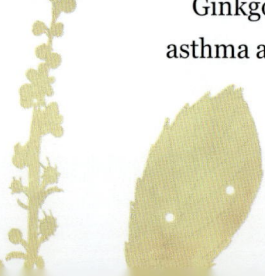

Eczema

There are different kinds of eczema but most commonly atopic eczema and seborrhoeic eczema is seen in children. There may be a familial trait which includes atopy or dietary triggers. If this is the case, long-term management may be needed. If there are certain exogenous triggers like clothes washing liquid, it may be that simple changes to lifestyle are needed. However, it will still remain the case that the child has sensitive skin and nourishing him or her in a way that aids skincare is good.

Factors to consider in a child with eczema:

Circulation – is the child often cold? If so, blood flow may not be nourishing the skin as much as in a warm child so adjust clothes and environment and encourage pungent or warming aromatic teas (ginger, turmeric, cinnamon, angelica).

Notice whether winter or wet weather makes symptoms worse.

Notice if phlegm producing foods do too, for example, dairy, or damp-making foods like nuts.

Note any foods or any products that trigger symptoms. A diet diary is helpful for this. Common triggers include gluten, dairy, sugar, salicylates, chocolate, some meats, nightshades (potatoes, pepper, tomatoes, etc.).

Supplements may include essential fatty acids, zinc, magnesium, B vitamins, and more. Taking fish or algal oils is a great idea. There are various ones which children like that are still fairly natural (eg. small capsules with added lemon oil) and you might get lucky with a kid who will swallow the oil no probs. Remember to find the right balance of omega 3, 6, and 9. Hemp and fish oil taken alternately are good for this. Address any inflammatory food reactions.

Plant allies

If scratching occurs then infection may follow. It is important to keep the skin as free from irritation as possible. Calming herbal creams are great here. They may include chickweed, lavender, and chamomile.

If there are weeping sores then try to keep the skin creams light, and if there are dry patchy presentations use a balm as a barrier. If the eczema appears hot and red, bitters and liver herbs are useful including vervain, skullcap, milk thistle, dandelion, artichoke, burdock.

SKIN-EASE CREAM

I like to use a hydrosol (lavender, rose, or yarrow) as my water content of the cream and blend with an infused oil of marigold. Add aloe gel, lavender, rose, violet, and essential oils of blue chamomile and ethically sourced frankincense.

SKIN-CALM BALM

Use marigold infused oil plus beeswax or shea butter as the ointment base (see Chapter 2). When it is cooling add in rose, lavender, violet, blue chamomile, and yarrow essential oils.

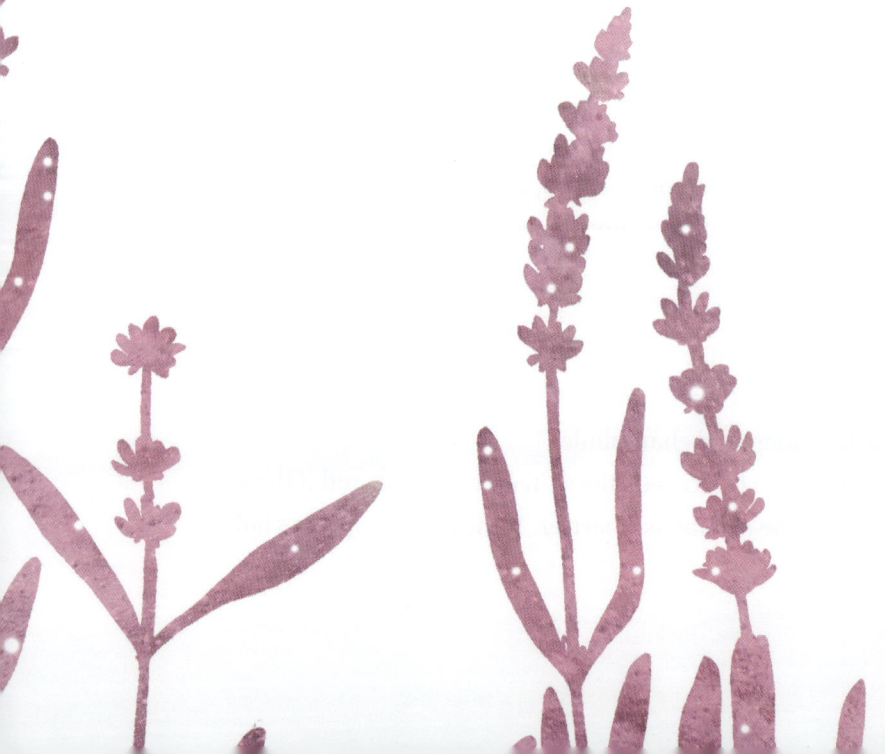

EMERGING BUDS: BABES AND CHILDREN

Remember to check the "Medicine making" section for all the base recipes from which you can start to make your own recipes up.

PLANT ALLIES FOR CHILDREN

Chamomile *Matricaria recutita*

Nature: hot and dry

Celestial body: Sun

Chamomile is one of the most commonly used herbs for children as it is gentle, soothing, calming, and effective. It is used as an anti-inflammatory, mildly bitter, an anti-infective, and nervine so is really helpful when dealing with children's ailments.

German chamomile and Roman chamomile may be used, the latter being stronger and more bitter so for children German chamomile may be more palatable. If you are growing chamomile, Roman chamomile is a perennial and German chamomile is an annual so you'll be able to tell the difference after the growing season if not before. It is very easy to grow.

Chamomile is often used with babies and children for upset stomachs, colic, and other digestive issues because it's very soothing on the digestive tract. It is useful for spasm, constipation, pain, and tummy upsets and therefore with its gentle action makes a really commonly used herb for kids as these kinds of gripes are very common.

As it is gentle it can also be used for baths and teas in babies and very young children. Chamomile is famous for its calming sedative action and is also quite uplifting so for kids who are irritated or grumpy this is especially good. If there is agitation or stress which is causing worry or insomnia, a simple chamomile infusion can be used. It is easy to make for children. A little honey may be added if desired.

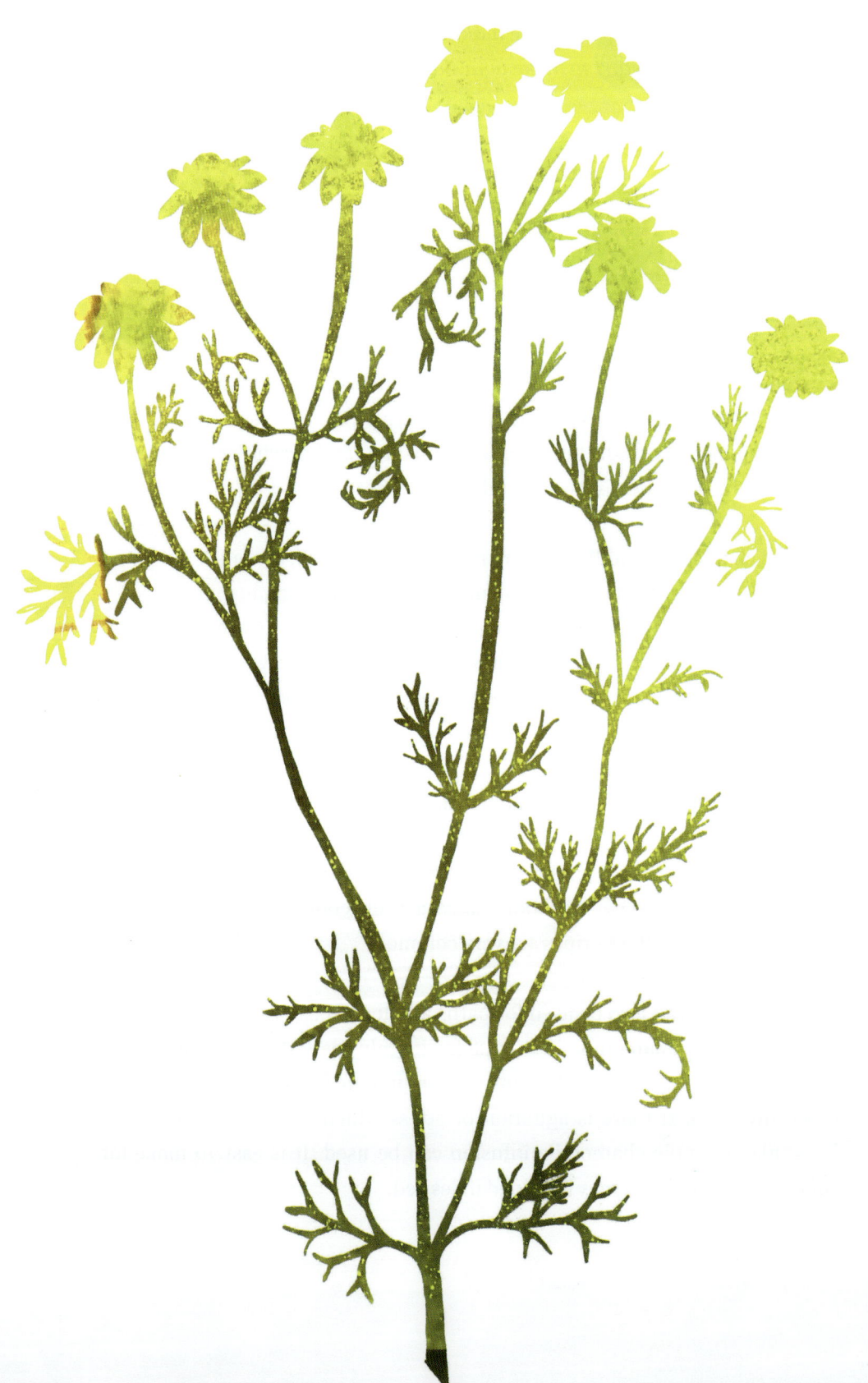

It's a great anti-inflammatory and anti-infective, the latter in part due to its volatile oils chamazulene (blue chamomile) and bisabolols, which help fight infection and increase healing of tissue especially in the gut.

As a first port of call it can also be used in coughs and colds as it promotes fevers and gently relaxes the bronchioles, helping the child be calm and breathe more easily. It is also one of the herbs that can be used in a hay fever remedy or an anti-allergy remedy along with other herbs such as plantain, nettle, or eyebright.

Chamomile is a lovely herb to add into creams for itching or irritated skin conditions in children. I also use it in toothpaste for my kids and as a gentle mouthwash as a tea. Despite its gentleness chamomile works really well to help the child increase immunity and is really important if your child is experiencing anything ongoing such as chronic coughs and colds, chronic asthma, chronic digestive upset, nerves or worry – it is a great one to have to hand in your apothecary.

As the sanguine humour is dominant in children a herb like chamomile which soothes and calms can be really useful. It is a herb of the sun so will have some gently warming effects which won't aggravate most sanguine (hot and dry) children.

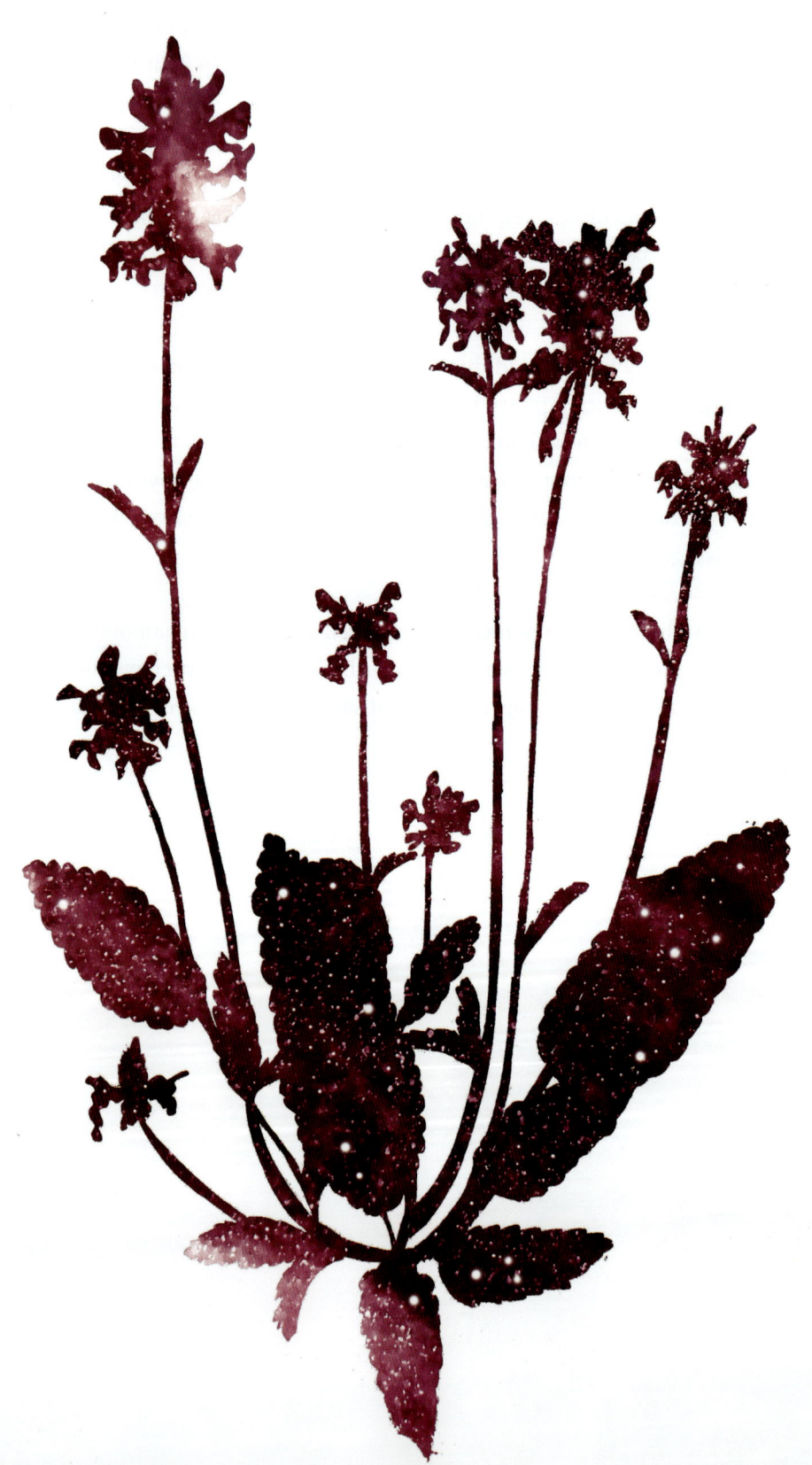

Betony *Stachys betonica*

Nature: dry and neutral

Planet: Jupiter

Betony is one of my favourite nervine herbs. It is particularly useful for children if they are worrying or stressed or can't sleep due to night terrors. Betony exerts a calming effect and helps relax the nervous system especially in stressful situations. It is also a specific for headaches and worrying thoughts so if children aren't able to express their fears but you can see they're agitated, betony can be really useful.

As betony is a tonic herb, with gentle action, it is particularly good for children who have a lot of fiery energy, for although sanguine is the dominant temperament during childhood, some kids are simply more choleric than others so calming and grounding action may be needed.

It is also really helpful for transitions such as a new school, moving house, or new friends, so lovely to keep in the apothecary for when your child needs it.

It exerts an effect on the liver and so for angry children can be helpful – in many cultures anger is seen to reside in the liver so aiding the liver is an important part of healing for those who are prone to anger. This is not to say that the anger is not necessary or valid, but it is just a way of coping with the anger while the root cause is addressed.

It is useful for kids with digestive upsets because it is an astringent and can help any inflammatory conditions such as colic, spasm, or too much wind in the belly causing pain and irritation in children.

Betony was traditionally worn as an amulet or bracelet and this is a lovely action for children – actually meeting and getting to know the plant then making a tangible medicine from it. Protection is a good thing and a medicine pouch or similar can feel very welcome by a child in need.

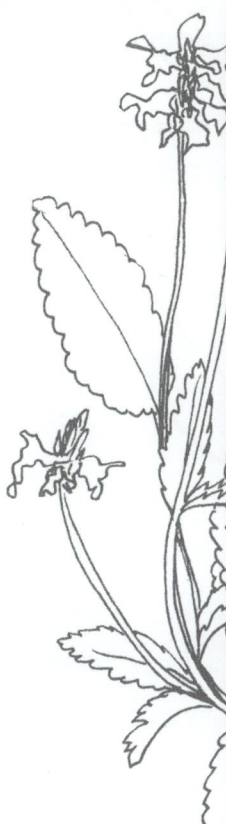

```
CALMING KIDDIE DROPS
Tincture or glycerite

Wood betony     2 parts
Lime flower     2 parts
Vervain         1 part
Rose            1 part

Give a few drops in water to calm when needed.
```

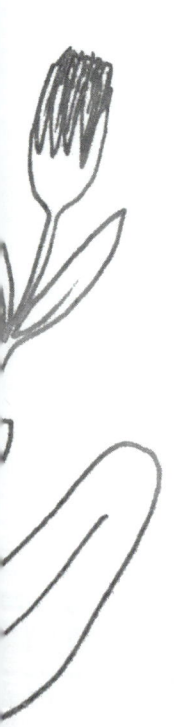

Marigold *Calendula officinalis*

Nature: hot and dry

Celestial body: Sun

Marigold is so helpful for children because it is so versatile. This herb is a great anti-inflammatory and it can be used for all kinds of skin problems, digestive issues, wound healing, and first aid. It is also an excellent lymphatic tonic which while gentle as an infusion has a brilliant effect on, for example, tonsillitis in children, or clearing toxins after infection. It can be taken as a gargle for sore throats and gum infections or as a mouth wash as it has excellent anti-infective qualities with its resinous content.

Alongside healing virtues, antibacterial qualities of marigold come in useful for nappy rash or sore genitals particularly if children wet themselves or have sore, itchy bottoms (worms, eczema, etc.). Marigold is also lovely as a strong tea in the bath and works as a general anti-inflammatory.

Marigold can also be used as part of a skin balm for insect bites and stings and cuts and scrapes from playing outside and having fun.

You can also get your children to pick the petals off marigold and scatter them on their salad. Once we did a cake with a bushcraft fire on top and marigold petals as the flames. It was lovely!

EMERGING BUDS: BABES AND CHILDREN

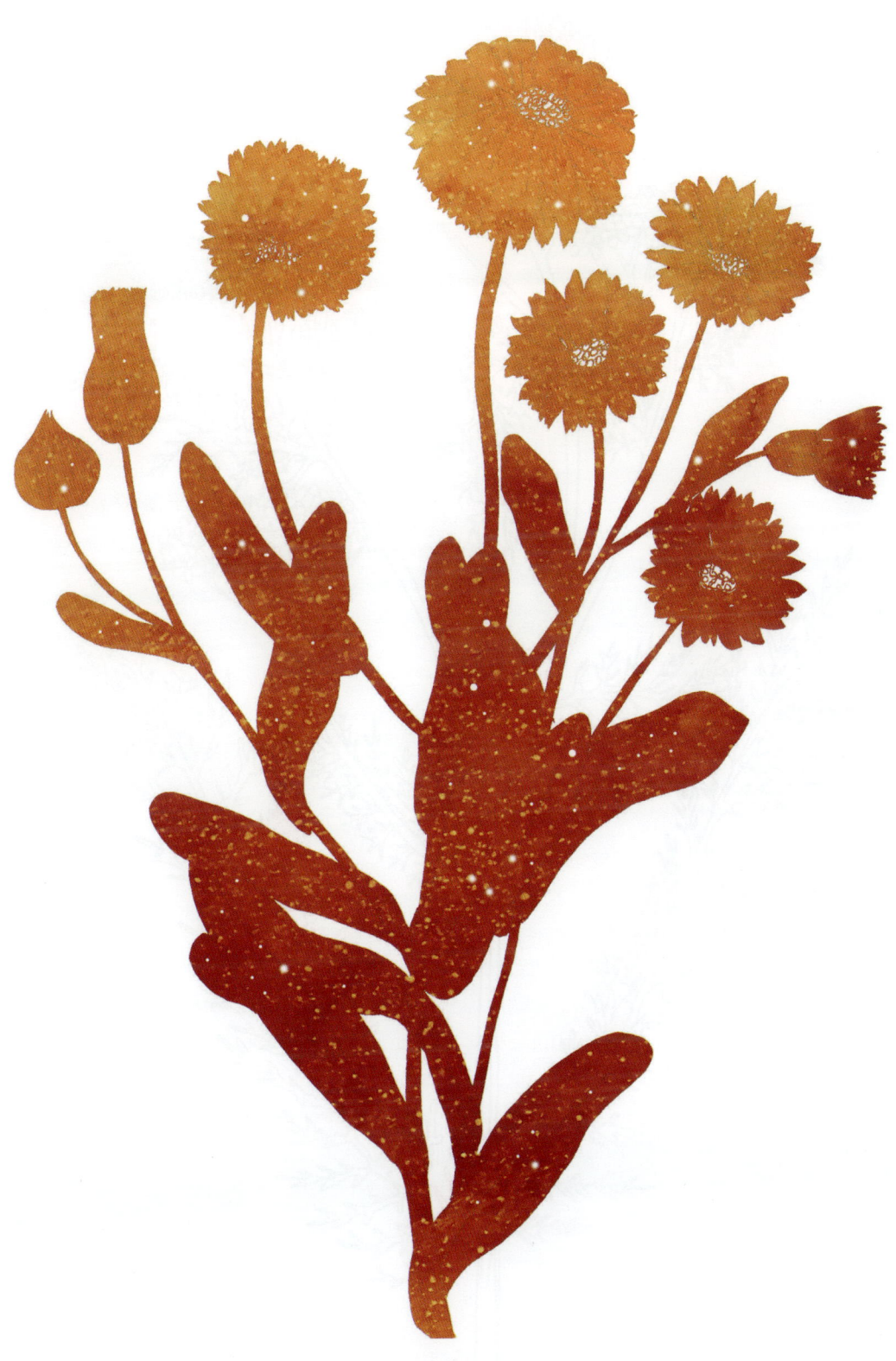

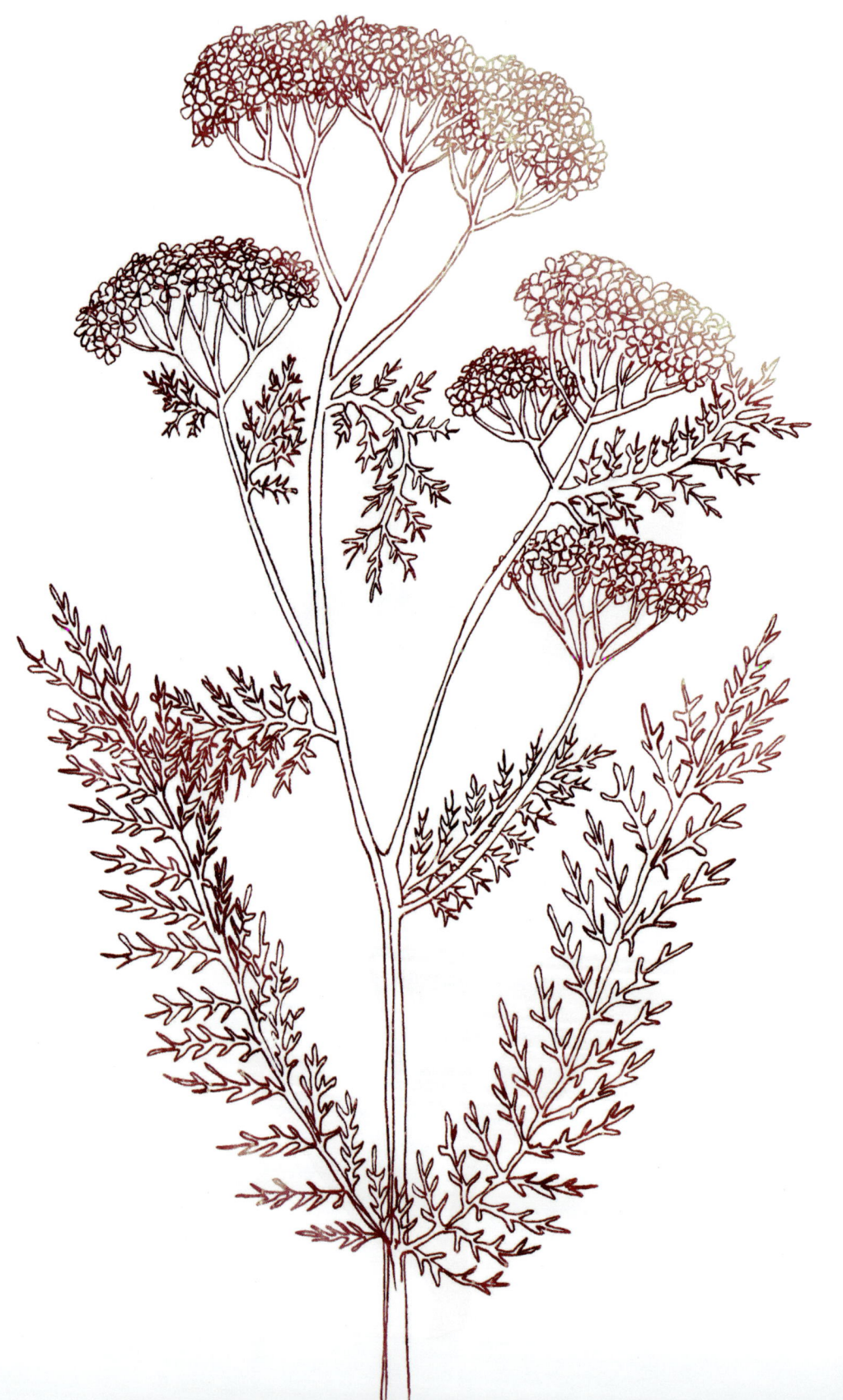

Yarrow *Achillea millefolium*

Nature: hot and dry

Planet: Venus

Yarrow is a protective herb. You can give it to children in a little amulet, pouch, or in their shoe, or keep a little in their bedroom. It is also a wonderful herb that can be used as a tea for very young children if they have fever or infection. It may be used as an infusion for warming and easing coughs and colds and getting the blood around the body as it is a circulatory stimulant.

Later in teenage years it is a fantastic herb for menstrual sluggishness manifesting as pain, cramps, and clotty periods. It is useful for cold or deficient kids who need a little push to get the blood moving, or those who always seems to have a snotty nose. It tastes good when combined with other herbs or a little honey and you don't need much at all. It is a little bitter so if left to steep may be more unpalatable. This bitterness, however, is excellent for digestive and skin conditions (skin often being reflective of the digestive system).

For adults yarrow is used in all kinds of conditions to move the blood, fight infection, and raise vitality. It is a digestive herb and, of course, the famous wound-healer of Greek warrior Achilles (hence its Latin name *Achillea*. Its other name *millefolium* means a thousand leaves which completely makes sense when you see the leaves!).

This herb is abundant and flowers for a few months so if you come across a big swathe you might like to try wild crafting a little for your apothecary.

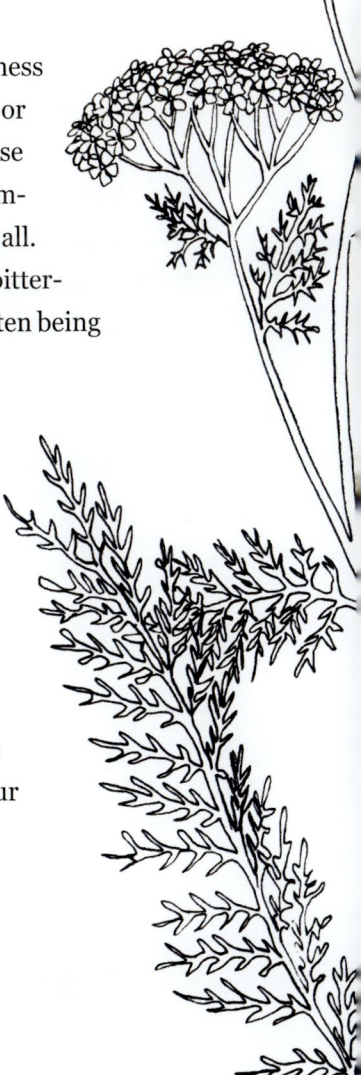

JOURNALING

You might like to explore what childhood means for you – which, if any, children are in your life right now, how your childhood was, and what your connections to plants were as a child. How do you connect with nature or the earth?

Draw plants that remind you of play, laughter, fun, silliness, love, or care. See if you can connect back in some way to your inner child. Your own age will determine how much work you want to do here. If you can, for each stage of your childhood, tune in to a plant that may have been predominant – for instance, when you were five you picked daisies, when you were ten you climbed an apple tree all the time, when you were sixteen you liked roses, and when you were eighteen you sat by a lake with rushes. Tune in to how these plants make you feel, what the landscape evokes, and how you might learn something from those experiences.

If you have kids who would like to engage with nature more, ask them to do drawings, prints, pressings, etc. of plants and begin a little book of plant secrets.

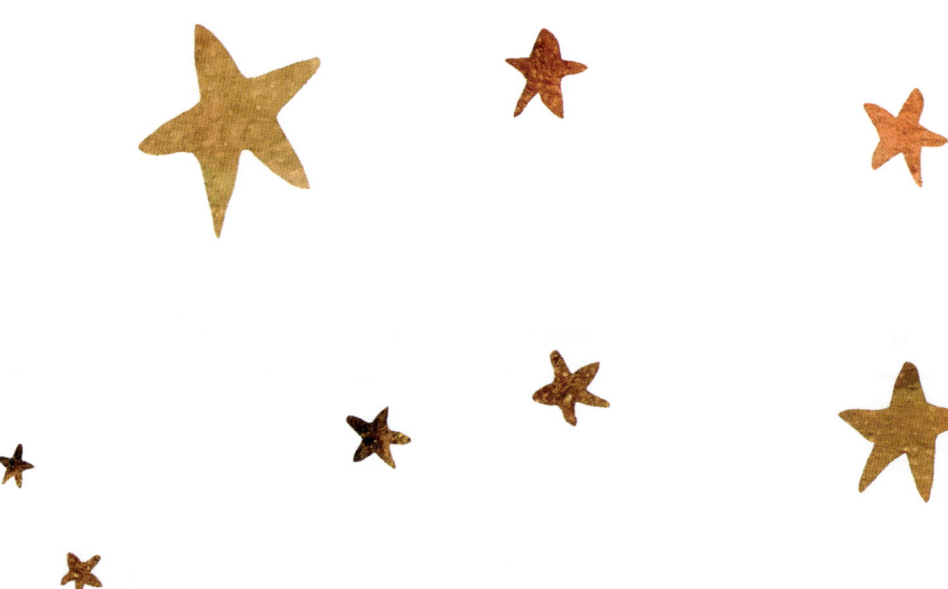

Mila, Claudia's granddaughter, with herbs

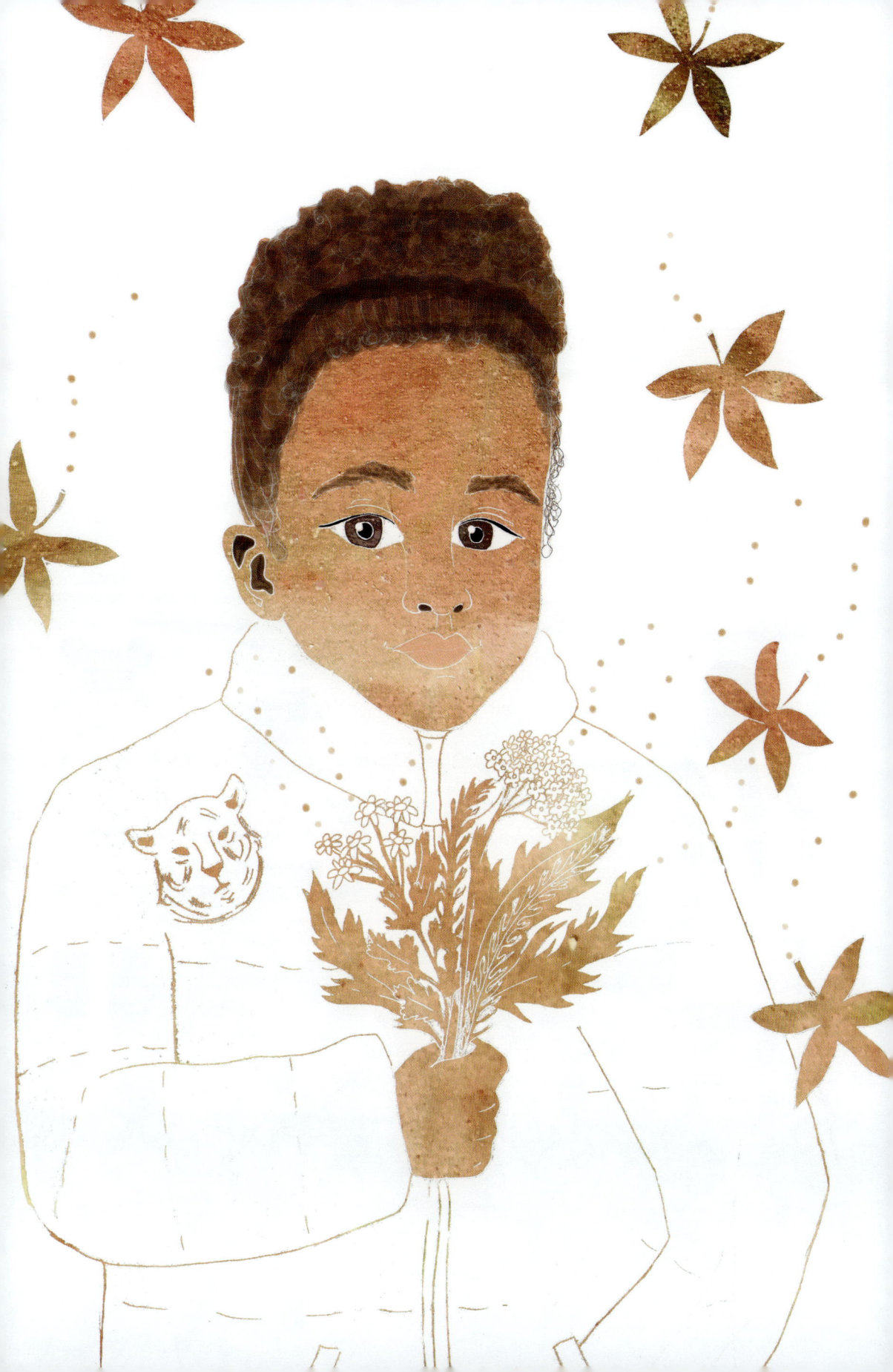

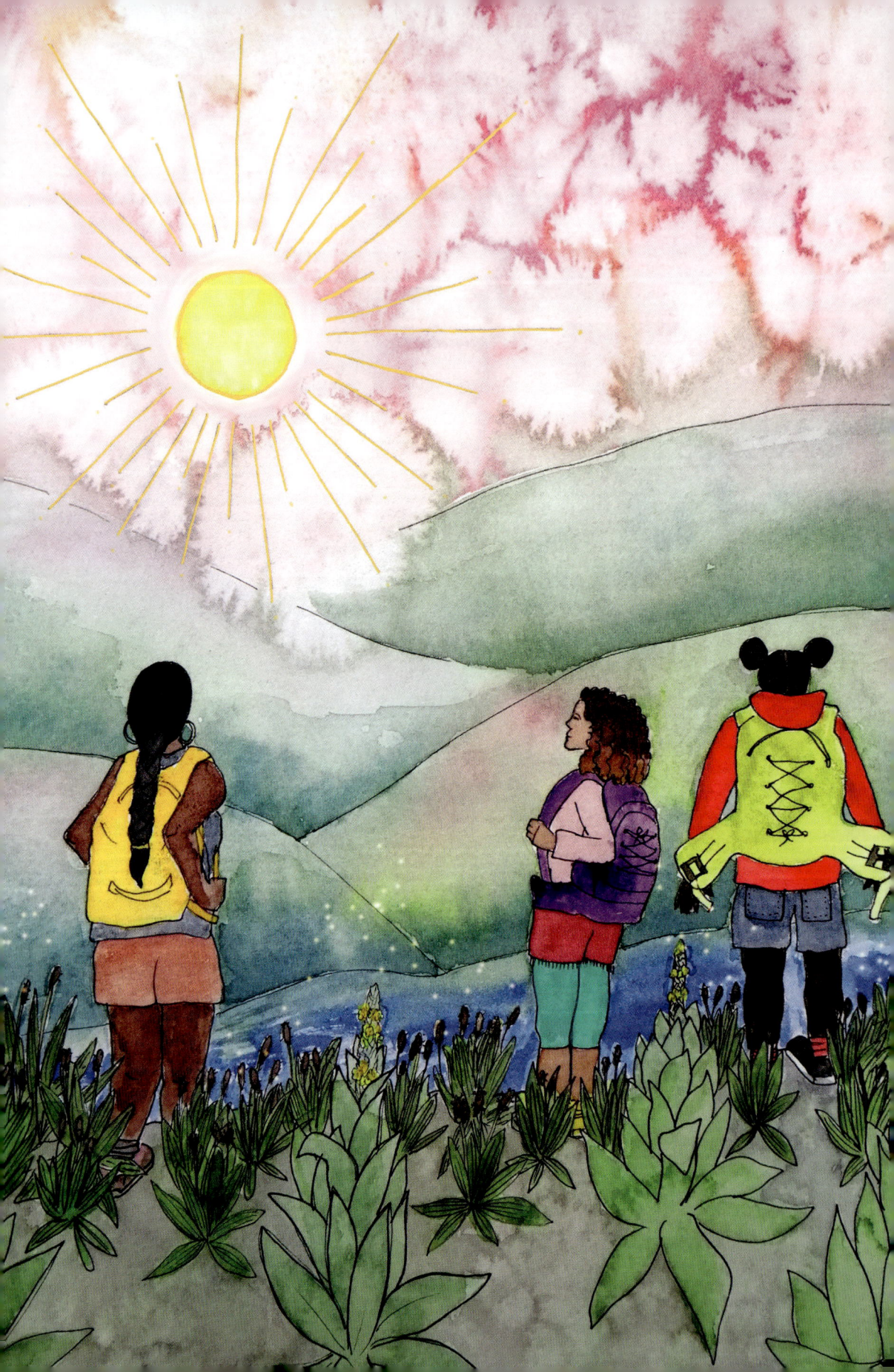

CHAPTER 5

OPENING BUDS: YOUTH

. . . always speak English outside the house or people will think you're a terrorist; here's how to fold dough into a samosa; here's how to make mattar paneer; here's how to make the perfect momo; here's how to make the perfect momo sauce; here's how to make a peanut butter sandwich for school so the other kids don't make fun of you; (. . .) here's how to cry during a Bollywood movie; here's how to smile and nod when a white boy makes jokes about eating with your hands; here's how to get good grades; always tell your relatives you want to be a doctor even if you don't want to . . .

An excerpt from "Brown Girl" by Indigo Mudbhary, winner of Top 15 Foyle Young Poets of the Year Award 2020

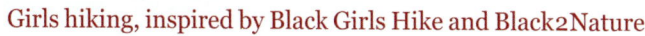
Girls hiking, inspired by Black Girls Hike and Black2Nature

ENERGETICS AND ELEMENTS

Youth is a testing time – so much to learn, so much to do, so much to become.

The choleric humour is dominant in young people as they grow out of childhood into adulthood. Transitions are huge at this time of life, puberty arrives, sexuality awakens, aspirations come into view, children seek their own identity, and life becomes, for some, a social affair. Summer is the dominant season of the choleric humour, with its high energy and life. Fire is the element of the choleric humour.

Choler is the fire of youth and may manifest in anger, moods, passion, new relationships, independence, frustration, charisma, activity, fun, dynamism, restlessness, drive. It may also show up in physical symptoms like red acne, angry eczema, digestive issues, and insomnia.

Choleric folk often respond to direction in their lives, to self-discipline, and thoughtful, boundaried, loving consistency from parents with lots of short-term goals and projects that can be completed. Youth and choleric types need exercise, movement, and expression. If you try to sit children or young people in a chair for too long and make them study, they most likely will begin to exhibit signs of imbalance, so a good balance and understanding of the fire of youth is super helpful.

Rewilding exercise – Move and envisage

If you are unable to walk or run, or even go outside, envisage how you can connect with movement – any kind of movement can be practised with intention. We all need to move as best we can to encourage blood and lymph flow; improve our digestion, lung, and joint health; and provide mental-emotional balance. It affects every system in our body. Find a way to move – your arms, fingers, neck, or whatever works for you, and look to the outside – through a window or in a green space and simply notice what you see, feel, and sense.

Walk – if you can

Often when we walk with intention we have an experience. That experience can be called upon when needed – the thoughts, feelings, and occurrences can all be journaled to keep this practice in mind.

For teenagers or young adults, journals can be a great way to recall experiences such as these small walks and be added to if the individual wants to share, discuss, reflect, or express.

A really simple walk is to just walk. Go out and walk then return and journal. Note anything that comes to mind. Then repeat with a specific intention in mind, such as, "Notice what you are drawn to on this walk" (eg. rocks, views, trees, tiny lichens, etc.). When home, journal again. These are very simple exercises and can ground a fiery teenager, channelling some energy.

Run to harness fire – if you can

Slightly more active exercises include running – if teenagers can run instead of walking, then note all they saw, they will be doing it in a choleric frame of mind instead of a calmer, more melancholic slowness. This may suit some teens very well.

Encourage teens to be in nature, with others as befits their social fire, or alone with a little heart-tending going on.

I like to nourish fire with fire. In a small group allow teens to come together in the woods, or a campsite or in the garden – wherever a small fire is allowed. Ask them to find or make the kindling and where possible allow them to create the fire themselves; they can also nominate a fire keeper who sees to the fire during the session. Encourage the teens to talk, use the fire for letting go – writing things they'd like to let go of on paper and in gentle ceremony burn it. Encourage gratitude for the fire and discussion about what fire brings up. This can also be done for all the other elements. Finish with some food or drink cooked or heated over the fire. A song is always nice too.

CONDITIONS

We will look at common conditions that affect our youth. We will also concentrate in this chapter on menarche and menstruation.

MOONTIME

Periods have had such a hard rap. I remember the day a tampon (organic and plastic free, but no, not a mooncup . . .) fell out of my bag only for my child to pick it up and wave it about. At first I was a bit embarrassed and then I thought "why?" Why are we sold the notion that periods should be hidden and that bleeding girls and women should be able to do all the things we normally do with a tiny pad in tight jeans?

It simply isn't the case.

In some cultures, a woman is not to be touched during her period, in others she cannot enter the temple or mosque, cannot cook, or is banished away. There is a need to cultivate an environment of respect, honouring this amazing time that, while it has its challenges, is essential to life and the cleansing of the womb.

Periods. Coming on. Moontime. Yoni flow. There are many ways to describe blood flow, and girls will feel a certain way about it – embarrassed, fearful, excited, grown up, cross, etc. This is a transition time from childhood to womanhood and it is a beautiful thing if you can honour a girl and make her feel that this natural, incredible process is just that.

Menarche, the onset of menstruation, used to occur around fourteen to sixteen years of age in girls – now the average age is twelve and a half, partly due to modern lifestyle and environmental oestrogen. Girls are starting their

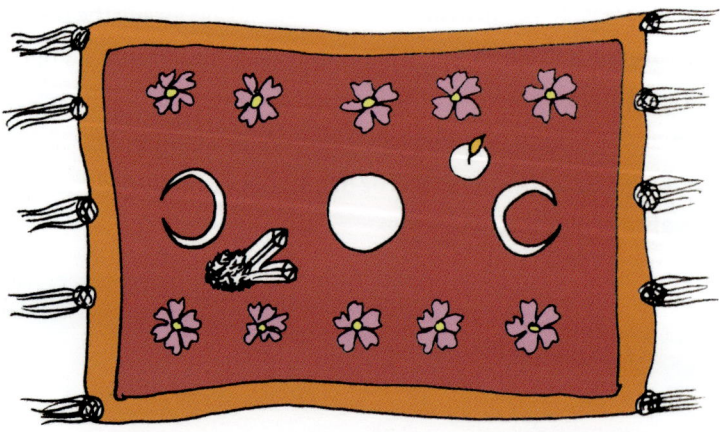

menstruation earlier and menstruating longer, and indeed living longer. We adults bear fewer children now than we used to on the whole and breastfeed for a shorter amount of time, if at all. Our diet is more refined, sweeter, and more plentiful and our environment has completely changed in all kinds of ways from transport to office jobs to technology in modern times.

With these changes it is possible that women may have up to ten times more periods now than women just a few generations before us. Women are having to cope with so much on top of menstruating every single month for longer than ever before. It is no wonder that more women than ever before are experiencing more gynaecological conditions.

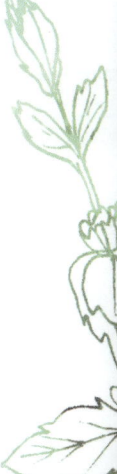

Rewilding exercise

When a girl first bleeds and feels ready to go outside, ask her to go to a tree or plant she feels drawn to – it may be that day, or in the following few weeks. When she finds one (a little help may be needed to guide her away if poisonous), ask her to start listening to that plant or tree, just for a few minutes.

Once she feels she's connected with it in some way, ask her to start finding out what that plant is. It may be a plant she knows or isn't familiar with in terms of name. She can do anything she likes – draw it, read about it once identified, press parts of it, listen more, rest by it, etc. Just get to know it. It's good if the plant in question is near her home so she can visit it frequently (or find another example of the same type of plant close to home).

It may become a plant she can associate with support for her Moontime. If you don't or she doesn't feel comfortable finding one in the wild for whatever reason, try a garden plant or see if you can find a herbalist who can help you or your girl do the same kind of connection work. For example, you might like to hold a rose ceremony which might include a rose tea tasting, rose chocolates, and rose cosmetics – it is all about nourishing and tending the growing young person. You don't have to be outside to connect deeply with nature, the earth, or self, but it is really healthy to be outdoors. Staying inside is entirely an option and much work can be achieved through tea tastings, listening, meditation, observing trees outside, etc. Singing is a fantastic way to connect, and learning songs or writing songs based around trees or connection is very powerful too.

A word on menstrual language and apparatus. We like to use the word Moontime for a period, as often we bleed in sync with the moon, or at least we can tune into the moon through cyclical periods, or Moontimes. We don't use the term "sanitary pads" or talk of it as "personal hygiene", we honour our flow and use moon pads or menstrual pads (often recyclable or home-made or made by women's co-operatives), yoni or moon cups or tampons (organic cotton, bamboo, or sponge). There is nothing unsanitary about it. Finally, the "tampon tax" has been dissolved in the UK as the government starts to become clear that looking after oneself during Moontime is a necessity not a luxury.

Tampons and Mooncups are used as plugs to stem the flow of blood into clothes. This interruption of flow may exacerbate period pain and may promote clots and "stagnation".Many people prefer pads or even free flow.

All over the UK, and I'm sure many other countries, red tents are popping up, giving women a space to meet and share time, stories of womanhood, and most likely (raw) chocolates. Once bleeding, a girl can join this beautiful movement and learn self-love and have some fun too. Throughout history and the world, women would enter the forest, the red tent, the sacred space when bleeding. This gave women time to rest, chat, share, connect with each other and the earth. This has been all but lost in modern society.

Yoni or vaginal steams or smokes are becoming widespread and young women are finding their way to understanding menstrual/yoni/vaginal health. In normal circumstances, the vagina is self-cleaning. Our yonis have an acidic pH balance and clear discharge from the vaginal canal is a normal occurrence at certain times of the month. Over-cleansing the vaginal canal may cause infection as can insertion of a whole load of items available for purchase designed to make women feel than their vaginas need to be cleaner, pinker, more this, less that (for example, vagina glitter making your discharge sweet and glittery, vagina lipstick making your labia a certain colour, scented tampons, and more).

Women are reconnecting with their most intimate bodily parts. Let's throw off the cloak obscuring menstruation, and female empowerment, and the making of it taboo by religion, cultural impetus, and social myth.

When a woman knows her cycle, she can tune in to the times of the month she knows she will be more energetic, and times she knows she might need a little time out, a little more nutritious food, a little more rest. She might also become aware of the moon cycles and whether she follows them or she may be able to tune in to her body and nature's cycles if she is not bleeding. Cycles help with rhythm and understanding so it is always a good thing to tune in to them. This is all great practice once bleeding has started. If she knows there is support out there, she can tune in to it whenever she needs to. There are lots of resources now in womancraft (tending women) and menstrual health including The Red School, and The School of Shamanic Womancraft.

A beautiful act is gifting a girl a moon bag or joining a moon daughters group. A moon bag holds various gifts pertinent to a girl's menarche and rite of passage. It may include moonpads and books, high quality ethical chocolate, home-made fresh perfume or cosmetics – creative, personal gifts that a girl will enjoy and use to celebrate her menarche. For it is a celebration!

Moon Daughters groups are for girls approaching or going through menarche and their mamas or close women friends or relatives. Together the girls explore different aspects of girlhood and growth – it can be done in many ways from different activities to sharing words or songs around a fire. It is similar to the rites of passage boys may go through in groups such as Journeyman which support this transitional phase.

Not all who bleed identify as a girl so tending each growing child or young person in their own way is really important – find ways to connect and honour as best suits each individual.

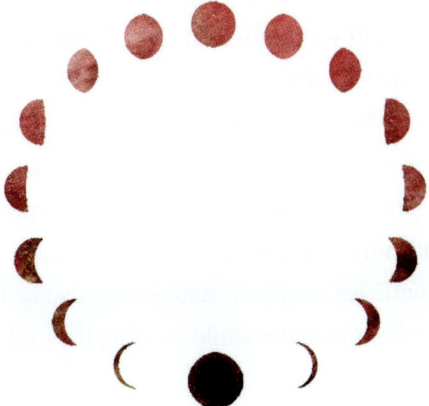

SYMPTOMS ACCOMPANYING MENSTRUATION

Menstrual cramps

Painful menstruation is common, and has become normalised in society, and for the most part is put up with by women. Pain is a sign of imbalance and may be accompanied by dizziness and nausea or vomiting, heaviness or pain in the legs, sweats, and fatigue. As herbalists we have to question why the womb is cramping in order to expel our monthly flow; this is not considered a "normal" physiological action.

Ischaemia of the uterus and/or cervix can also contribute to spasmodic pain. There may be constipation and/or diarrhoea before and during the period. Care should be taken to assess what is happening when a girl or woman gets period pain.

Exercise and diet may eradicate all cramps in menstruation and a healthy relationship with your cycle may really encourage this connection. If you can't find a way to calm or experience menstruation without cramps there are herbs that help.

The pain may be secondary dysmenorrhoea which is more common after childbirth or when women reach their thirties. It is often connected with other gynaecological conditions such as endometriosis, inflammation of the uterus, and PMS.

Painful periods may be helped by exercise, a change in diet, and different posture. Supplements such as fish oils or algal oils can help with prostaglandin pain. Calcium, magnesium, and probiotics may also be of benefit. Hot baths or hot water bottles may ease cramps. Relaxing the spasm increases circulation which helps to nourish the womb and move the blood. Large clots are a sign of menstrual stagnation – herbs such as ginger and feverfew can be really useful here. Hydrotherapy (hot-cold water alternations), herbal baths, and postural changes may also yield positive results.

In general, liver herbs are recommended (bitters, hepatics) as the liver is often a little more under pressure due to hormone imbalances and metabolism. It is also the seat of anger – for any PMS symptoms, supporting the liver is essential. Uterine tonics and hormone balancers for some girls will be needed and nervines, anti-inflammatories, and lymphatics may also be indicated. Pain mixes can be made as acute relief medicine while treating the underlying cause.

Plant allies

Antispasmodics – crampbark or black haw, valerian, German chamomile.

Bitters – vervain, burdock, artichoke .

Nervines – rose, valerian, vervain, chamomile, pasqueflower (this is only prescribed by a herbalist).

```
NO CRAMPS TINCTURE

Crampbark        55 ml
Valerian         40 ml
Ginger           5 ml

Take half a teaspoon of the mix in a little water as
soon as the girl notices pain (1 teaspoon for an
adult) and again half an hour to 1 hour later if pain
has not subsided.

Rest should also be encouraged.
```

Constipation or loose stools

Menstruation can affect the gut so be gentle with yourself or your daughter and eat healthily, encouraging the intake of plenty of fresh veggies, fruit, slow-releasing carbohydrates (millet, buckwheat, quinoa, wild rice, sweet potato, etc.), healthy sugars, and avoid fried foods, chemical additives, etc.

Herbs can be used but diet is key. I find gentle infusions of nervines and carminatives taken the week leading up to moonflow can help keep the gut healthy during menstruation. These include chamomile, vervain, burdock, marigold, fennel, lemon balm, lime flower, bitters (good for constipation – eat them!), and mints.

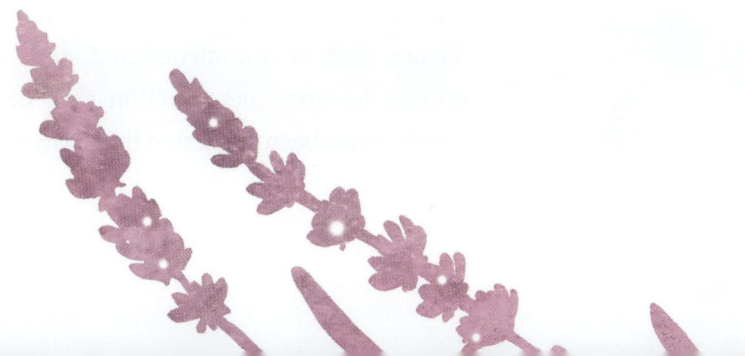

Mugwort is a beautiful herb for constipation around menses; it is a bitter and moves stagnancy and is also a womb herb. Sip the tea with a little honey or make a glycerite of mugwort buds and leaves.

Mood changes (PMS, "PMDD")

These symptoms can be seen in young women and older girls as well as more mature woman. Crying, irritability, and moodiness are all symptoms which can appear just before or during menstruation but usually the onset of menstruation relieves the symptoms. There is a lot of emotional stigma attached to "hysteria" before periods and it can be belittled. Don't let this be the case. Something is causing these feelings and must be acknowledged rather than ignored or ridiculed. This cycle of mood changes and associated symptoms ceases upon menopause (induced or natural).

Symptoms can include:

> Anxiety, anger, depression, irritability, social withdrawal, crying
> Breast tenderness
> Headaches
> Swelling (usually in the extremities), but this might be more common when older
> Bloating

There are also associated cravings for carbohydrate foods or chocolate (check zinc and magnesium levels and consider gut bacteria).

This is common in adults too and will affect teenagers at different stages. Hypotheses of what causes these symptoms include different hormone levels (eg. excess or deficient oestrogen and deficient progesterone), prostaglandin or neurotransmitter dysfunction, HPA (hypothalamus pituitary adrenal) axis dysfunction, nutrient deficiency, diet, environmental and stress factors, negative attitude towards menstruation (self or societal). More recently, it has been suggested that CNS neurotransmitters respond to cyclical hormonal changes – oestrogens increase serotonin and dopamine levels where progesterone might do the opposite.

Plant allies

Hormone modulation – chasteberry, vervain, lavender, rose, skullcap, passionflower.

Adaptogens – check with your herbalist if these are suitable. Ashwagandha, Siberian ginseng, rose root, schisandra, nettle, dong quai.

Anxiolytics/anti-depressants – vervain, St John's wort, lemon balm, Cali poppy, passionflower.

Bitters/hepatics – vervain, gentian, dandelion.

Lymphatics – marigold, cleavers.

```
CALM AND NOURISH TONIC
Vervain
Passionflower
Lavender

Equal parts, 5-10 drops as necessary just before symp-
toms of PMS start and throughout the luteal phase
until bleeding begins. This can be taken daily
if desired.
```

Headaches or migraines

Regular headaches or migraines just before or during menstruation are most likely due to the oestrogenic and progesteronic influences over CNS neurotransmitters, making them a premenstrual symptom. The withdrawal of oestrogen in the luteal phase of the cycle (between ovulation and menstruation) precedes a migraine and seems to occur in particular in women who have higher levels of oestrogen in the follicular stage.

Premenstrual headaches often have a gradual onset, sometimes triggered by stress and typically last twelve to twenty-four hours and can be very irregular in frequency. Premenstrual migraines may be preceded by auras, and the onset of pain is often in the afternoon, again triggered by stress, menstruation, and certain foods. They typically last for eight to twelve hours but may last up to three days, and the pain can be constant and intense and throbbing.

There is a lot that can be done, from working with the menstrual cycle in general and balancing hormones, to dealing with stress, attitude, sleep, anxiety, inflammation, spasm, etc. Supplements that may help include magnesium, coenzyme Q10, riboflavin, vitamin b12, vitamin D, calcium, and EFAs.

Plant allies

Feverfew – This plant has been used for headaches for over 300 years! Feverfew can bring down the frequency and intensity of a migraine and relieve the accompanying symptoms. Teas or strong infusions are recommended and may also help with painful periods.

Ginger – All over the world where ginger grows it is used for pain and nausea. Ginger acts as an anti-inflammatory through the inhibition of enzymes and prostaglandin synthesis, therefore helping to relieve painful headaches.

Peppermint oil has traditionally been applied to the head for tension headaches. Such a simple action as rubbing it on the temples in a base cream or oil a few times in an hour can relieve headaches.

> DROPS FOR PREMENSTRUAL HEADACHES (TINCTURE)
>
> ```
> Skullcap        2 parts
> Chamomile       2 parts
> Feverfew        2 parts
> Crampbark       2 parts
> Lavender        1 part
> Ginger          ½ part
> ```
>
> Use 10 to 20 drops of the mix in water from the first sign of discomfort and take up to 4 x daily.

Breast tenderness

Breast tenderness is so common that it is almost considered a normal part of the menstrual cycle. It may be indicative of changes in diet (more coffee, less veggies, etc.), stress, posture, lack of exercise. Depending on the age of the girl or woman, different herbs can be given but a good basic tea is marigold, to be drunk liberally.

Breast massage is also really important if there is tenderness as the breasts (like the prostate) are made largely of fatty tissue so need to be moved to encourage lymphatic flow. Massage helps the lymph to drain excess or stagnant fluid so alone can prevent tenderness. Massage is so important and is used in Ayurveda for breast lumps.

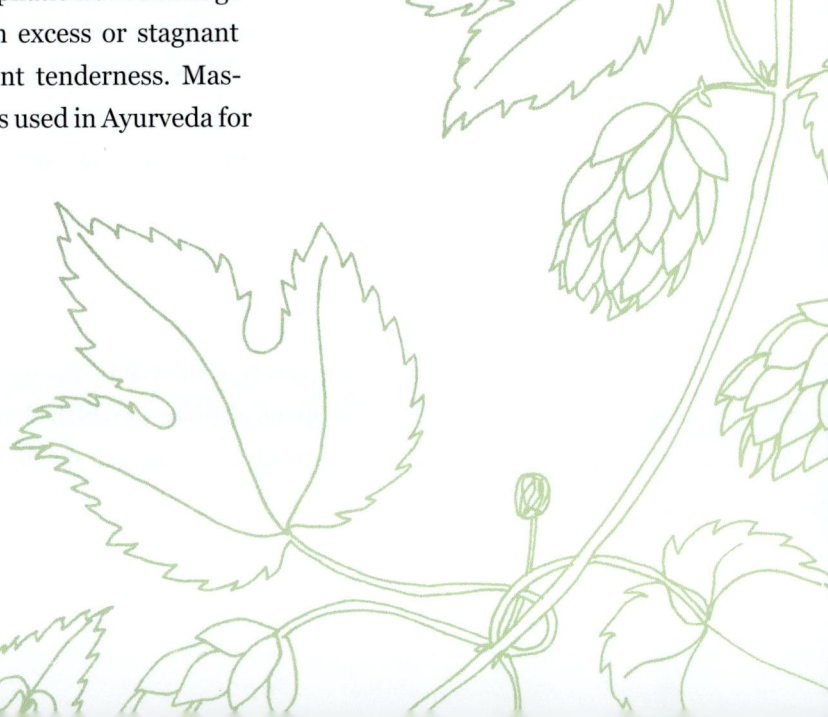

```
TENDER BREAST TEA

For breast tenderness a tea mix with marigold can be
given and drunk freely throughout.

Marigold          2 parts
Cleavers          2 parts
Nettle            1 part
Rose              1 part

Infuse 1-2 tsp of the tea blend for 5-10 minutes and
strain. Enjoy.
```

Acne

Androgens (hormones) increase in puberty as part of normal sex development and this is often when acne starts. It can affect anyone and is usually a miserable affliction because our faces are seen. Our faces are our presentation of ourselves – they are the "interface" between the outer and the inner, and in modern society, which seems to thrive off marketing beauty and aesthetic ideals, acne can be hard. It may range from small and infrequent pimples to constant painful cystic acne.

In many older girls and women androgen levels haven't increased past normal levels, but 5-α reductase is elevated at the sebaceous gland which implies a sensitivity to androgen. This means that women who have acne as a teenager may well have acne until well into their forties.

I have scarred skin from acne when I was young. I had no idea what to do about it – nor that there was anything to be done – and when I was taken to the GP by my well-meaning mother, I was given antibiotics which changed my gut bacteria and caused bloating I'd never experienced before and never really recovered from. Then I was put on the contraceptive pill for my spots, which I despised, and discovered I wasn't really into the orthodox approach. I wish someone had told me about eating well and cleavers!

If androgen excess is part of a bigger picture then further work needs to be done but if there are no other obvious signs of underlying conditions, you can seek to improve skin function and hormonal balance. Cruciferous vegetables such as broccoli, cabbage, and mustard leaves are very useful for clearing and recirculating steroid hormones.

Plant allies

Anti-inflammatory – witch hazel, lavender, liquorice, marigold.

Anti-infective – echinacea, lavender, tea tree, thyme.

Nervine – lavender, skullcap, chamomile, vervain.

Adaptogen – ashwagandha, liquorice.

Alterative – burdock, barberry, yellow dock, figwort.

Lymphatic – cleavers, marigold.

Hepatics – dandelion, oregon mountain grape, barberry, burdock, docks.

Hormone modulation – chasteberry, vervain, dong quai

If there is a hormonal element as is so common for both boys and girls it is best to see a herbalist who can do a thorough consultation.

A cleansing diet, lots of fresh air, exercise, and a supportive framework of friends where possible really help.

```
ACNE INFUSION
Cleavers
Marigold
Vervain
Nettle

Equal parts of each. Drink this tea liberally.
```

Moods – particularly for boys who don't "talk"

While girls may experience mood changes as a premenstrual symptom, any teenager may be prone to mood changes – hormonal or otherwise – which may be present and difficult to cope with. While times are changing, boys often have no one to talk to about their feelings as the patriarchal male model is one of individual independent success and dominance. These kinds of emotions can be very isolating and confusing.

While therapy or close role models, diet, lifestyle, and love can help, herbs may be chosen to relax the youth. Many nervines may be suitable. All teens may have the same or slightly different worries and mood changes.

It could be a simple change like cutting out dairy to which the child/teen is sensitive and so releases adrenaline every time it's eaten, slowly depleting the adrenals while staying in the sympathetic nervous system (fight or flight) mode . . . if you think of cycles, the body isn't able to rest and digest. This is exhausting if frequent.

All young folk can benefit from nervines which can really help with mood shifts of various kinds. It is great to see a herbalist as they can give specific herbs that work with each individual teen – with a hormonal element, a dietary question, an emotional challenge, trauma, and so on.

Cooling nervines include vervain, violet, hops, and wild lettuce. Other useful actions include protecting the heart or liver from excess heat – these herbs might include motherwort and lemon balm for the heart and dandelion and burdock for the liver.

```
IF THERE IS YOUTHFUL ANGER PRESENT, THEN TRY A
TEA CONTAINING:

Vervain
Violet
Dandelion root
Artichoke
Rose

Equal parts, infuse 1-2 tsps for 5-10 minutes, strain.
Drink 2-3 cups daily.
```

> IF THERE IS A SCARED, EMOTIONAL YOUTH, TRY A TEA CONTAINING:
>
> Milky oats
> Rose
> Violets
> Lemon balm
> Motherwort
>
> Equal parts, infuse 1-2 tsps for 5-10 minutes, strain. Drink 2-3 cups daily.

Anxiety

Anxiety is one of the most common presentations in clinic. Often parents want a consultation for their children for a digestive issue, a skin condition, juvenile arthritis, or menstrual issues, for example, and while we look at those conditions, it is often anxiety that is triggering them or accompanying the condition.

With so much stress and the burden of judgement weighing on people's shoulders nowadays, anxiety can be crippling for youth and adults alike, creating a personality that the beholder does not recognise. Excessive anxiety can cause a child to freeze and their worry can be tangible ("I'm worried about . . . my exams, parents splitting up, bullying, identity, social media pressure") or intangible ("Something is making me feel ill and I can't verbalise or visualise it fully"). Symptoms can be vague or specific and include fatigue, difficulty concentrating, brain fog, muscle sensitivity/tenderness, irritability, insomnia, teariness, glumness, restlessness, lack of appetite, mood swings, digestive issues, and disassociation. Clinical symptoms include sweating (diaphoresis), headache, tachycardia (racing heartbeat), and trembling and panic attacks may ensue.

Generalised anxiety disorder (GAD) is poorly understood and usually associated with adults but more and more we are seeing our teenagers suffer with anxious conditions. Various areas in the brain appear to be involved as does neurotransmitter deregulation. Hormonal influence is a possible cause as are stress factors on the body. Claudia suggests GAD is a "manifestation of late-stage capitalism with pressures from the media to look a certain way, to perform and to be successful". We have so many pressures on our shoulders in Western society.

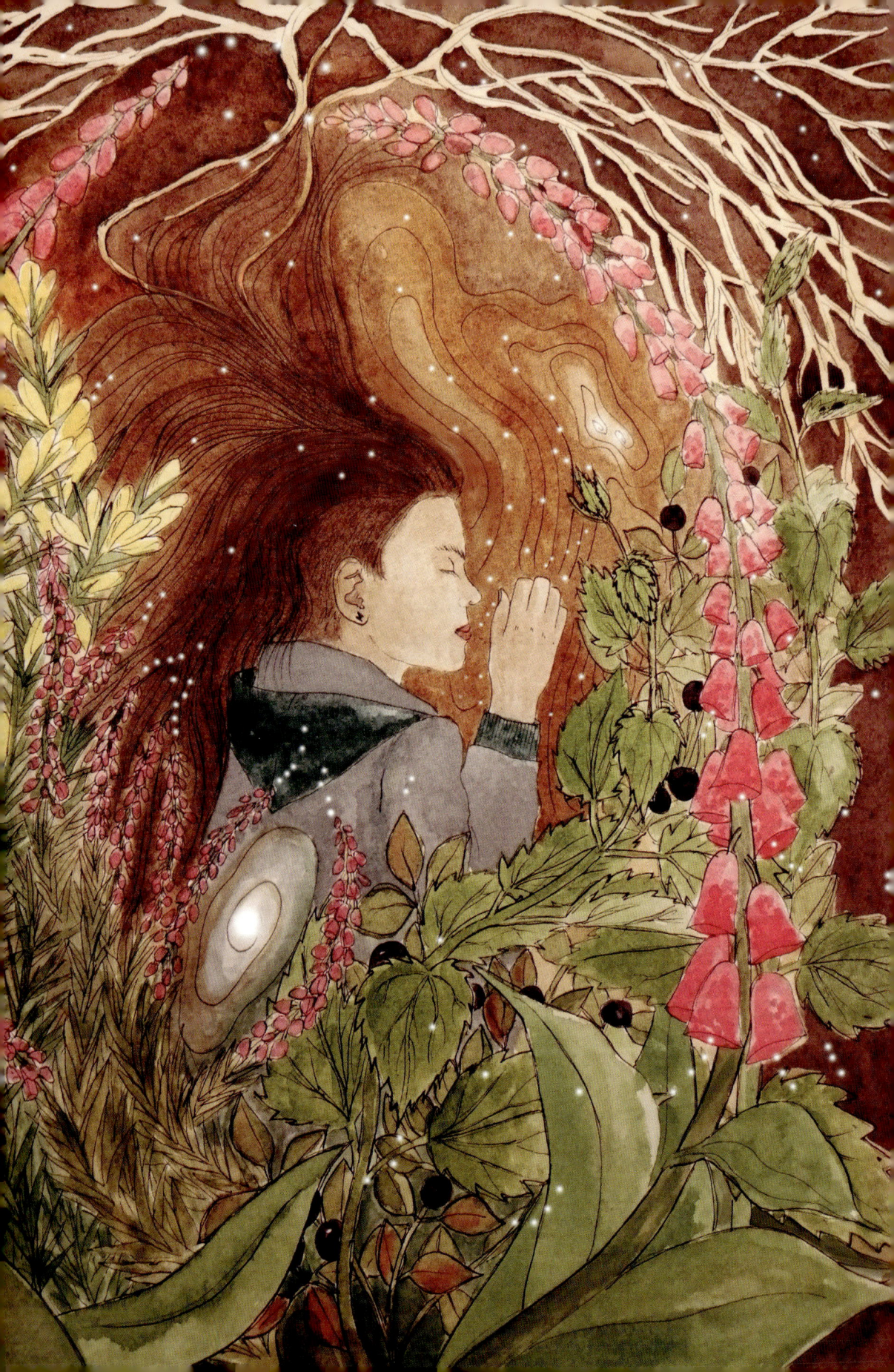

Plant allies

In terms of herbs, it is very much down to the presenting symptoms and nature of the individual. We all present our anxiety differently and often choleric youths present with extreme behaviour or totally mask it all in bravado or over-confidence or sullen moods that are attributed to "teenage angst" as if it were a trivial matter. It can be tricky to spot.

Anxiolytics, nervines, sedatives, and adaptogens all have their place:

Anxiolytics – passionflower, lavender, pasqueflower (prescribed by a herbalist), lemon balm, valerian.

Nervines – oats, vervain, skullcap, St John's wort, damiana, chamomile, rose.

Sedatives – Cali poppy, hops, passionflower, valerian.

Adaptogens – ashwagandha, motherwort.

```
CLASSIC ANXIETY FORMULA TINCTURE
Lemon balm      2 parts (eg 100ml)
Pasqueflower    1 part  (eg 50ml)

3-5ml 2-3 x daily in water
```

Fatigue

This is so common. It is true that teenagers need more sleep. In this modern world with blue screens and a lot of sitting around, we aren't stimulating the body in the same way. Each child should be walking every day, running, playing, doing sports – most children in Britain simply do not move enough. With exercise and expression comes fatigue at night time and good sleep (in general). Without good amounts of exercise, restlessness, insomnia, and fatigue can present. This isn't the only cause of course but well worth taking note of for choleric youth.

Stealth pathogens, stress, anxiety, diet, nutrition, muscular conditions, and more can affect a teenager's energy levels. Bodily changes are also going on

In His Wild: my little fire wren held by the earth

with lots of growth, hormonal changes, and transitions into "who we are". Support through group work, nature connection, and the arts is also of great benefit.

If fatigue is due to a chronic condition or underlying pathology, please seek help from a herbalist, or GP for diagnosis, as the root cause needs addressing.

Plant allies

Herbs to help with depletion – adaptogens like ashwagandha, liquorice, or borage.

Herbs to calm and relax – vervain, valerian, chamomile, milk oats.

Herbs to stimulate energy or uplift – ginsengs, lemon balm, orange blossom, ginger, nettle.

Herbs to clear stagnant accumulation – marigold, cleavers, dandelion, burdock, dock, vervain, yarrow.

```
NOURISH TEA

Nettles
Milky oats
Oatstraw
Liquorice
Marigold

Equal parts. Infuse 1-2 tsps of the tea blend for 10
minutes; strain and drink liberally.
```

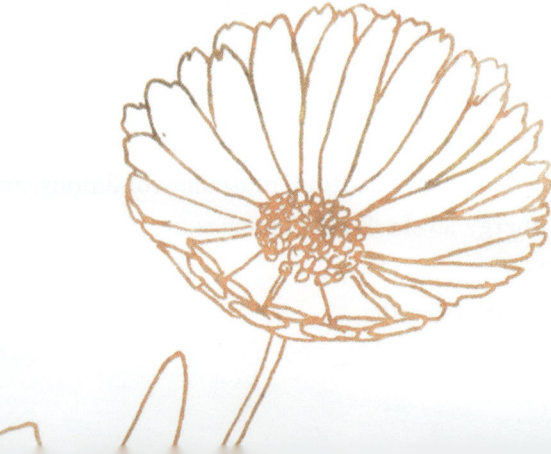

PLANT ALLIES FOR YOUNG FOLKS

In general herbs that work well for the choleric humour include cooling and softening herbs like marshmallow, plantain, and violets. The same goes for foods – soft cooling fruits and lots of water.

Nervines and restorative herbs also really help teenagers along with anti-inflammatories for certain conditions.

Cleavers *Galium aparine*

Nature: phlegmatic

Celestial body: Moon

Cleavers is a cooling and slightly moistening herb which is a prime lymphatic tonic. It will clear toxins through encouraging the lymph and it will clear damp heat that may be stagnant and cause acne or rashes. It is helpful as a spring cleanse with a cold water infusion being made of its aerial parts. Juiced cleavers is also really useful. Juice the aerial parts before it flowers and pour into an ice-cube tray. Freeze this and take out a cube at a time for adding into smoothies. It is easy to store and maintains the fresh cleavers magic. Drying cleavers is OK and teas can be made but it is much more vibrant as a fresh plant infusion, or cold infused dried plant tea, juice, or tincture.

Cleavers can help where there are lumps, like swollen lymph nodes and cysts and heat like acne and eczema. It is an abundant herb in the spring and well worth getting to know. The roasted seeds are good in place of coffee but will stick to anything!

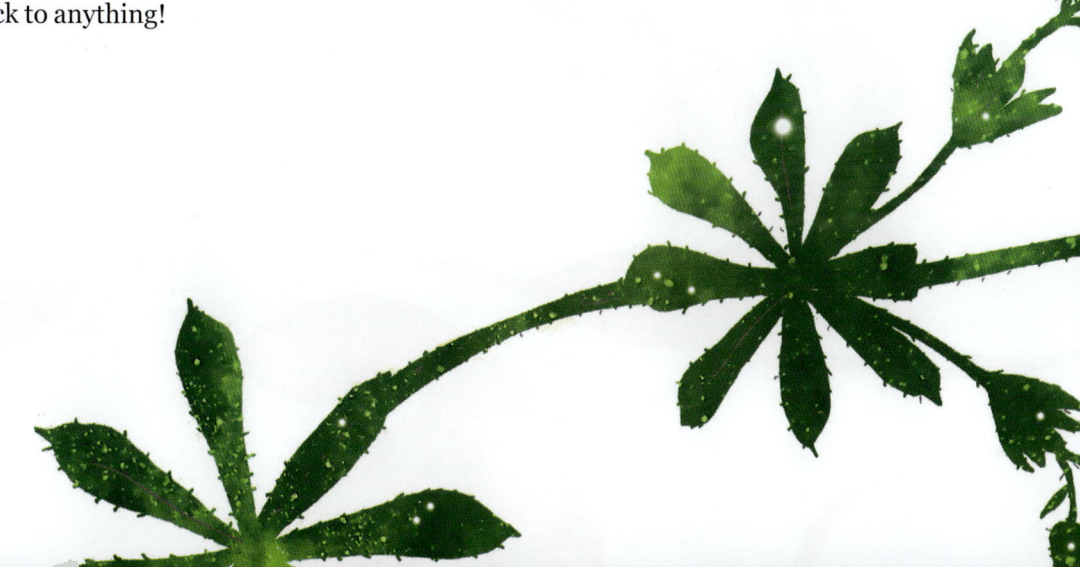

Passionflower *Passiflora incarnata*

Nature: cooling, drying

Planet: Venus

Passionflower is calming, cooling, and drying. It is often used in cases of anxiety and is a fantastic herb for the apothecary to soothe worried minds and bodies. It releases tension from the body, and indeed the head, so headaches from too much studying or worry are eased. Nervous tension or depression from anxiety or agitation are also eased with passionflower. Other nervous signs like palpitations, twitches, and stress are reduced with a tincture or tea of the beautiful *Passiflora incarnata*.

In terms of traditional Chinese medicine, this herb is described as suiting those with a constitution where yang energy surfaces a lot – tension, passion, anger, excitement, etc., all the qualities of choleric youth. This is a calming herb and brilliant for our young adults.

Passionflower is contraindicated in pregnancy.

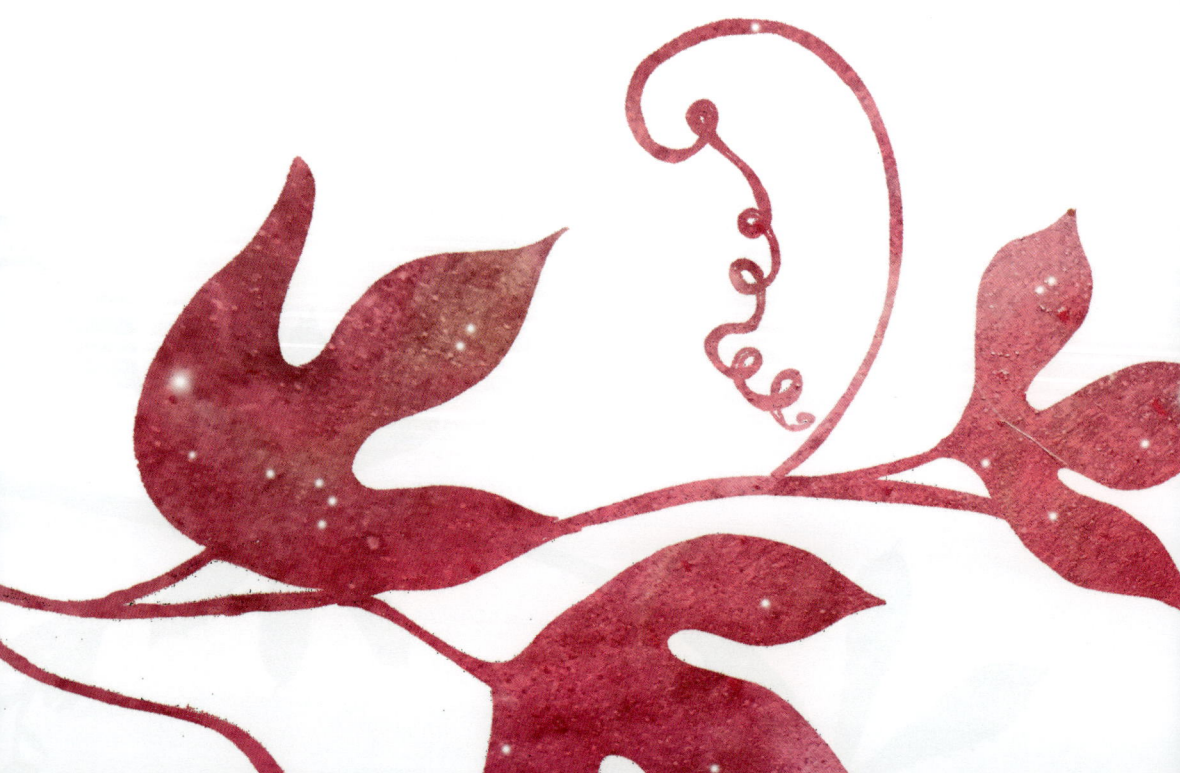

Skullcap *Scutellaria lateriflora*

Nature: cooling

Planet: Saturn

Skullcap is a commonly used nervine in the herbal world. It is easy to grow and does well in the UK climate. It is a nervine first and foremost, calming the body and soothing the mind. It is often given for headaches and head tension and for stresses of all kinds – physical, emotional, and spiritual. It is one of my favourite herbs for insomnia when mixed with valerian, vervain, or wood betony depending on the insomnia of the person.

It is a soothing night remedy for teens, safe, cooling, and slightly drying. It is also a herb which helps with studies as it promotes clear thinking and focus. Often a small dose of skullcap tincture was taken before many an exam in herb school! Just to calm the nerves and focus a bit better. Skullcap relieves agitation and also helps to bring us down to earth; where the excitement of new discoveries in youth might take us to all kinds of adventure, skullcap can keep us a little more grounded. It is a lovely tea with linden and rose for any agitated student or hyperactive teen.

Violets *Viola odorata*

Nature: cooling

Planet: Venus

Violets are moistening and cooling and absolutely gorgeous. If you find them in spring and catch a whiff of their sweetness you are in for a treat. Sweet violets (as opposed to dog violets) are famed throughout the world, as rose is, for their wonderful scent. Violets are generally safe for everyone and are high in rutin which strengthens blood vessels.

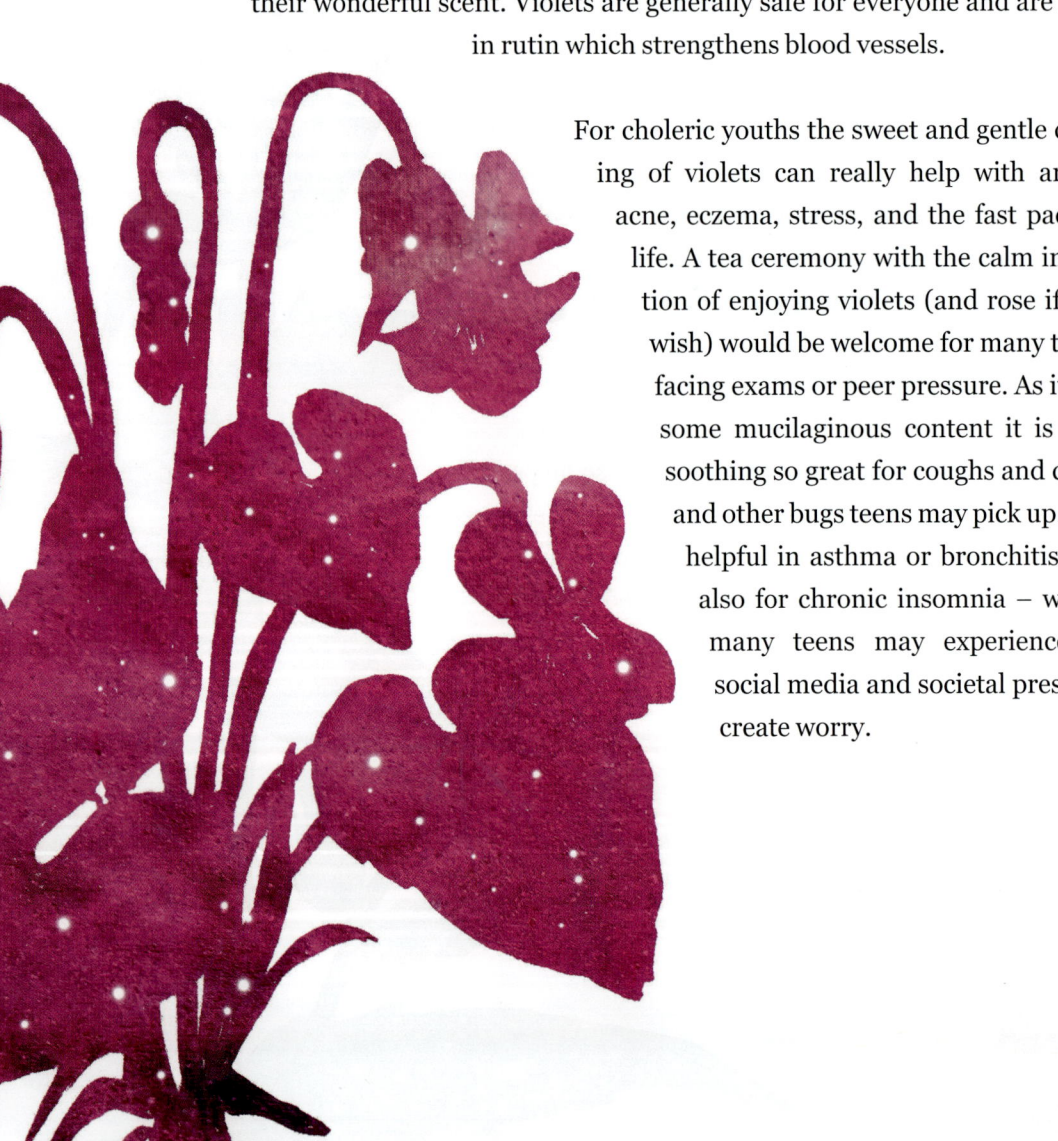

For choleric youths the sweet and gentle cooling of violets can really help with anger, acne, eczema, stress, and the fast pace of life. A tea ceremony with the calm intention of enjoying violets (and rose if you wish) would be welcome for many teens facing exams or peer pressure. As it has some mucilaginous content it is also soothing so great for coughs and colds and other bugs teens may pick up. It is helpful in asthma or bronchitis and also for chronic insomnia – which many teens may experience as social media and societal pressure create worry.

JOURNALING

It would be great to journal about what new adventures life is taking you on, how you perceive your place in them, and how much you value them. In terms of rewilding, think about how your ventures are becoming you and serving the earth and yourself. Try a tea of skullcap to journey into these thoughts and focus on the plant and your journey. Note what comes up and how you feel.

Also choose a cycle you'd like to tune in to – perhaps the moon cycle. Note down if you feel any changes before the full moon, or on the new moon, etc. If you are bleeding, note when you feel the best and see if that correlates to a part of your moon cycle. If you are not bleeding, see if there is a part of the moon cycle that you prefer and tune in to that every month. Cycles are so important in our lives! If you can, design a ceremony that suits you – for example, a gratitude ceremony on the full moon when we can see the world in a different light. Whatever comes up for you, see what happens, experiment, and play.

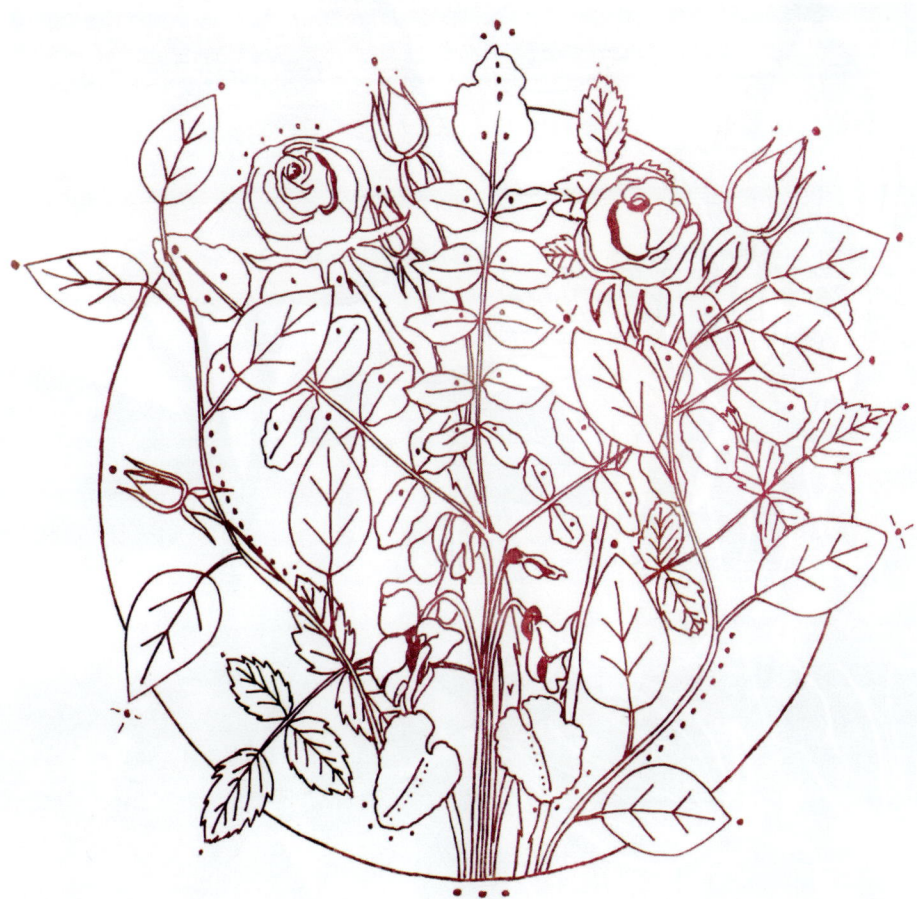

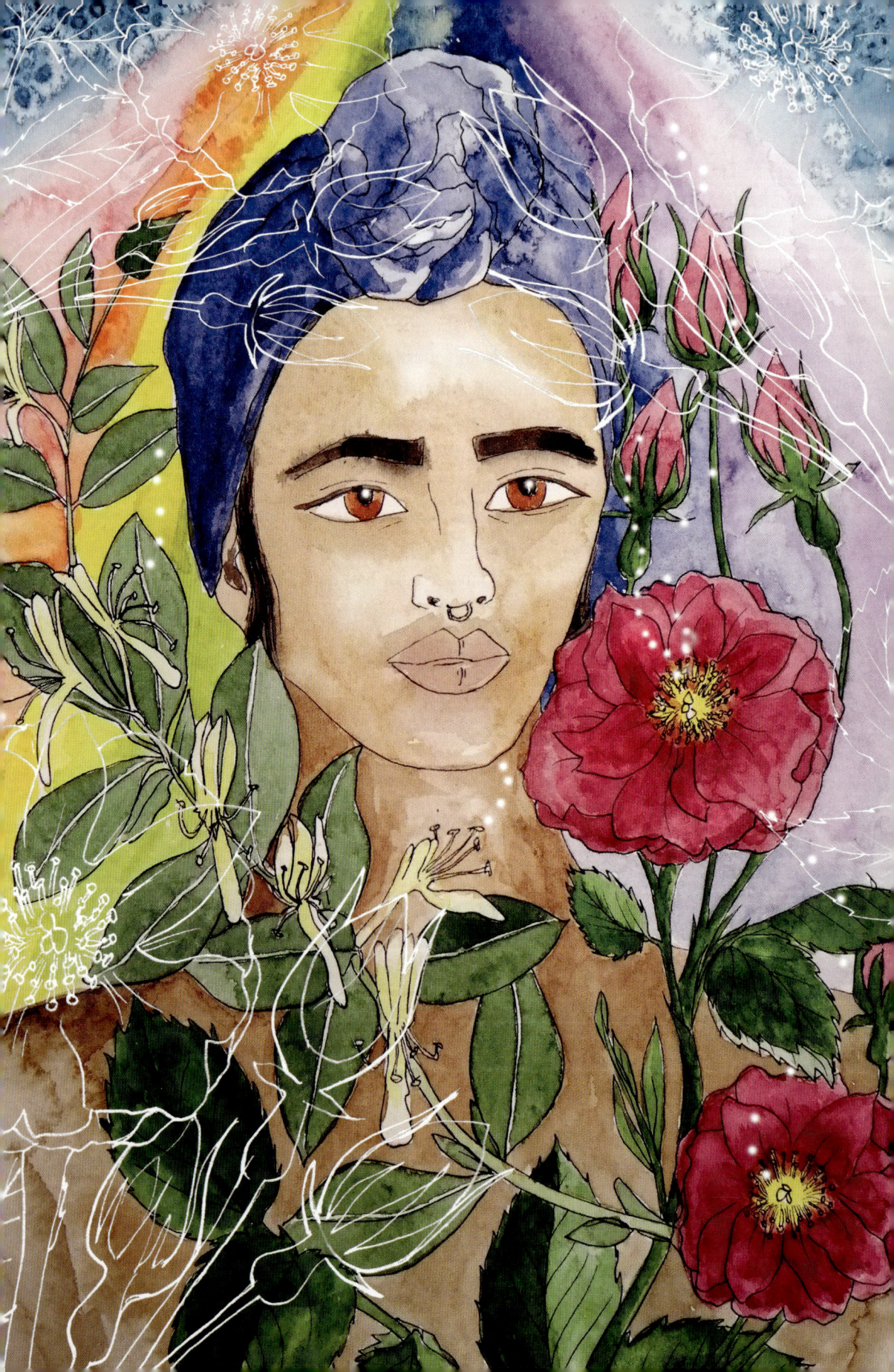

CHAPTER 6

FROM BUD TO BLOOM: TRANSITIONS

Don't you know yet? It is your light that lights the worlds.

Rumi

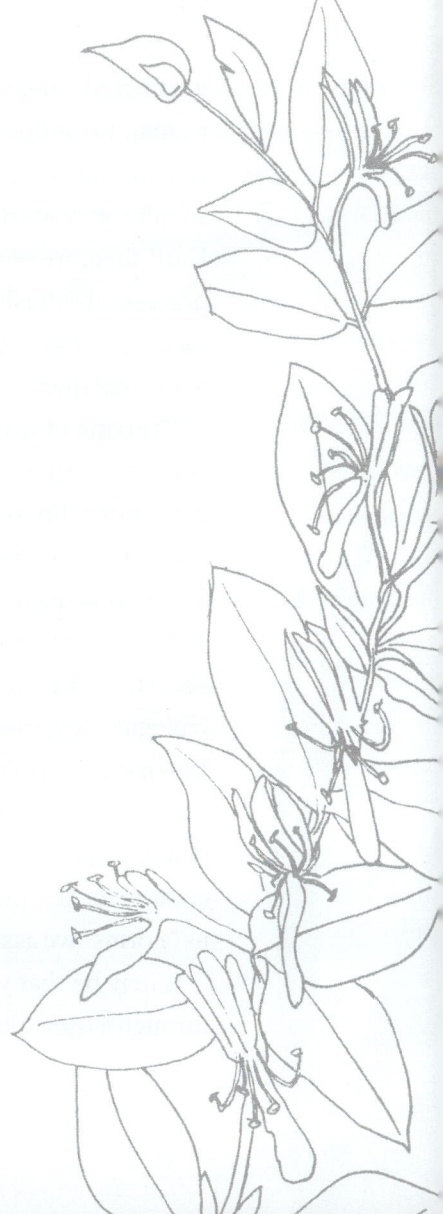

Beauty with roses and honeysuckle

"**B**eauty is in the moment of transition, as if the form were just ready to flow into other forms," said Ralph Waldo Emerson a while back (1800s). And so it is. Beauty, always in flux and transition and making new magic as it evolves, changes, and expresses itself. Beauty is within and without and does not adhere to one path.

Caught in the glass prism, light scatters into rainbows and shows itself to be more than we, perhaps, thought. Just as the light presents itself in multiple ways, folk transition in as many ways as are needed or desired – it is not a linear axis of one to another, each with the same or similar outcomes, it is a transition special to the individual and rooted in the expression of that person only.

Transitions are difficult – from gender to growth (puberty) to decline (moving towards the end of life), from singledom to relationship or vice versa, from woman to mother or grandmother, from husband to widower, the list goes on. As constructs of patriarchal alignment begin to be dismantled, greater joy and wonder may start to flow as we learn different, healthier ways to transition. Until then, we can each find our own resilience, magic, and wild time in the process of smashing (as Claudia says) patriarchy, colonialism, capitalism, racism, and systemic misogyny to rebuild an inclusive non-linear open vision of life together.

Thinking of gender as binary (he/she) is common in mainstream Western culture and there are many countries where expressing anything but cisgender heterosexuality is illegal. However, things are changing. In many cultures the diversity of genderism and sexual identity is, or was, far more fluid, broader, and embracing of difference.

At the time of writing there are over 80 genders reported (as opposed to sixty-three which some of you may be familiar with). Gender is not the same as biological sex, though it is common for folk not to distinguish between the two. Biological sex isn't binary, nor is gender, or transgender which essentially transcends binary confinement. Indeed, even trees, such as the UK's oldest tree – a magnificent yew – changes biological sex. There are many variations on presentation of genitalia. Genderisation is a toxic affair for the most part, teaching us "norms" we assume rather than allowing us to discover ourselves.

It may be that you are identifying with a gender not assigned to you, going through a transition as you identify with a different gender, you are non-binary, or you do not identify with gender at all. You may feel that social constructions of gender binary do not feel appropriate, safe or a reflection of yourself.

When I wanted to educate myself more about supporting trans and non-binary folk, as a herbalist, I didn't find much. I have drawn on my experience of working with people who have anxiety, gut conditions, and skin issues... I work with people.

Trauma often resides in the tissues of anyone who does not identify with their birth assigned gender, or anyone experiencing transition. This trauma may be labelled "gender dysphoria" by the mainstream. Claudia recently described hearing a trans activist state that this person, in fact, had "gender euphoria", which I was delighted to hear. Claudia has been an amazing ally and friend in educating me about colonialism, Eurocentrism, and different ways of life. Having her support reminds me of the help we all need in any stage of life transitions – from (non) gender to grief.

Before the arrival of European settlers, many Indigenous cultures were not confined to a masculine/feminine duality. Europeans brought with them the loss of respect of and safety in Indigenous freedom. Today trans, intersex, and non-binary people, in particular non-binary women of colour, are subject to psychological, physical, economic, institutional, and sexual assault.

Herbs and empathetic herbalists can be a source of support. Herbs support the body through the medical/biological transition gently and energetically, adjusting as the journey evolves. When using herbs, we aren't limiting ourselves just to a reductionist course of hormonal support. Herbal medicines can buffer side effects, promote liver detoxification, hormonal excretion, and emotional support. Our plant allies can become part of the journey of healing and growing.

Emotional or energetic support can be given to all those who feel detached, disengaged, or traumatised by their assigned gender or societal expectations. Support can be given as nervous system nourishment and adaptogenic buffering to ease the stress of chronic pressure, worry, and sadness. More specific hormonal support can be given when a transition is being experienced and herbal support is desired. Using solely herbalism to transition may not bring about the desired effects but may instead support the journey.

ENERGETICS

What are the energetics of transition? Whether young or old, each individual will have a constitutional make-up that is choleric, sanguine, melancholic, or phlegmatic, and most likely a mix of a couple of dominant types. In transition I think it's worth thinking about your constitution and how easy or difficult it may be for you to change.

By this, I'm thinking of melancholy and the earth element. Earth is solid, dry, and cold – so change is a little harder, or slower. Yet earth supports and holds, which is so needed. If you are earthy, you can bring this side of you into your self-care. If you aren't, you might like the support, if possible, of someone who is.

Air and sanguine qualities may allow an easy change but may bring worry and nervousness too, even frequent change as air keeps dispersing seeking equilibrium. If you are airy, or sanguine, you might like to ground yourself just a little with earthy, experiential hands-on actions such as: growing your own medicinal plants, sticking your hands in the earth, being in the forest. Finding teas that ground you and music that supports you.

If you are choleric and are into doing, you might experience rage and frustration, alongside passion and swift action. As you transition, which may be for your whole life, watery practices may balance out and aid you to flow, or become still and find the essence of what you seek. Deep waters are within all of us and accessing them may take a little calm, slow time. Nervine herbs can help here, as can little rituals of the day such as a tea ceremony, plant journey, or meditation.

If you are watery, by this I mean sensitive or easily able to access emotions, and can flow, remain calm, and experience emotion, even feel your way through life, you may find transitioning can be overwhelming when faced with the constructs of patriarchy and its pervasive domination in this society. It may be good to support yourself with grounding, warming aromatics and evening fires.

We don't always think to take herbs when we are "fine". It is often something that comes to us when we are not "fine". Sometimes the battle of trying to be someone others expect and not ourselves (or vice versa) seems so great that a cup of chamomile tea is all we can do when the melancholy threatens to keep us stuck. Other times, the choler can erupt and we stand up and rebuild and make changes and undergo what we need to. Or the water of emotions overwhelms us or gently guides us into flow. Air can keep us light and in transition so we don't get so stuck in one paradigm.

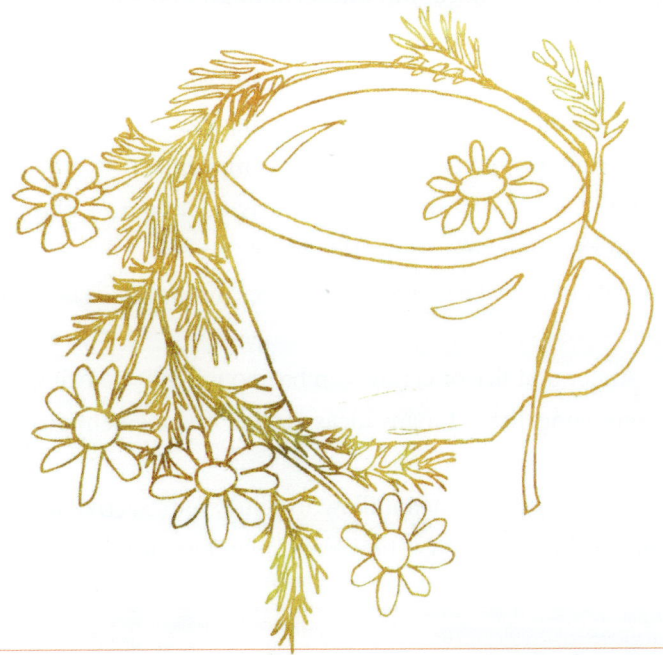

Rewilding exercise – Calling on all the elements

If you are in transition or struggling with the tide of change or rigidity, connecting with all the elements is a beautiful way to find out what resonates for you, what temperaments you might be predominant in, and what you might need to bring about balance.

Take the time to think about what calls you – do you like the ocean, the mountains, the heat? This will already tell you something of what you need and how you might find balance. For example, I always seek out the highest mountains and the sea, and yearn for them. I am mostly fire and earth so it seems natural and right that I look for huge skies and great swathes of ocean. In fact my favourite ocean is a blustery one where sea air fills my lungs.

Outside, somewhere you feel calm, begin to draw upon the elements.

If you start with earth, you need only find soil. Touching the soil or grass or forest floor, etc., and visualising pulling up the earth energy into your body will help you remain grounded; if you prefer, you can visualise your energy moving gently downward into the earth to ground you – different folk will like different visualisations.

Breathing the air into your body can be done anywhere but somewhere fresh and vibrant would be ideal. You can try calling the wind too. This is a lovely exercise and allows you to feel the air on your skin.

When by water – spring, stream, canal, lake, river, or ocean – allow the energy of the water to enter your being. Do you like the cool calm waters or does the profundity of the lake make you feel a certain way? See how each element resonates with you.

For fire, the sun or a lit fire or candle can be enough. As you bring each element into your being, listen for any ideas of what that element provides you or how you react to it.

By bring into your being, I mean allow to enter your sacred space of being – noticing, feeling, thinking – however it manifests for you.

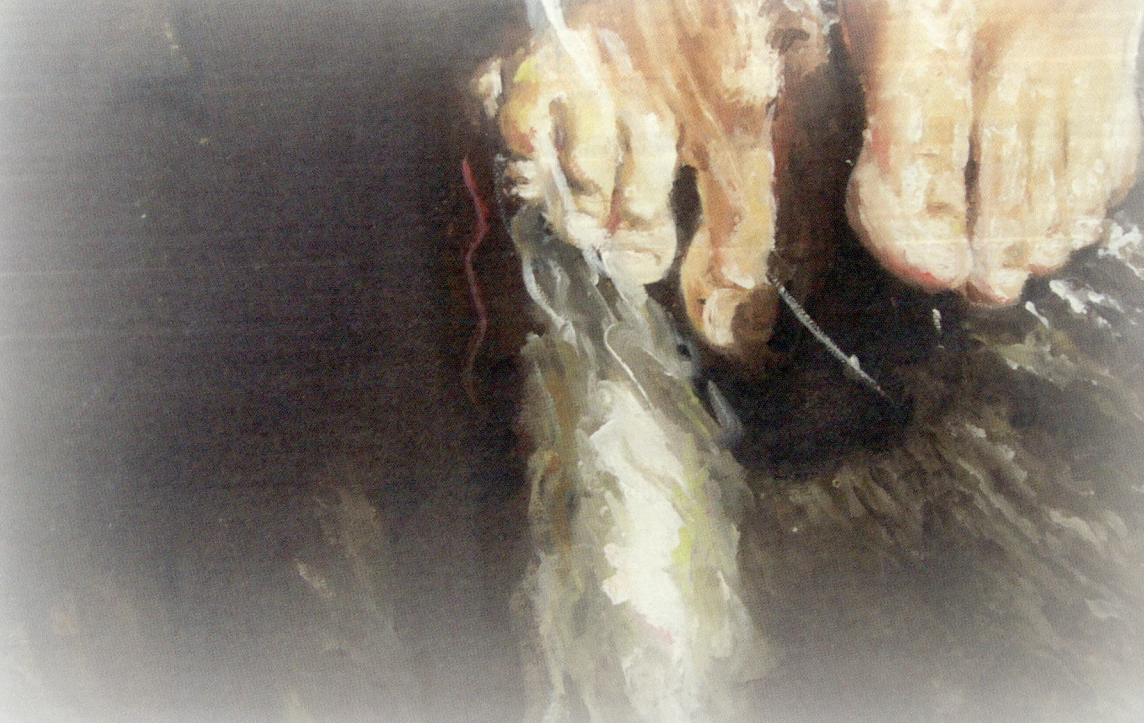

TRANSITIONS AND PLANT ALLIES

Supporting someone in transition requires a holistic approach working with each individual rather than simply looking at hormonal health and profiles. That said it is useful to understand the ways in which herbs can influence hormones and how plant allies may work in the wider context of herbal healing for each person.

Hormones and their effects can be a really big part of any transitioning herbal protocol as one's change in physical appearance can be really important to the individual. A hormonal protocol may be a supportive one or a radical change-making protocol with drugs, herbs, surgery, and more.

Biology has been taught to many of us in the following way: all mammals generally start off as female in the womb. In utero the typical differentiation into male and female occurs at around eight weeks and at twelve weeks a cis female will have all of her eggs that she will release during her lifetime in her tiny womb, which is incredible to think of.

We all have the same hormones in our bodies and they basically act in the same ways but with differing effects following the gamete development and gender distinction in terms of growing reproductive organs. Much as we don't all share the same organ growth, some of us are born with differing chromosomes from what is typically considered when talking about people, that is, XX or XY.

People have varying chromosomal expression such as X, Y, XXY, XXYY, XXX, XXXX, XXXXX, and we also find polysomy or monosomy in fungi, insects, plants, and mammals; it is nothing unusual and yet most of us don't know much about it.

There are some physically male presenting folk with XX and physically female presenting folk with XY chromosomes. Sex determination only really started in the 1940s with testes being attributed to maleness. Now the presence of a Y chromosome is the medical determinant – not whether you have ovaries, breasts, or slender hands.

If we think of the differences in our anatomy, we can easily see that each person is different so it should come as no surprise that we are a people of diversity in all manners.

Common endogenous hormones (name and action):

> Follicle stimulating hormone (FSH) increases oestrogen and sperm production.
>
> Luteinising hormone (LH) increases progesterone and testosterone production.
>
> We all have cholesterol, an essential component of steroid hormones.

Plant allies

Herbs may influence hormonal effect through buffering, potentiation, enhanced detoxification of hormonal excess and recycling. Herbs often support orthodox drugs effecting and maintaining transitional change.

Actions of herbs that may ease or maintain transitional hormone states include the following – note that this is a fairly reductionist synopsis and not necessarily indicative of the whole of plant medicines and their effects on the body, mind, and soul.

> **Steroidal saponins** – these are plant steroid precursors (building blocks).
>
> **Phytoestrogens** – are plant oestrogens that bind to human oestrogen receptors (can contain isoflavones, lignans, and genistein). Some bind weakly and some bind tightly like endogenous oestrogens. Phytoestrogens are not all the same even though they are commonly described as one thing.
>
> **Phytoandrogens** – these bind to testosterone receptors in the body and are androgenic.
>
> **Phytotestosterones** – these molecules are the same as endogenous testosterone and act like it in the body.
>
> **Phytoprogesterones** – these mimic progesterone action in the body and help maintain hormone levels. They may increase breast tissue when applied topically.

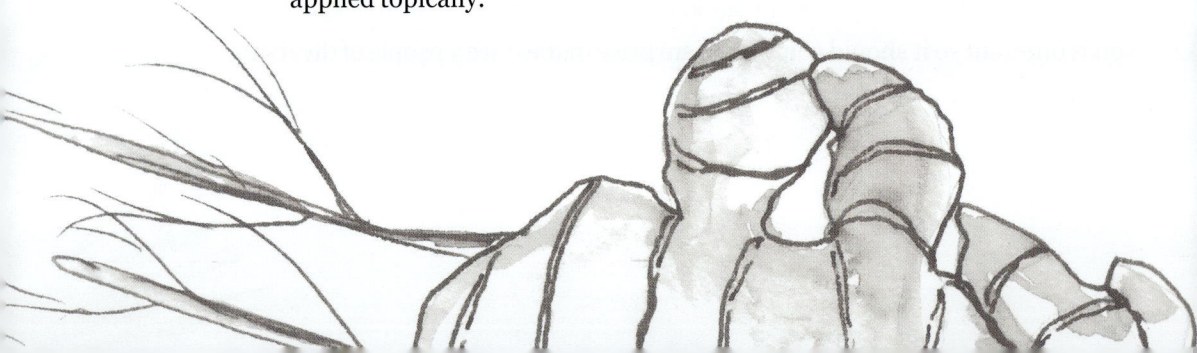

Testosterone production blockers include chasteberry (dose dependent), saw palmetto, and scute root (*Scutellaria baicalensis*). Androgen receptor blockers include spearmint and liquorice. Oestrogen blockers include nettle root and leaf, passionflower. Foods include honey and propolis.

Aromatase inhibitors – aromatase is an enzyme that under normal circumstances converts testosterone into oestrogens; inhibitors allow testosterone to stay in the blood stream and not be converted to oestrogen. These include: selenium (in brazil nuts), melatonin (in pistachios), zinc (shellfish, pulses), grape seed, green tea, citrus flavonones (orange and grapefruit rinds), tomato skins (tomatoes!)

Elimination of oestrogen can be supported with hepatics and lymphatics. Probiotics, fibre, lignans (broccoli), magnesium, fish oil, phytoestrogens, B vitamins, and cruciferous vegetables can help prevent oestrogen dominance. Possible feminising herbs include wild yam, fenugreek, dong quai, red clover, alfalfa, chasteberry, saw palmetto, spearmint, Chinese skullcap, raspberry leaf, nettle, marjoram, fenugreek, fennel, hops, anise, sage and many more phytoestrogens which protect the body from xeno-oestrogens and excess endogenous oestrogen. Phytoestrogens bind with oestrogen receptor sites in the body. They also increase levels of SHBG which binds to free oestrogens, protecting the body from excess oestrogens while decreasing aromatase enzyme which prevents testosterone from turning into oestrogens thereby maintaining more testosterone in the body.

Progesteronic herbs include chasteberry and lady's mantle. Androgenic herbs include sarsaparilla, damiana, ashwagandha, ginseng, oat straw, rosemary, fleeceflower, plantain, cleavers, ginger, star anise, garlic, pine pollen, chasteberry, prickly ash, horny goat weed, Siberian ginseng, astragalus, nettle root. It's important to note that beer, hops, plastics (that we all need to avoid) and xeno-oestroegens are oestrogenic.

Kao krua (Pueraria mirifica), white peony root, and soya oils have been popular in trans communities. NB. there is potential for adverse effects at high doses.

The above is a list of herbs with the potential to affect hormone balance in the body. When we work with people, Herbalists try not to be reductionist – we formulate blends that support each person with gentle nudges to aid what that

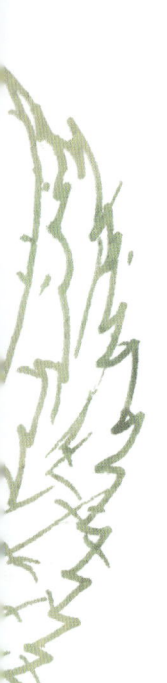

person needs or seeks. I hope this shows how plant medicine may assist each person going through a transition as well as supporting them in so many other ways. Transitions benefit from a holistic approach alongside targeted herbs or drugs. Supporting and tending each person and their many complexities are important.

Other types of plant allies which may help transitions

Adaptogens may be needed because of the constant stress created by the process and the ensuing excess levels of adrenaline and cortisol which suppress androgen production and disrupt endocrine function. The kidneys and adrenals need to be tended as they produce 90% of all testosterone in the body. Gentle kidney tonics include cornsilk, nettle seed, and marshmallow while lovely adaptogens include liquorice, ashwagandha, rose root, or nettle seed.

Nervines may be needed to make sure the nervous system is nourished and the individual is relaxed which then allows the body to get on with everything else it's dealing with. skullcap, oat straw, or passionflower are lovely.

Alteratives cleanse the blood and increase pathways of elimination without decreasing the effectiveness of synthetic hormones. I like nettle, burdock, and possibly red clover depending on what is indicated for the individual.

Hepatics (liver herbs) metabolise testosterone and other steroidal hormones through the liver detox pathways. These include milk thistle, artichoke, and dandelion. Bitters will also help the body when going through any hormonal changes (so also menarche, menopause, puberty, and other states of change). These include milk thistle seeds, dandelion, burdock.

Self-care for those undergoing or maintaining transition may include trying to maintain a good immune system and encourage lymph flow, hydration with electrolytes, and consuming healthy oils which provide cellular building blocks for healthy hormone production. Make sure any injection wound sites are kept clean. Encourage uterine massage and lymph scrubs to keep things from stagnating. Use bitters and aromatics to maintain health in the liver, digestion, and blood. Inspire regular gynaecological check-ups, including blood work for hormone levels.

Testosterone hormonal replacement therapy is more effective than oestradiol HRT. This is because we all share the same embryonic starting point – this can mean the transition from male to female can be more subtle as qualities such as voice tone remain similar even if testosterone is blocked.

Knowing the processes that are involved in transitions helps us find ways to support the individual when we seek herbalism as our path to health. There are also, so importantly, emotional factors that will need support and understanding. There is little information out there but due to the diligence and work of a few contemporary herbalists it is becoming more and more accessible.

```
SELF-LOVE ELIXIR

    Macerate rose petals or whole flowers
        (organic or wild as typical cut roses
         are sprayed heavily) in honey or
         vegan alternative (nothing too
         flavoursome if you want to catch the
         rose scent). Leave for 2 weeks.
    Strain and add the same volume of
brandy, whisky, or vodka. Take drop doses
when in need of a little self-love.
```

```
NOURISHING JUICE, USEFUL FOR TRANSMASCULINE FLOW
AS IT IS POTENTIALLY ANDROGENIC

3 celery stalks
½ cup of organic corn
½ cucumber - remember the goodness is in the green so
don't peel cucs!
½ cups green leaves - including nettles
A few berries of choice for extra antioxidants

Juice together in a masticating (cold press) juicer
and enjoy. If it's really unpalatable for you, add
half an apple.
```

ELEMENTAL ELIXIRS

LISTEN TO THE WATER

Betony flowers
Meadowsweet flowers
Willow flowers
Borage flowers

Pick the flowers of each plant. Some grow by the water and some are full of watery energy for flexibility and flow. Pop a few of each into a bowl of water – think which water you would like or have access to – tap, filtered or spring? Allow to sit in sunshine for 3 hours.

Strain and gift back plants in ceremony to earth or water or have as tea. Add brandy (or vodka) so that your ratio is 1:1 water to brandy (vodka). If you don't want to add alcohol, you can preserve for a few months in cider vinegar. You can also take some drops just as water, so make tiny amounts. You can transition this remedy too – moving through the seasons with little adjustments. When willow flowers are dying back, you could use willow leaves or another plant coming into flower, such as figwort, sea holly, or marshmallow – all of which have an affinity with water.

Bottle – a pipette bottle is good. Take 1–3 drops as needed.

For a little grounding, an earthy tea is good:

> ROOTING TEA
>
> These are all roots but you can blend a formula that feels earthy to you – I particularly like elecampane root and in my mixes I add nettle leaf, marshmallow leaf and flower, and rose as I feel that works for me.
>
> | | |
> |---|---|
> | Liquorice | 1 part |
> | Elecampane | 1 part |
> | Angelica | 1 part |
> | Burdock | 1 part |
> | Dandelion | 1 part |
> | Valerian | ½ part |
>
> 1 tsp per cup of boiled water, infused for 5-10 minutes. Once dried, you can grind the roots or if you prefer (I do), cut them up into small pieces before drying – they dry faster and are easier to store and make into remedies if you have little room.

I give gratitude for the hard work of herbalist and nurse Kara Sigler (the San Francisco Herbalist) who put a lot of effort into researching this area of care and whose work I read and have used as part of the base protocol in terms of transgender herbal possibilities and protocols. See the "Resources" section.

Plant allies for any kind of medical transition should be taken under or alongside the care of a herbalist and specialist if you can. However, if you are transitioning, feeling it out, or have transitioned, there are many herbs you can take to support yourself. Below are a few of the beautiful herbs that may become allies.

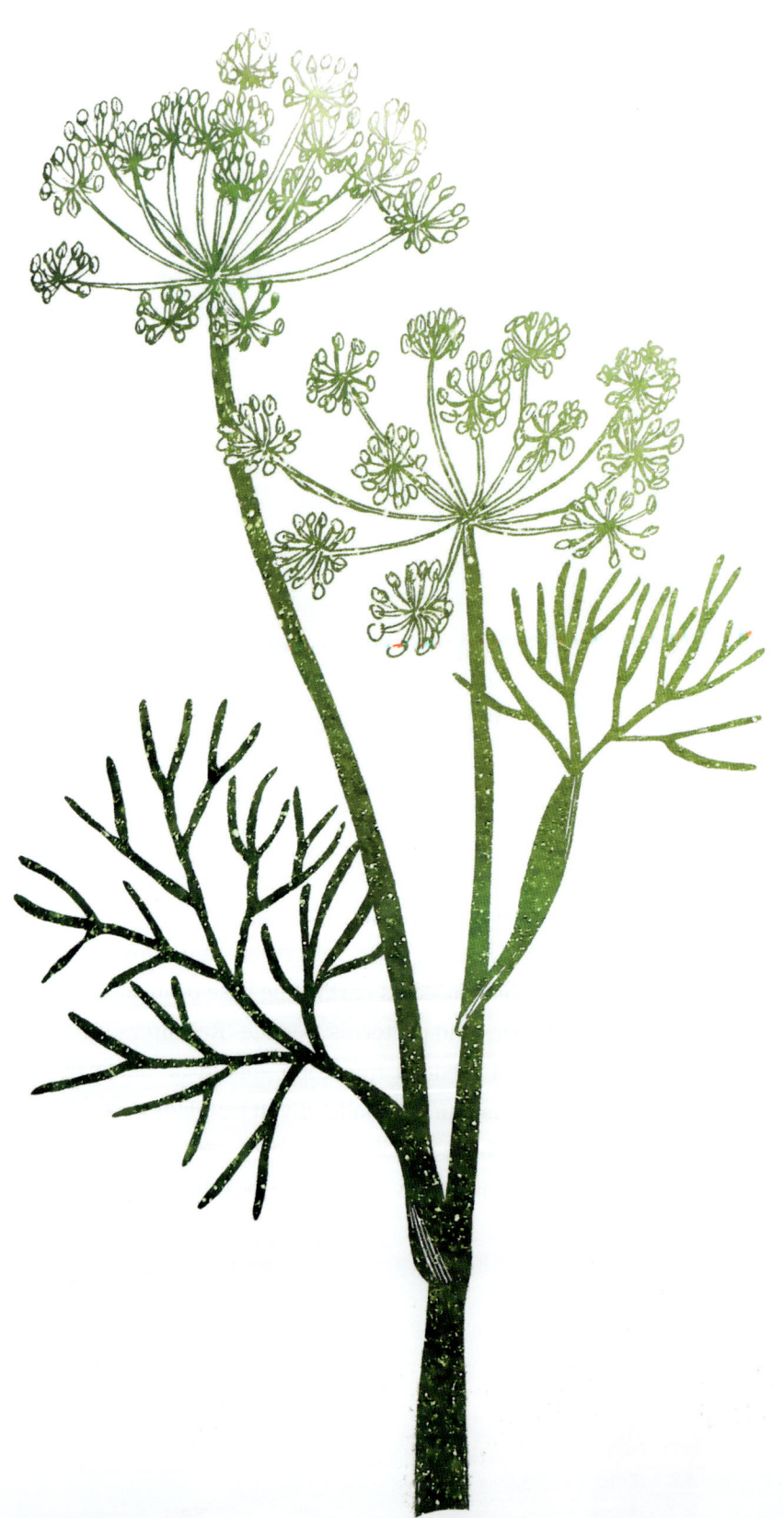

Fennel *Foeniculum vulgare*

Nature: warm and dry

Planet: Mercury

Fennel seed is an uplifting, easy-going ally to have in the cupboards. The seeds also look beautiful in a jar, waiting to be nibbled, made into tea, or added to food for fennel's warming aromatic loveliness. Fennel is so easy to come by, and grow.

It is a refreshing herb that tends to clean the palate and refresh the digestive system. As a carminative, any digestive issues causing bloating may be eased and as a warming aromatic, respiratory conditions may be helped.

Fennel is also very much an endocrine system herb used to regulate the menstrual cycle and support fertility. Both fennel tea and the lovely fennel essential oil (diluted in a carrier oil) have an antispasmodic effect, so that spasm from digestive upset or bronchial constriction can be eased. Painful periods and uterine spasm caused by decreasing oxytocin and prostaglandins are also eased. While taking fennel breast tissue may increase likely due to the oestrogenic volatile oils.

In terms of energetics fennel, as a warming aromatic, is warm and dry. It is harvested in autumn after the heat of the summer and its main constituent is its volatile oil which is brought out by heat.

Fennel is a herb that is nourishing, calming, and soothing. Its gentle uplifting qualities are lovely for those who have been hurt or are in need of gentle self-love or plant ally compassion. It is a great herb to take if you are finding it difficult to be intimate or connect with your own sensuality. For this reason, I think it is beautiful for those in any kind of transition. It is taken in small drop doses as an elixir for those transitioning from female and as teas and tinctures or hydrosols for those transitioning from a man. It is a welcomer of the new.

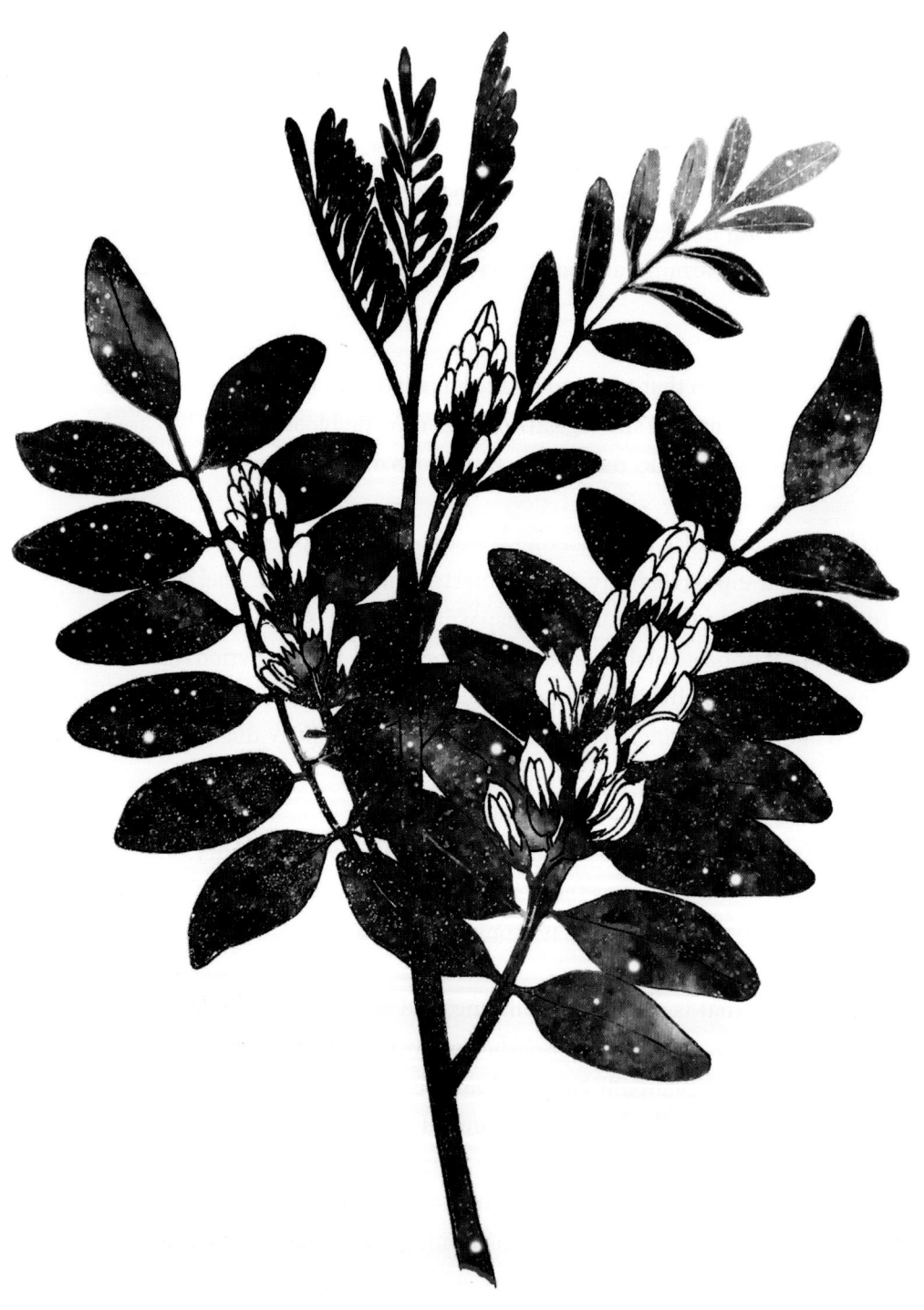

Liquorice *Glycyrrhiza glabra*

Nature: sweet, soothing, moistening, cooling

Planet: Mercury

This herb is so diverse in its use. It has an effect on most systems in the body and is rightly highly prized and known throughout the world. It is a well-used adaptogen and supports the adrenals which will of course be affected in any time of change, transition, trauma, or hormonal imbalance caused by stress.

Liquorice supports the adrenals so that they can work more efficiently and less cortisol is needed by the body; the adrenal support also means that the cortisol to DHEA levels in the body are improved and by maintaining good levels of unbound DHEA, progesterone production is helped, thereby reducing the likelihood or presence of oestrogen dominance. It is used often for PCOS, menstrual irregularities, cystic breast tissue, endometriosis, fertility, and more.

Liquorice is also protective, nourishing, sweet. It is an anti-inflammatory and demulcent and soothes the body. In traditional Chinese medicine it is known as the great "harmoniser", reducing hyperprolactinemia and androgen levels.

Contraindicated for high blood pressure.

Liquorice root is often connected to the base chakra, to the root, to sexuality, and to release fear of change.

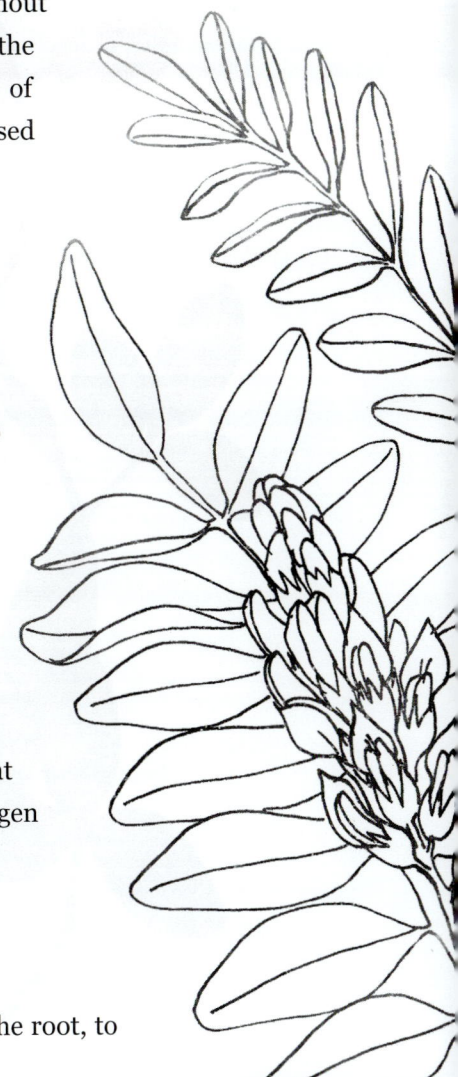

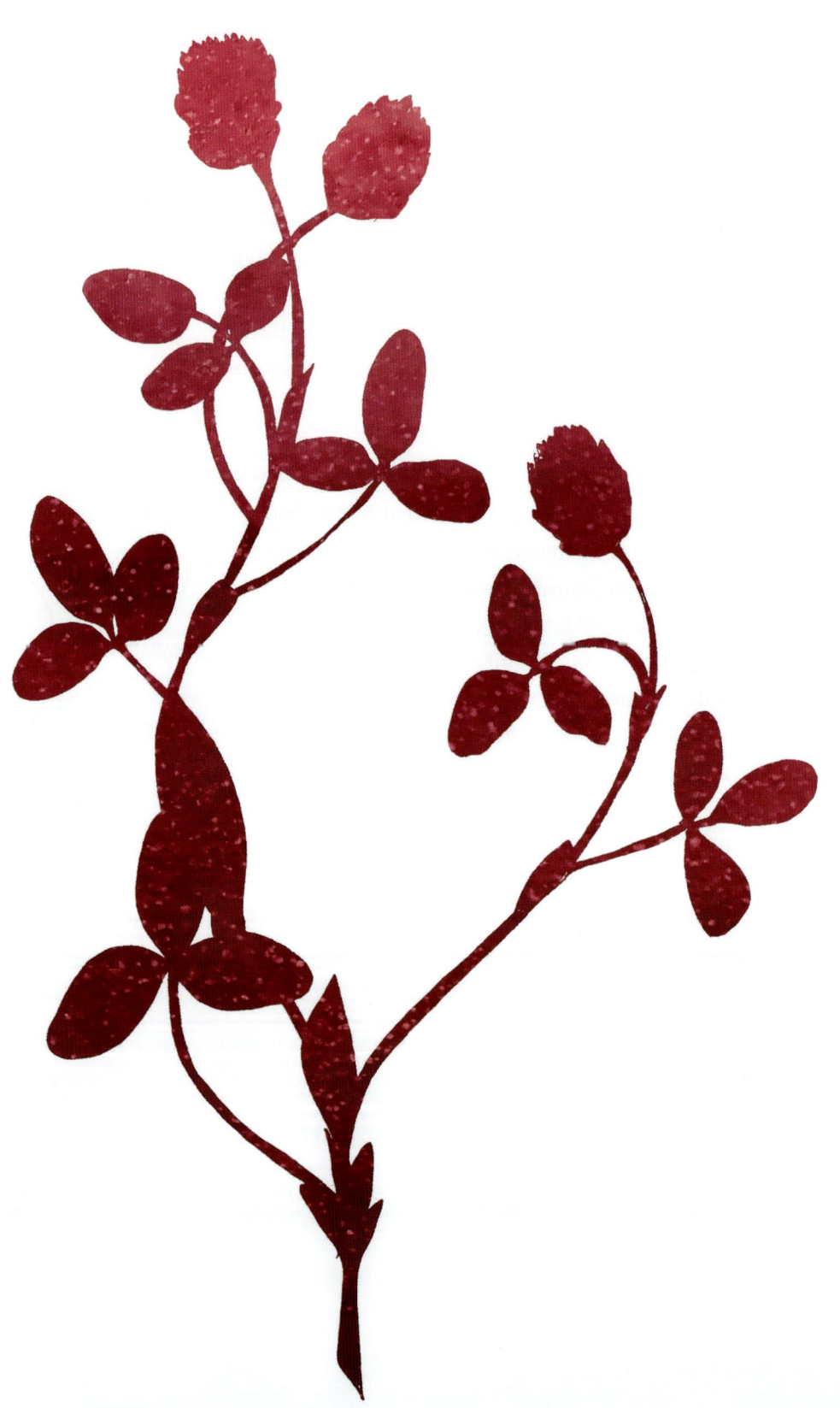

Red Clover *Trifolium pratense*

Nature: sweet, salty, cool

Planet: Mercury

Red clover is an alterative and moves blood around and is well known for its phytoestrogenic properties due to its isoflavone content. This herb is one of the most commonly used by the general public in the Western world.

As an alterative it is useful for stagnant conditions and skin conditions, "cleaning" the blood. It is also incorporated into different blends for people who have a form of cancer.

Red clover has been used in times of menopause as a natural alternative to HRT and is also used for fertility. It is useful in hypercholesterolaemia and hormonal acne or acne due to a lack of vitality. It is used for vaginal dryness and mastitis.

Just as red clover is traditionally used for growths in the body such as tumours and cysts, it is also used for emotional overgrowth where you just can't seem to shift stuck emotions. It is nourishing while allowing a kind of release or opening or letting go to occur. It is also really helpful for vitality when the weight of the world is on your shoulders.

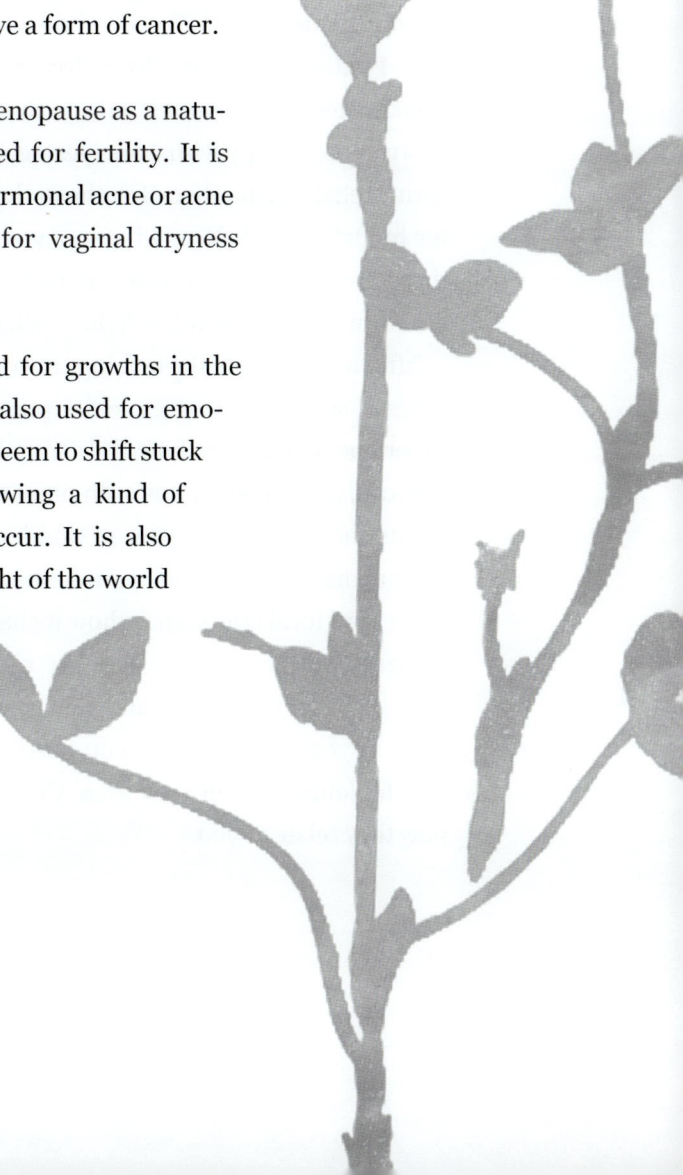

JOURNALING

Transitions, in all their forms, can be hugely stressful. Breathing may be the most important way of feeding the body in times of stress. Even more calming and nourishing may be breathing under a canopy of trees. So for this exercise, try to find a canopy of trees rather than a solitary tree, even if it's just a small copse.

Enter the copse or canopy with an intention to connect; this will most likely bring a sense of calm in itself. You can start the process as soon as you leave your home. You could practise the art of meeting the trees from a distance and then move a little nearer as your perspective changes as described in Chapter 1.

Once you are under the canopy, or branches, find a place to rest. Deeply breathe in the air and fill your whole body with the freshness from the tree canopy. Find a spot to lie down (or make yourself comfortable) and without thinking too much about it, take in the tree canopy with all your senses.

Study the canopy with your eyes, see how the branches and leaves intertwine with or elude each other. Breathe in the scent of forest floor and leaves, or winter branches, or lichen, whatever you find. Listen. Are the birds singing? Is there a wild scuttling or insect noises? What is the biome of the little copse you are within doing? How it is living? What can you feel?

After a while, note these things in your journal and repeat the exercise many times – see what changes, write poetry, songs, words, do drawings of your experiences, and note how the canopy changes and how that makes you feel. You can, of course, do this with more than the canopy. You can do it with any plants and little microcosms of wonder. Choose what you are drawn to. Journaling about the places near your home is a great exercise because you will get to know your local landscape – how it changes and what it needs.

Plants will grow where they are needed. Thorny, stingy, or painful plants may grow over areas of land that need protecting. Fruit or medicinals may grow in your area because you need them. Take a look around and find out which plants grow in your area. Create a journal of local medicinals and see how they relate to you.

Passionflower – a perfect flower

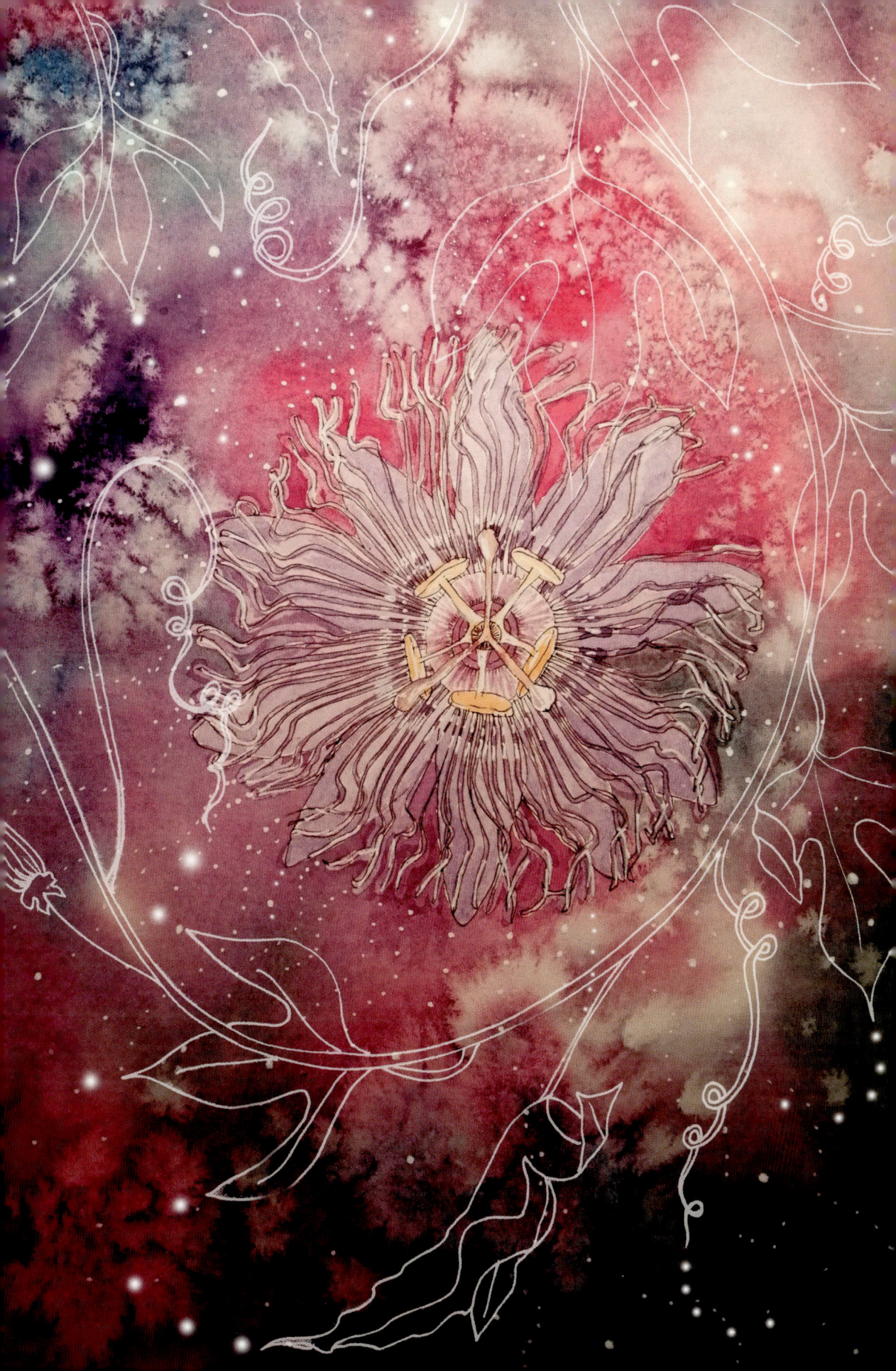

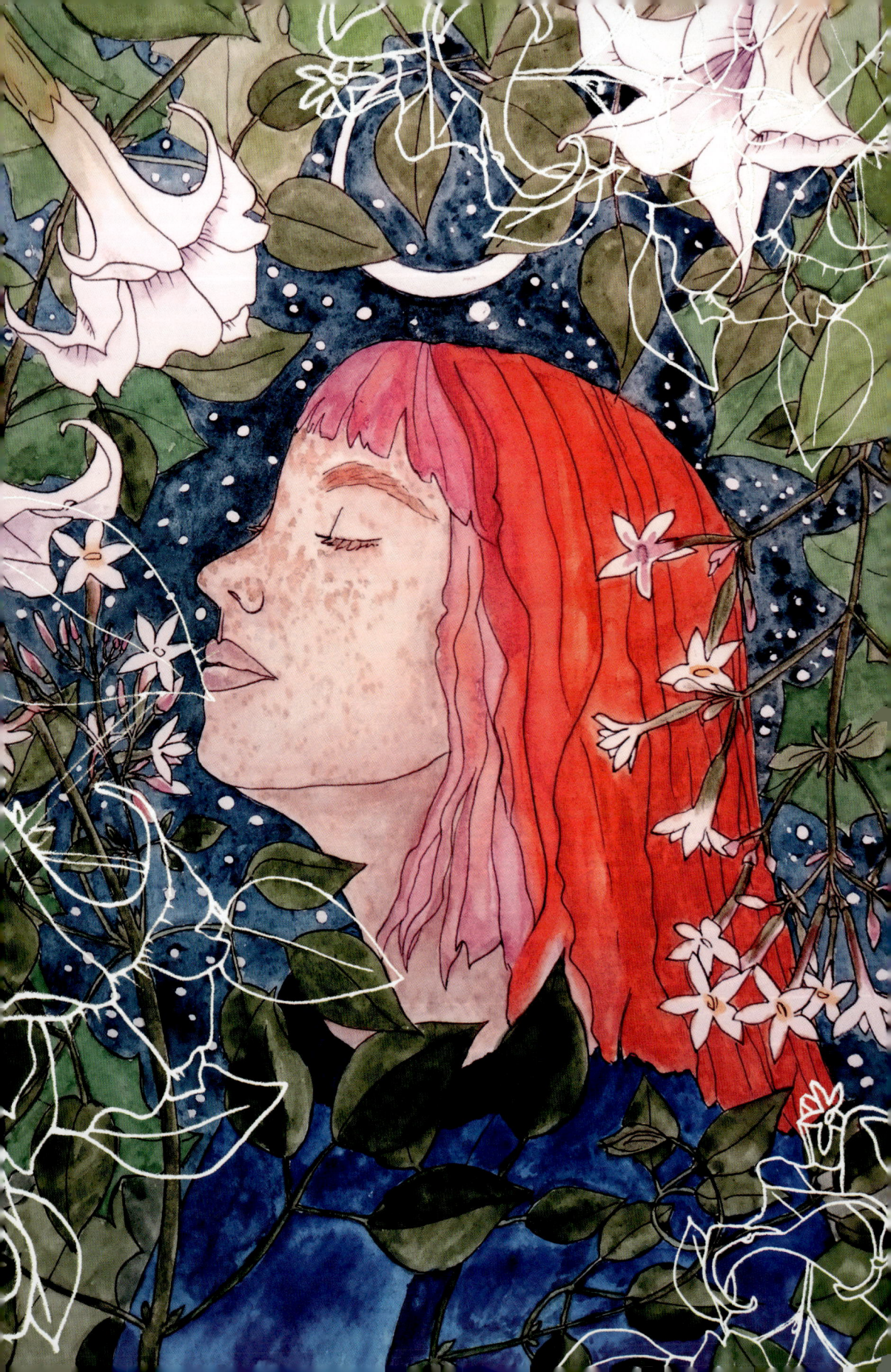

CHAPTER 7

BLOSSOM: WOMEN

Woman
Women
Wombyn
Womyn
Womxn
Wemoon
We Moon
Witch Moon

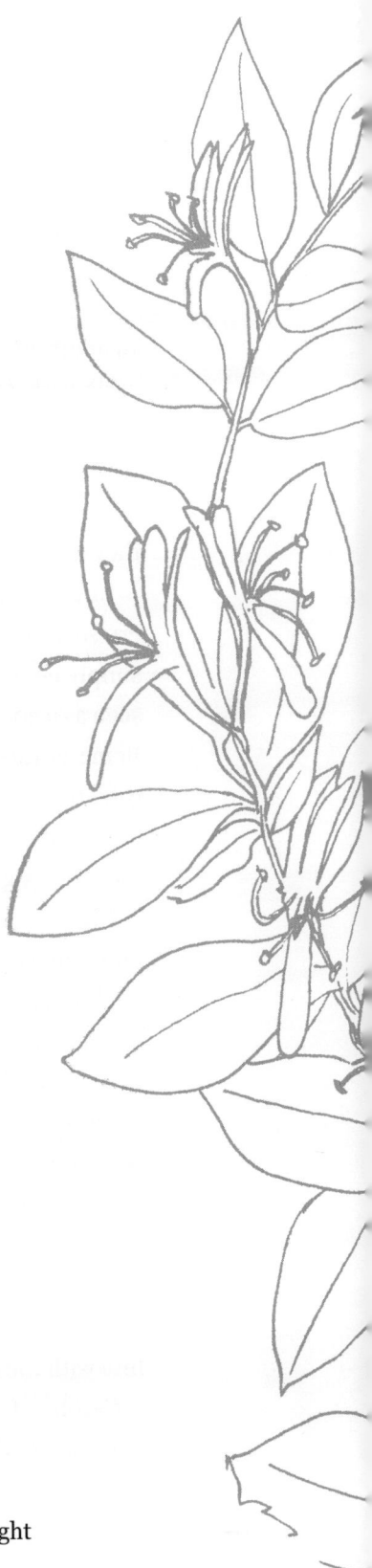

Womxn with jasmin and thorn apple in the dark of the night and the light of the moon

In this chapter we will concentrate on women and wild medicines. Having looked at menarche and menstrual conditions in youth – we will look at fertility and women's gynaecological conditions along with menopause and the journey into cronehood.

ENERGETICS AND ELEMENTS

In adult life, the melancholic humour begins to dominate. It is the humour of earth with its cold and dry qualities. It is aligned with autumn and the calming of the high summer fire energy (choler). When I think of autumn, I think of trees, changing but standing tall, pushing the energy into their fruit and finally letting go in preparation for a winter slumber, safe in the sacred knowledge they will replenish their roots and push forward again come spring.

Interestingly this humour is the one that is least regarded in modern Western society; it is the one that simply is, that allows or requires the individual to simply be. In modern society, thinking is key, a sanguine trait. Doing things is seen as a good thing, a choleric trait. Being is undervalued, a melancholic trait. Being is rather misunderstood yet so deeply needed in a time of industrial catastrophe as the human tries to further tech and the earth suffers. Our dominant system of patriarchy does not value melancholy and has aligned it with the most stigmatised of health conditions – depression and mental illness.

Direct work with the earth requires a balance of humours (thinking, doing, and being) but is dominant in the melancholic humour, as are respecting healthy earth traditions and quiet introversion and reflection which lead to action once more. Melancholic work is a quiet but deep affair to be valued with integrity and wonder.

Autumn is not as valued as spring and summer by many folk, and similarly, as the energy shifts towards the earth temperament, women may recognise a melancholic affinity as the dominant system of our time (patriarchy) is built around men and values the male energies of thinking and doing, despite endless calls for equality. In writing that "Representation of the world, like the world itself, is the work of men; they describe it from their own point of view, which they confuse with the absolute truth," Simone de Beauvoir speaks the truth.

Caroline Criado Perez in her book *Invisible Women* says, "the lives of men have been taken to represent those of humans overall. When it comes to the lives of the other half of humanity, there is often nothing but silence. And these silences are everywhere because when we say human, on the whole, we mean man."

Women in particular have to deal with more adversity while being ignored, just like the beautiful melancholic temperament. Sadness and stubbornness are traits of the earth temperament and yet a deep reverence for our land and an empathy that extends beyond is also intrinsic in earthy folk.

Earth is cold, and in traditional Chinese medicine is also aligned to the yin characteristics which are female, receptive, dark, and deep. Yin elements are the water and moon (fertile, cycles, emotion, imagination as traits).

The shift into adulthood for a woman may bring children and practicality or knowledge, gentle wisdom and understanding, or a solidity, a finding of oneself that leads to empowerment. Menopause can be a hard and long transition too, from the fertile (for many) days of womanhood to becoming a crone. All this is a journey through life in the melancholic stage of the journey but also growing towards eldership and crone wisdom.

Rewilding exercises

Nourishing exercises for times of melancholy (not depression) include allowing time to simply be outside. Taking time is important. Allow a while outside and simply find somewhere comfortable – sitting, lying, standing, resting against a tree, it doesn't matter too much where you rest. The key is to simply be there. Be present, gently aware of what is around you and attuned to "being" within and without. This may take some practice. The art of not thinking is simple. And so difficult. Concentrating on your breathing or a tree, water flow or natural beauty (rock, stick, flower, etc.) may help. If your thoughts do flow, let them come back to you, to your breath and to the object of gentle focus.

Repeat daily.

You may also like to bring a little doing to this task. Not much, mind! Gently place your hands or feet on the earth, preferably soil, forest floor, field, meadow, rock, sand, rather than concrete or man-made grounds. As you breathe in, visualise the healing energy of the earth entering you – you might choose rooted nourishment or seedling potential. As you breathe out allow what does not serve you to be absorbed by the earth and composted. Grief, anger, resentment, scattered thoughts, worries, guilt . . . any of these may be composted if needed. Sometimes we need to be processing these emotions – and other times it's better to let go. I think of the lyrics written and sung by Aurora Aksnes: "When, when I am down, I lay my hands upon this ground."

Then I put my hands in the ground too. And. Just. Be.

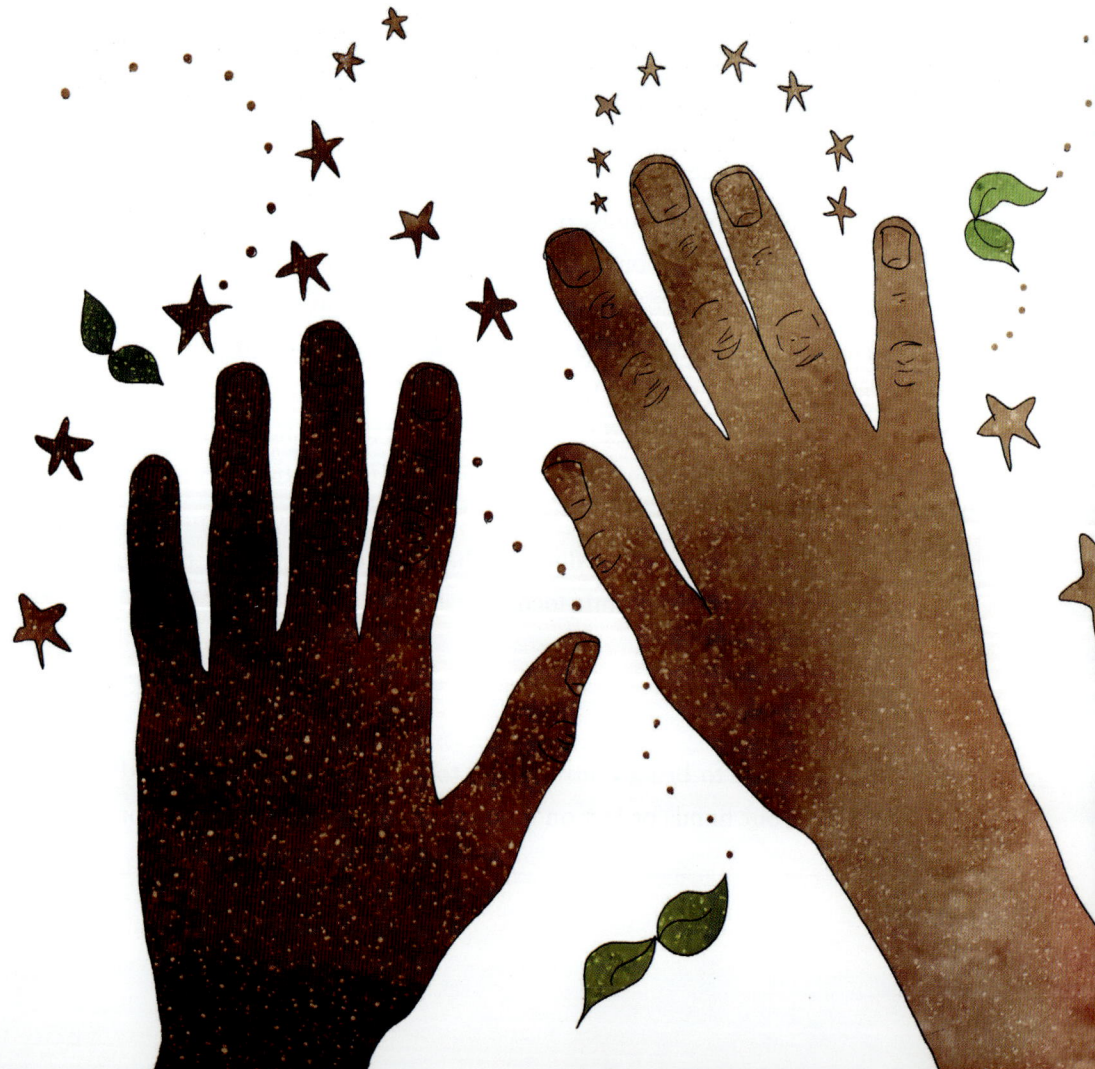

CONDITIONS

Let's look at common conditions including fertility, pregnancy and related conditions, gynaecology and menopause. We will look at fertility and gynaecological conditions, and gynaecological complaints.

FERTILITY

Women come to clinic, my clinic at least, way more frequently than men and often present with gynaecological conditions. Often these conditions are entwined with other things going on for that woman – emotional issues, complexities or losses, different bodily illnesses that ebb and flow through menstruation and menopause, anxiety, social stigmas . . . all sorts. A woman's worth was once judged on her ability to conceive and that notion hasn't left our collective consciousness.

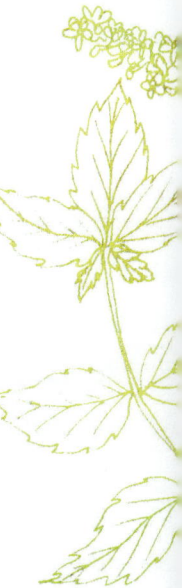

Some women hold deep trauma around not having children. Some around having children. As our communities have been deconstructed and dispersed and the capitalist fantasy in which success is measured by monetary gain and materialism reigns, so our understanding of care has waned. Care is something we all need and yet many miss receiving and giving it.

Of course this doesn't pertain only to women and fertility but it has had so much impact on women and how women value or perceive themselves. In terms of fertility, the emotional context is huge. There is a lot of work being done by many women in different cultures to redress the suppression and conditioning women have faced for too long.

As children, some girls will be conditioned to think in certain ways, simply because they are girls and society has decided that pink headbands on bald babies are appropriate (see Hannah Gadsby's filmed performance of Nanette). Obviously it's deeper than that but the path of what is expected of you as an individual has already been set in some ways.

While life expectancies are affected by system oppression, a woman's life expectancy in general is longer now than ever before. Even so, due to all the change over the last century in terms of lifestyle, food, work, and stress, let alone prolonged oestrogen exposure, radiation, and carbon emissions, women are presenting with more fertility issues and gynaecological conditions than ever before.

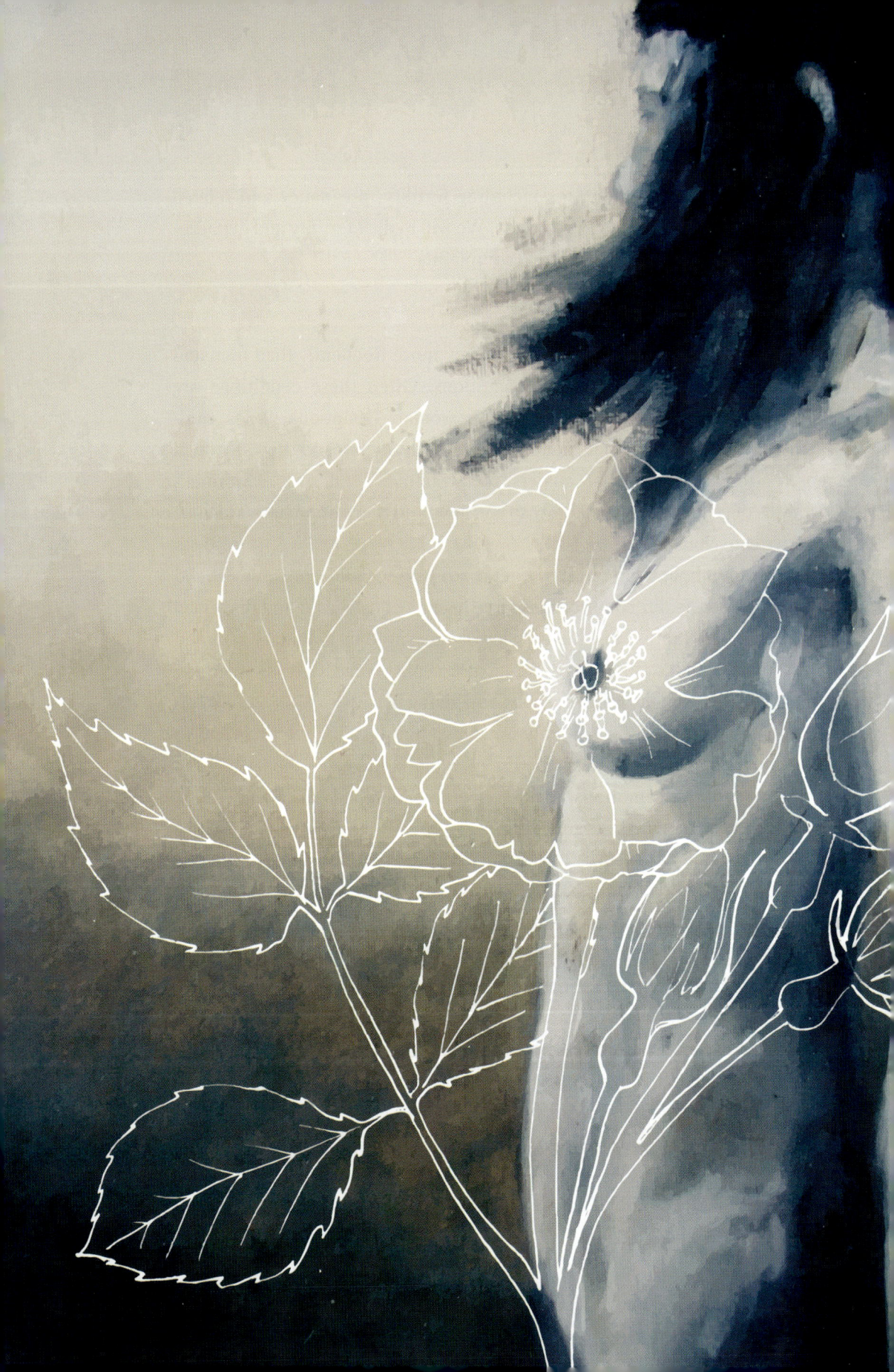

> "I am a woman
> I am an infertile woman
> I do not know anyone else who has gone through this,
> So my truth sits hidden in the folds of my tongue."
>
> By Kat François in Fertile

So many people are struggling with fertility and conception at the moment. If a couple tries to conceive and doesn't manage it within twelve months of unprotected sex, "infertility" is diagnosed. This word alone carries implications of "failure" and "barrenness", an "inability".

Either partner and sometimes both partners may be facing fertility challenges, further investigations can be done to figure out the underlying causes or influences of being unable to conceive. There are many reasons for not conceiving; in fact the list is so long with many conditions having a potential effect on our fertility from autoimmune conditions to gynaecological conditions to hormone imbalance or liver conditions. Tests to check ovulation and hormones are common and it is worth finding out if there are any known causes contributing to lack of conception or difficulty carrying full-term. Knowing your body, as a woman, and its fertile cycle (signs of ovulation including temperature and discharge, etc.) is very, very worthwhile.

Consideration of underlying physical, emotional, mental, or spiritual blocks must be made as there are so many issues which we subconsciously, or otherwise, enact or suppress. These might include grief, shock, pain, worry, fear. All or any of these may hinder conception.

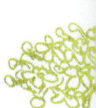

If there are issues with ovarian function or cervical mucus, there is usually a hormonal element needing balancing. If a woman is experiencing no periods because she has been on the contraceptive pill, for example, there are herbs to encourage the regulation of normal cycles, such as chasteberry.

If there is no known reason for not being able to conceive then a general cleanse/detox may be indicated and some tonifying or nourishing. Adaptogens and tonics may help here.

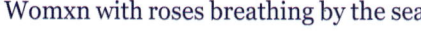

Womxn with roses breathing by the sea

Plant allies

Hormone regulation/fertility tonic – dong quai, shatavari, peony, saw palmetto, raspberry leaf.

Immune support – echinacea, thyme, liquorice, albizia.

Anti-inflammatory – liquorice, marigold, nettle.

Liver support – schisandra, milk thistle, dandelion, vervain.

Stress relief – schisandra, dong quai, vervain, oats, lemon balm, betony, rose, skullcap, ashwagandha.

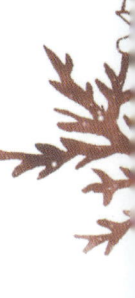
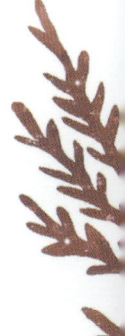

Raspberry leaf is a lovely herb, it is gentle yet effective, strengthening and toning, and has a relaxing effect on the pelvic muscles. As a partus-preparatory herb it is commonly used in the last trimester to prepare for birth but may be used at other times – see your herbalist.

Tea of raspberry leaf is delightful combined with nettle and rose – this is my Wild Woman tea blend and is useful at any time of life but I particularly like it for nourishing folk in deficient states.

Lady's mantle is a uterine and vascular tonic with a hormone balancing action and progesteronic effect which promotes fertility. Tea or tincture is good.

Black haw and crampbark both act as pelvic antispasmodics and help the uterine muscle to relax and promote uterine and ovarian circulation, thereby helping to keep the womb nourished. These herbs can also help strengthen the uterus after miscarriage in preparation for future conception.

Dong quai is a wonderful female reproductive tonic, increasing vitality and blood flow, thereby nourishing tissues and reducing any stagnation. It is contraindicated in those who have a history of spontaneous miscarriage.

Shatavari is an Ayurvedic nutritive tonic for the reproductive system in general. It is excellent in promoting a sense of well-being and connection to oneself in terms of sexuality. It is adaptogenic and regulates menses. Excellent for stress or immune-induced fertility difficulties.

Chasteberry increases progesterone and luteinising hormone while nourishing the corpus luteum. It is very helpful for women who are prone to miscarriage due to low progesterone.

Note: if taken to promote fertility, chasteberry must also be taken in the first trimester and then reduced slowly to avoid a drop in progesterone which could result in miscarriage – consult a herbalist for support here.

Saw palmetto can be great for nourishing the uterine cavity – it nourishes the uterine cavity and assists reproductive activity. It is warming and gently stimulating and can aid libido while reducing inflammation around the ovaries.

Rosemary or yarrow can be used to increase circulation to the pelvis, increasing uterine blood flow and decreasing stagnation. Marigold can also be used to lessen pelvic congestion and is of course an anti-inflammatory.

Fertility issues due to loss of libido can also be quite emotionally stressful for many people. Damiana is an aphrodisiac, sexual stimulant, antidepressant and also promotes well-being – so really great to take at such times.

Example blends:

```
FERTILITEA

Lady's Mantle           2 parts
Raspberry leaf          2 parts
Nettle                  2 parts
Mugwort                 1 part
Rose                    1 part
```

Infuse 1-2 tsps for 5-10 minutes, strain and enjoy.

Drink this blend every day – especially on the full moon which holds such energy and wonder, lighting the night with potency.

Good food, nourishment, and a good night's sleep are essential for both parties when trying to conceive.

The yoga pose, "The Cobbler's pose", or Supta Baddha Konasana is lovely to open the pelvis and decongest the area. Claudia reminded me of this and I remembered I often call the lying down version "the goddess pose" as it feels very opening and often vulnerable, but so well supported by the earth and if one can relax (support with pillows or cushions as needed) I find it feels very connective with spirit all around. There is also a menstruation sequence by Gita Iyengar, which is a great resource freely available online.

PREGNANCY

Herbal safety in pregnancy is important and talking with a herbalist may ease any worry if you have access to one or can find one. Bloom tea is a lovely blend of herbs that are safe in pregnancy. It is calming and tonifying and delicious.

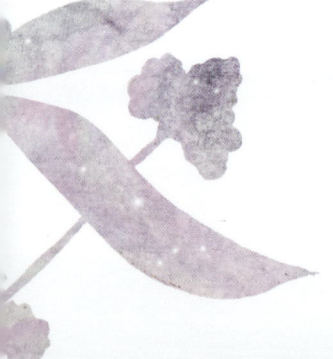
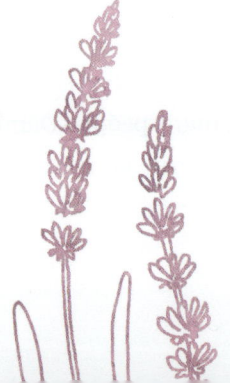

```
BLOOM TEA
Linden              1 part
Chamomile           1 part
Lemon balm          1 part
Spearmint           ½ part
Lavender            ¼ part

Infuse 1-2 tsps for 5-10 minutes, strain and enjoy.

Drink to ease nerves and relax.
```

It's important to note that racial disparities affect pregnancy outcomes. Dying in childbirth is five times more likely for a Black woman than for a White woman.

As a general rule, we avoid herbal medicine in the first trimester of pregnancy unless indicated or very gentle such as chamomile or ginger tea with honey. Tinctures and high doses are not recommended.

CONDITIONS AFFECTING A WOMAN IN PREGNANCY

Nausea and hyperemesis gravidarum

If you are experiencing morning sickness, there are lots of things you can do. It can be very mild to severe and even debilitating, when it is known as hyperemesis gravidarum – basically serious throwing up.

The feelings of nausea and any accompanying vomiting usually pass after eighteen weeks into the pregnancy, but not always. It can mean a woman misses work a lot during that time so the socio-economic aspect is serious for something that is passed off as merely transient and inconsequential a lot of the time.

Morning sickness describes a pattern of waking and feeling nauseous – this is often to do with blood sugar levels but it isn't confined to that time of day by any means. Hormonal changes can affect the digestive system too, so women with pre-existing digestive issues like GORD are more susceptible to vomiting or hyperemesis.

Avoid any triggers such as low blood sugar, certain smells and foods, and try

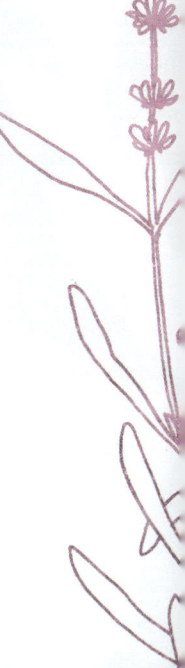

to lessen phlegm at the back of your throat (cut out dairy if this exacerbates it). Drink plenty of water or herbal teas and keep hydrated and try eating small regular meals so that your blood sugar doesn't drop too much.

Plant allies

Ginger tea, or ginger tincture in drop dose diluted in water, can be really helpful. Some herbalists make ginger candies for the woman to chew if she is lacking energy and experiencing nausea.

Dried ginger has more shogaols than fresh (which has more gingerols), and is therefore more anti-emetic. Some people make ginger biscuits, for example, with the dried ginger as powder which can be really useful.

Peppermint and ginger are also great herbs for any heartburn felt in pregnancy and they make a tasty tea with a bit of pep should you be tired.

Bitters such as chamomile and dandelion can be useful too, and taken as tea or in drop dose.

Anaemia in pregnancy

Anaemia (low iron levels) is fairly common in pregnancy and as iron is an essential mineral for the body, it is vital that the pregnant woman has enough. In addition to an iron liquid supplement such as Floradix, there are a few herbs which are very helpful in anaemic women.

Plant allies

Nettle is so nourishing and it is the primary iron source from herbs for many herbalists, but it also combines well with other iron-rich herbs like alfalfa, dong quai, and peony; the latter two enrich the blood in traditional Chinese medicine.

The roots of yellow dock and dandelion can be made into a lovely iron tonic which is safe in pregnancy and also contains molasses (also high in iron) as its syrupy base. Infusions of the roots are easily prepared and drunk during pregnancy, and they can be flavoured with mints or ginger, etc. depending on what the person likes.

```
IRON-RICH RECIPE, DANDELION AND DOCK ROOT
IRON SYRUP

Chop 50g of both herbs

Decoct the roots in 8 cups of simmering water

Reduce the water until around 1 cup is left (do not
use a lid)

Strain and add ½ cup of molasses and mix well

Bottle, label, and keep refrigerated for up to 2 weeks
while taking 1-2 tablespoons once or twice daily.
```

Varicose veins in pregnancy

As a younger woman, you may never have seen a varicose vein before but they are very common in pregnancy, especially for melancholic and phlegmatic types and those whose circulation is a little sluggish. They may appear as haemorrhoids in the rectum and as distended veins in the groin or legs and be uncomfortable or painful or may simply be visible with no discomfort.

It is thought that oestrogenic and progesteronic receptors of the saphenous veins may be the reason why veins succumb to varicosing in pregnancy. Treatment is similar to non-gestational varicose veins with topical applications of horse chestnut and infusions of gentle astringents.

Plant allies

Topical applications for varicose veins in pregnancy include:

>   Arnica cream
>   Horse chestnut infused oil or cream
>   Witch hazel water – I often add this to a cream blend
>   Oak bark powder (finely powdered) in a cream
>   Yarrow tea or tincture applied externally
>   Yarrow essential oil can be added to creams

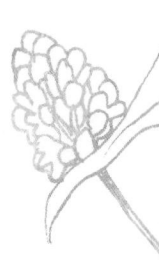

Nettle and bilberry tea

Rutin is a good supplement to take but can be found naturally in apricots, buckwheat, cherries, and grapes amongst other foods

There are many other serious conditions affecting pregnant women, including gestational diabetes, pre-eclampsia, ectopic pregnancies, breech presentation, herpes virus, pruritic urticarial papules and plaques of pregnancy (PUPPP), hypertension, and more.

Post-partum care

For pregnancy in general, raspberry and nettle leaf infusions in the last trimester are a fantastic way to tone up the uterus in preparation for the birth and for the womb after the birth.

Birth and post-partum care can be complex and there are serious complications which can arise. These conditions need greater exploration than can be provided here.

When a baby is born, a woman needs tending. Her placenta needs delivering (following vaginal births) and all kinds of pain, bleeding, clots, or infection may be present, so observation of mama and baba is key. I know from my own experience that "I don't feel right" after giving birth has indicated huge clots, oncoming haemorrhages, and septicaemia so it is well worth noting how a woman feels after birthing.

Plant allies

Aloe gel, diluted myrrh tincture, and infusions of echinacea, marigold, chamomile can all be really helpful to wash the vagina with. Padsicles (a covered icy pad) can be used for bleeding or supporting inflamed vulvas and can also act as a vehicle for herbal application by adding aloe gel with lavender essential oil to the pad and allowing the vulva to sit on it.

Breastfeeding and associated conditions

Note: Many herbs are contraindicated in breastfeeding as they can be passed to the baby via the milk and are too strong or aren't indicated for a baby. There are a few safe and commonly used herbs that are presented here for each condition and while not at all exhaustive, they are useful to know.

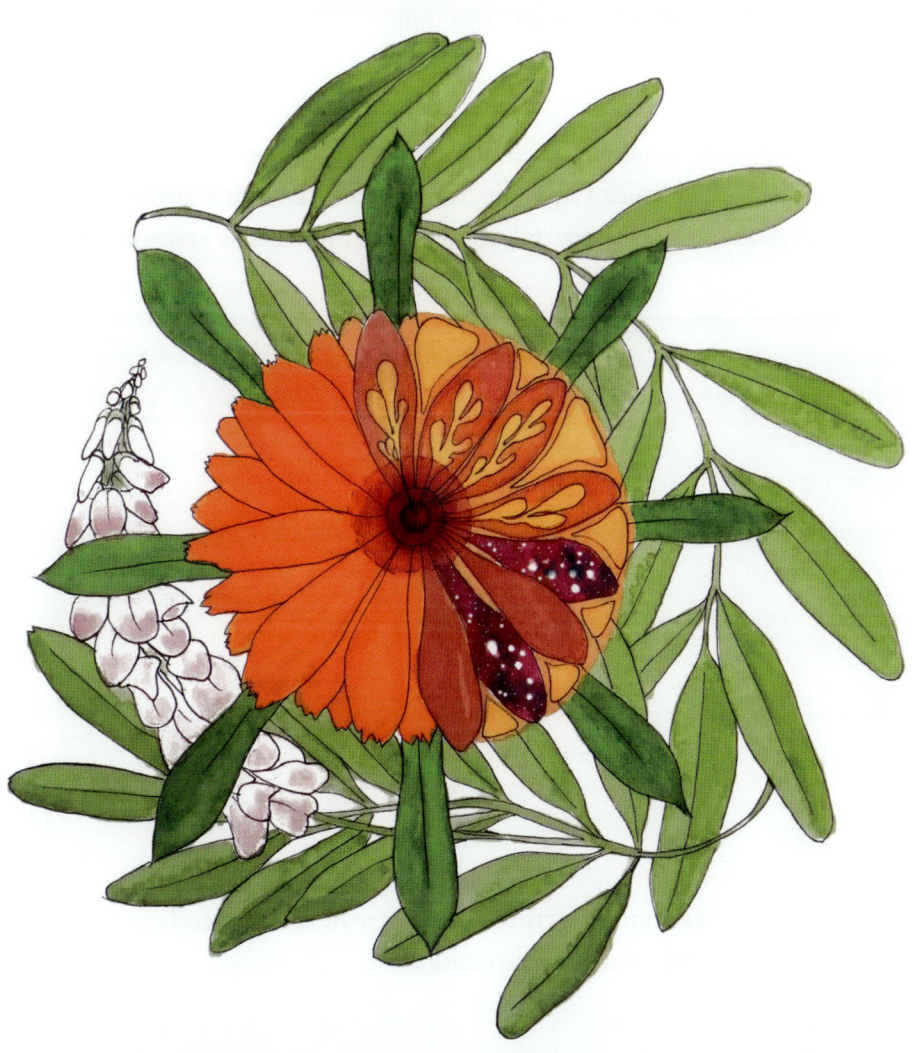

Marigold and goat's rue – two galactic breast plant allies

Low flow breast milk

This is actually the most common reason women give up breastfeeding despite being able to nourish their babies adequately. The despondent feelings that arise if the baby is fussing or attached constantly to the nipple can make a mama think she is not giving or producing enough milk.

If mama is eating enough and is relaxed so that her let-down of the milk is occurring, baby is latching on properly and nothing else abnormal is going on, galactogogues can be used as teas or tinctures depending on the herbs. Galactogogues are herbs that increase breast milk.

Plant allies

Vervain, fennel, dandelion, fenugreek, goat's rue, and oat straw are all galactogogues. Tincture or tea can be made; the latter can be drunk liberally and help a mother relax, produce more milk, and ease her into a new journey with baby.

```
BESTIE BREASTEA

Oat straw        1 part
Lemon balm       1 part
Marigold         1 part
Goat's rue       1 part
Lavender         ½ part
Fennel           ½ part

Brew 1-2 tsp of the tea blend per cup for 5-10 mins,
strain, and drink liberally.
```

It is also useful to eat grain porridges which are nourishing and can help boost milk production while mama gains energy.

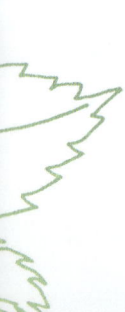

Mastitis

Mastitis can be excruciating and is the second most common reason for giving up breastfeeding. It can be accompanied by high fever and can lead to further infection so is well worth dealing with as soon as possible.

Encouraging milk flow is a good idea, wearing looser bras or no bras, nursing more often if possible, applying hot and cold water over the breast alternately (hydrotherapy) or hot flannels to help release more milk, pumping excess milk or massaging the breasts are all encouraged in mastitis.

Plant allies

The single best remedy (this is a phrase my mentor, Christopher Hedley used a lot! I would always take note when he said it) for mastitis must be the white or savoy cabbage leaf. A leaf the size of the breast can be tucked into a nursing bra or top overnight and incredible as it sounds, mastitis has often gone by the morning and you have limp cabbage leaves for your compost.

Grated potato may work better for some women – same deal, pop it into the nursing bra or on the breasts if you are lying down and leave for at least 20 minutes.

I like these two remedies because they are very cheap and very accessible.

A strong ginger and chamomile infusion can also be applied to the breasts as a soaked cloth at a temperature which is comfortable for you.

If there is sign of fever or infection, echinacea, lemon balm or catnip can be taken as a tincture at a dose of up to 5ml every 2–4 hours for 24 hours if needed.

Sleep remedies like hops, lemon balm, and passionflower can be taken to ease the woman into sleep, if needed, and are fine for short-term usage while breastfeeding.

Cracked or sore nipples

Cracked and sore nipples are common in breastfeeding but can become so bad that a mother stops breastfeeding as it is too painful. Keeping nipples pain-free is very important so mama can carry on breastfeeding if she has chosen to. Tending the nipples also prevents any thrush in the cracks being passed on to the baby as she or he suckles.

To tend nipples, bras and pads can be avoided so the nipples get exposed to dry air; check the baby has a good latch (MOBS or midwives can help with this), treat baby and/or mother for thrush, wash bras regularly in cases of infection if you do wear them.

Plant allies

Marigold is my go-to and great ally for breasts in general! Marigold balm is very useful and I usually include it in most new mama herbal care packs. A rinse of diluted 96% tincture can help if infection is present as it is very resinous. chamomile ointment (balm), cream or rinse (tea) can also be used (see Chapter 2 for a basic recipe).

GYNAECOLOGICAL CONDITIONS
Polycystic ovarian syndrome (PCOS)

It is possible to live with PCOS without any symptoms, however cysts can be reabsorbed, can swell or erupt or become malignant, so it is important to keep an eye on them.

Ovarian health in general can be supported by a healthy diet with lots of anti-inflammatory foods and supplements such as EPA and DHA (essential fatty acids).

Supporting the liver and kidneys is a great idea in the case of polycystic ovaries or PCOS as they help the body with detoxing in general and also with the reabsorption of cysts when they break down.

Avoid inflammatory foods like coffee, alcohol, gluten, etc. which are all stressors on the liver. If there are cysts, castor oil packs may be of great benefit. These are excellent for different kinds of lumps and work through transdermal absorption.

PCOS is the syndrome of polycystic ovaries – when symptoms start to occur in the body due to the cysts. It is the most common endocrine condition in women of reproductive age and there are multiple reasons why PCOS occurs in one or both ovaries.

PCOS is defined by hyperandrogenic characteristics and lack of periods where other causes have been ruled out. Other traits of the syndrome may include insulin resistance, increased LH:FSH ratio (high LH and low FSH), and hyperlipidaemia.

Common symptoms

Scant, irregular, or infrequent periods

Androgen excess may be expressed as hirsutism, a deeper voice, male pattern baldness, and breast reduction

Increased oestrogens as excess androgens are converted to oestrogens

Ovarian pain

Ovulation pain

Ovulation failure leading to difficulty conceiving

Obesity or failure in losing weight (if needed)

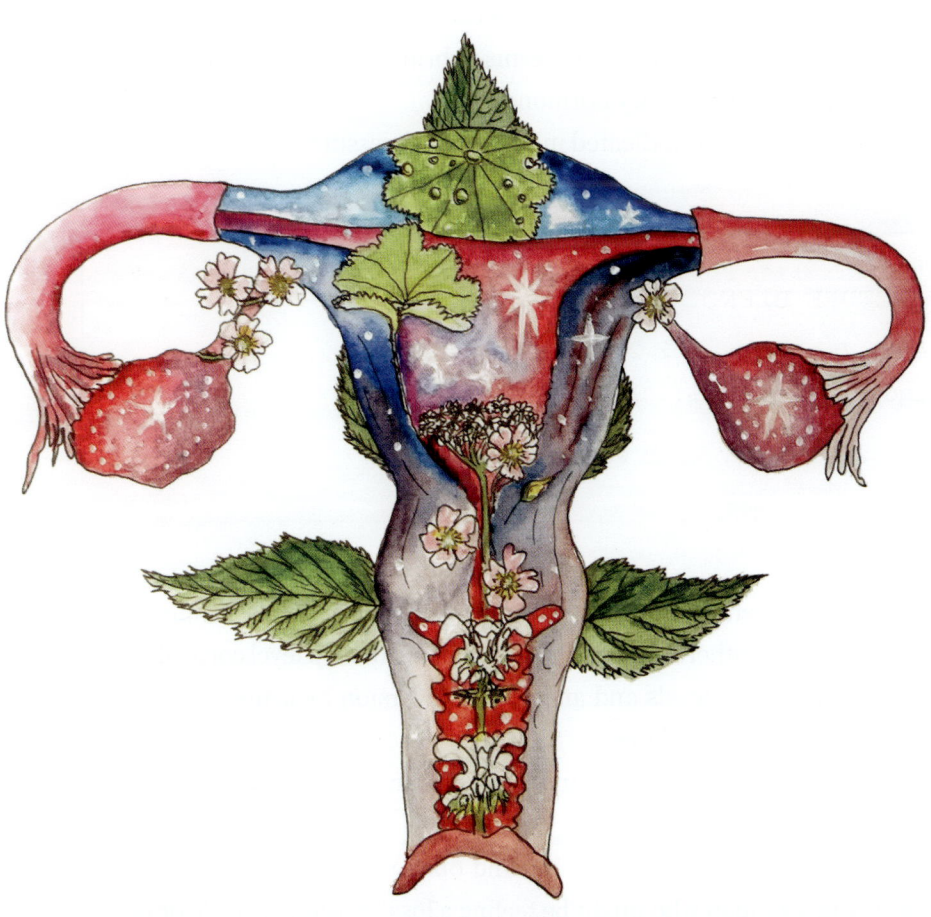

Galactic womb and plant allies

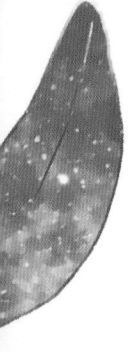

Plant allies

In terms of herbs for PCOS, any symptoms such as pain, acne, hair loss may be addressed with suitable herbs while the root cause is also assessed and managed through herbs, diet, and lifestyle. As with many hormonal conditions, professional help is recommended and a herbalist can work with you to bring the body into balance.

Chasteberry can be used for hyperprolactinaemia and low progesterone levels as the herb is indirectly progesteronic.

Peony and liquorice is a commonly used blend from traditional Chinese medicine. Peony can inhibit the production of testosterone and stimulate testosterone conversion to oestrogen through aromatisation. Liquorice can reduce the amount of serum testosterone; its phytoestrogens can also block androgen receptors. This blend seems to bring about a synergistic effect which helps balance the pituitary hormones.

Liquorice is contraindicated in high blood pressure.

```
TINCTURE BLEND

Peony (white)   1:2  2 parts (eg 50ml)
Liquorice       1:1  1 part  (eg 25ml)

5ml twice daily with water before food
```

Many adaptogens help regulate blood sugar levels, aiding insulin resistance. Schisandra, eleuthero, and other adaptogens can help level cortisol release and ensuing prolactin levels and androgen conversion by acting on the HPA axis and bringing it into balance.

Vervain supports the liver and gently balances hormonal fluctuations so is very useful in PCOS.

Rose can feel deeply feminising and open up the feeling of self-worth and beauty in a woman who might be feeling a loss of beauty (inside or out). There are many different types of rose each with their own vibe. I like to use *Rosa damascena* or *gallica* but sometimes I use whatever I'm drawn to in a rose garden.

Fibroids

Fibroids are benign lumps of fibre found in the uterine cavity and affect a quarter of women over 35 years old. Fibroids may not cause symptoms even when fairly large but they must be tended, especially if a stalk is present. They may contribute to fertility issues or may cause heavy bleeding during menstruation and if they are large, can cause frequency and urgency of urination, congestion, and bloating.

Fibroids are oestrogen dependent so are mostly present in menstruating women and almost always shrink after menopause. Pregnancy reduces the risk of fibroids where obesity, coffee, high blood pressure, and talcum powder may increase the risk.

Plant allies

Heavy bleeding caused by fibroids may be eased with lady's mantle, shepherd's purse, yarrow, white deadnettle, and raspberry leaf.

Herbs used to reduce the size of the fibroid include thuja, damiana, and marigold; vitamin C may also be useful.

Herbs to reduce oestrogen excess include peony, cinnamon, and chasteberry.

Consult a herbalist if you have fibroids.

Endometriosis

Endometriosis is one of the most common gynaecological conditions and can be very disabling, but only recently have proper studies into its effects on women across the nation been undertaken.

In healthy women, the endometrium, which lines the uterus in preparation for conception, is expelled during menstruation if pregnancy doesn't occur. In endometriosis, this tissue starts to grow in other parts of the body – usually in the pelvic cavity.

The most common areas of abnormal growth include the ovaries, fallopian tubes, outer area of the uterus, bowel, ureter, and bladder, and respond to hormonal shifts, proliferating and shedding as the normal endometrial tissue does. This internal bleeding aggravates the local tissue and can cause scarring and adhesions creating mild to severe pain. At worst it can also cause difficulty in conception.

Local oestrogen and prostaglandin presence is increased in abnormal tissue due to aromatase action not seen in normal endometrial tissue. Chocolate cysts also form in around two thirds of women with endometriosis. Endometrial tissue starts to grow on the ovaries and so the ovaries envelop the growths and try to contain them, forming cysts.

As these cysts grow, commonly during each menstrual cycle, they can cause pain with dying cysts causing scarring on the ovaries, irritation or damage in the pelvic cavity.

The pain of endometriosis can be the most obvious and crippling symptom. Fainting, diarrhoea, flooding, difficulty conceiving, painful intercourse, and more can present with endometriosis.

Aside from balancing hormones, nutritional issues should be tended to; these include magnesium deficiency, essential fatty acid deficiency, lower caffeine consumption, lower alcohol intake, and of course it is necessary to address levels of stress in the woman's life.

Plant allies

Dong quai is a prime herb for endometriosis – that is not to say it is for everyone, but it has a great many uses in this condition. It is antispasmodic, tonifying, and analgesic and has immunomodulatory and anti-inflammatory actions. It is indicated in traditional Chinese medicine for blood stasis which is exactly what is going on in endometriosis.

It has been recorded that feverfew was used by European colonisers (Eclectics) for menstrual irregularities and is often used as an anti-inflammatory. It inhibits prostaglandin formation (causing inflammation and pain) and COX 2 enzyme (which helps form prostaglandins) and eases pain.

Ginger is antispasmodic and anti-inflammatory and helps with dysmenorrhoea, especially if the pain is eased with heat, and also inhibits prostaglandins.

Gotu kola is anti-inflammatory, anti-infective, and anti-proliferative. It is used to prevent scar tissue formation. It is also used as an adaptogen.

Vervain is useful for regulating menstruation and getting the liver moving. A good "moving" combination is vervain and yarrow: this combination will help with sluggishness and blood stagnancy while promoting better hormonal balance.

Anti-inflammatory effects through the suppression of the key enzymes which promote pro-inflammatory molecules in the body have been demonstrated in a blend of liquorice, St John's wort, plantain, and marigold.

Rehmannia and white peony are often coupled in traditional Chinese medicine and show good antispasmodic and anti-inflammatory effects. Prostaglandin inhibition and smooth muscle relaxation were also demonstrated in studies.

Consult a herbalist for an in-depth personalised consultation to see what is going on for you or the woman in question, but know there are avenues of help out there.

Pelvic inflammatory disease (PID)

The symptoms of pelvic inflammatory disease are broad and painful; it is an almost catch-all term, describing chronic, acute, or subacute inflammation in the pelvic area. This condition tends to worsen over time but may also vary greatly from mild to severe in terms of pain. Symptoms include lower back ache, abdominal cramps, abnormal vaginal discharge, fatigue and/or weakness, heavy menstruation, shorter menstrual cycles, pain during intercourse, fever, lymphadenopathy in the groin, nausea and/or vomiting, and mittelschmerz (pain on ovulation).

Inflammation and presentation of pain and discomfort are most likely caused by bacteria moving up from the vagina – this risk is augmented when the cervix is opened, for example through childbirth, miscarriage, abortion, IUD fitting, or a D&C (dilation and curettage). Symptoms may come and go for years but can be debilitating in flare-ups. Intercourse and relationships can be affected, as well as self-confidence and self-care so sufferers need to make sure to tend themselves.

Plant allies

Herbal antibiotics such as yarrow, barberry, garlic, and others (chosen to suit the individual) may be given and used for acute or chronic conditions. Poultices or hot packs may be really useful to target the area. Castor oil packs over the lower back or abdomen may help reduce the congestion and inflammation.

A herbal formulation for the pain itself might be similar to one for a premenstrual headache:

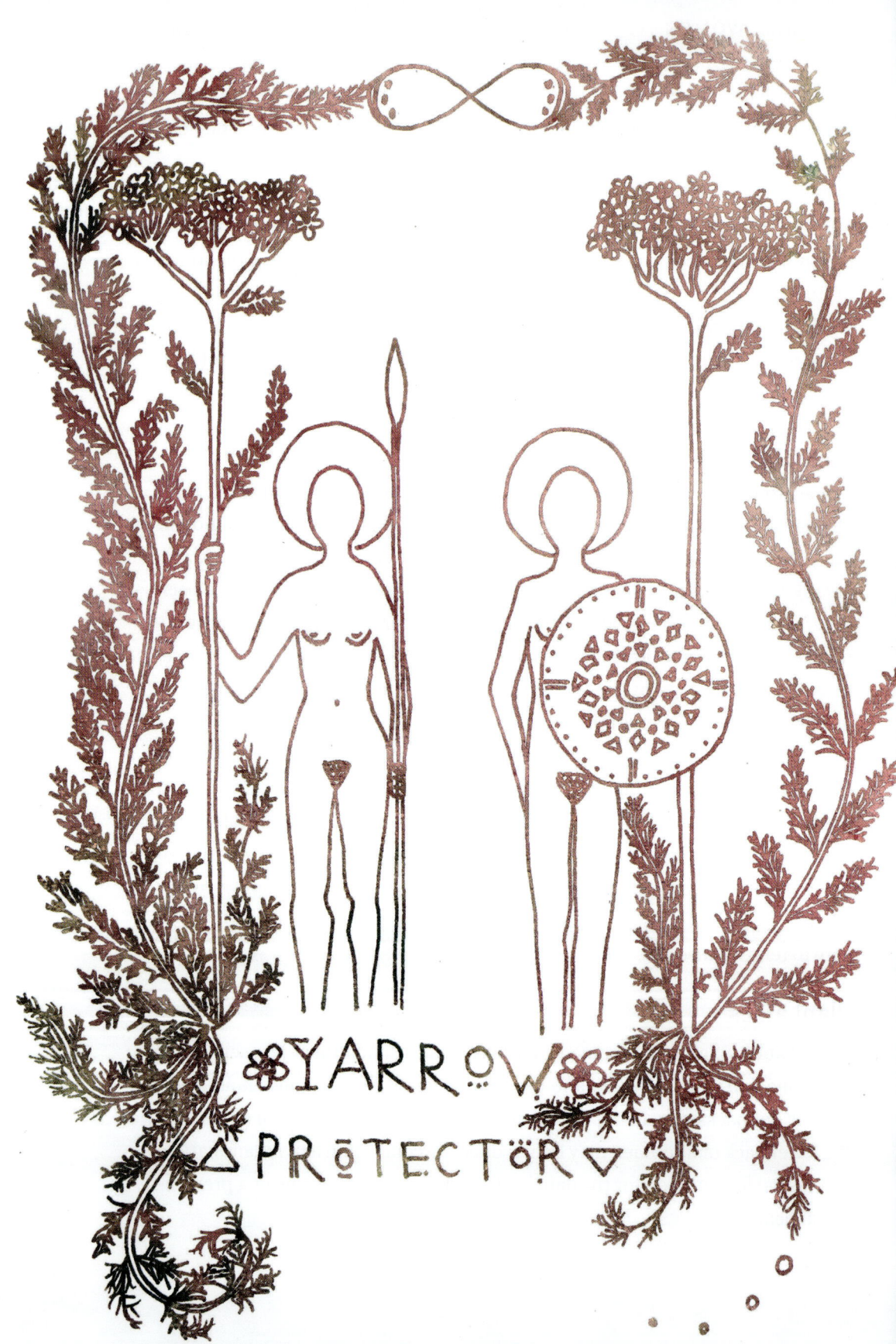

```
MOON PAIN MIX (TINCTURE)
Crampbark       1 part (eg 50ml)
Ashwagandha     1 part (eg 50ml)
Yarrow          ½ part (eg 25ml)

5ml twice a day with water before food.
```

There are so many options to consider, however, that a formula like this is really just treating the symptoms not the root cause. Anti-inflammatory herbs, adaptogens, carminatives, hepatics, demulcents, and more may also be used by a herbalist depending on what is going on.

CRONEDOM

Menopause is a slow-moving transition from fertility to elderhood. Women generally experience three stages of menopause: perimenopause, menopause, and post-menopause.

The first stage, perimenopause, can last up to eight years and begins when ovulation starts to decline. The whole process doesn't often start before forty years old and is usually finished by around fifty-eight years old.

HRT and mainstream treatment of menopause

Menopause is, unbelievably, classed as a "condition" or a disease. It is a natural transition marking the end of a woman's fertility. There may be accompanying symptoms due to a range of factors, not least the change in hormones, as women from different cultures have different experiences.

Hormone replacement therapy (HRT) is frequently prescribed to alleviate symptoms of menopause in the West. There are risks associated with its consumption including breast cancer and thromboembolism. Many women seek alternatives to HRT and look to herbs and diet. Herbalists often have the privilege to work with women going through menopause and it becomes an evolving journey into the wisdom years.

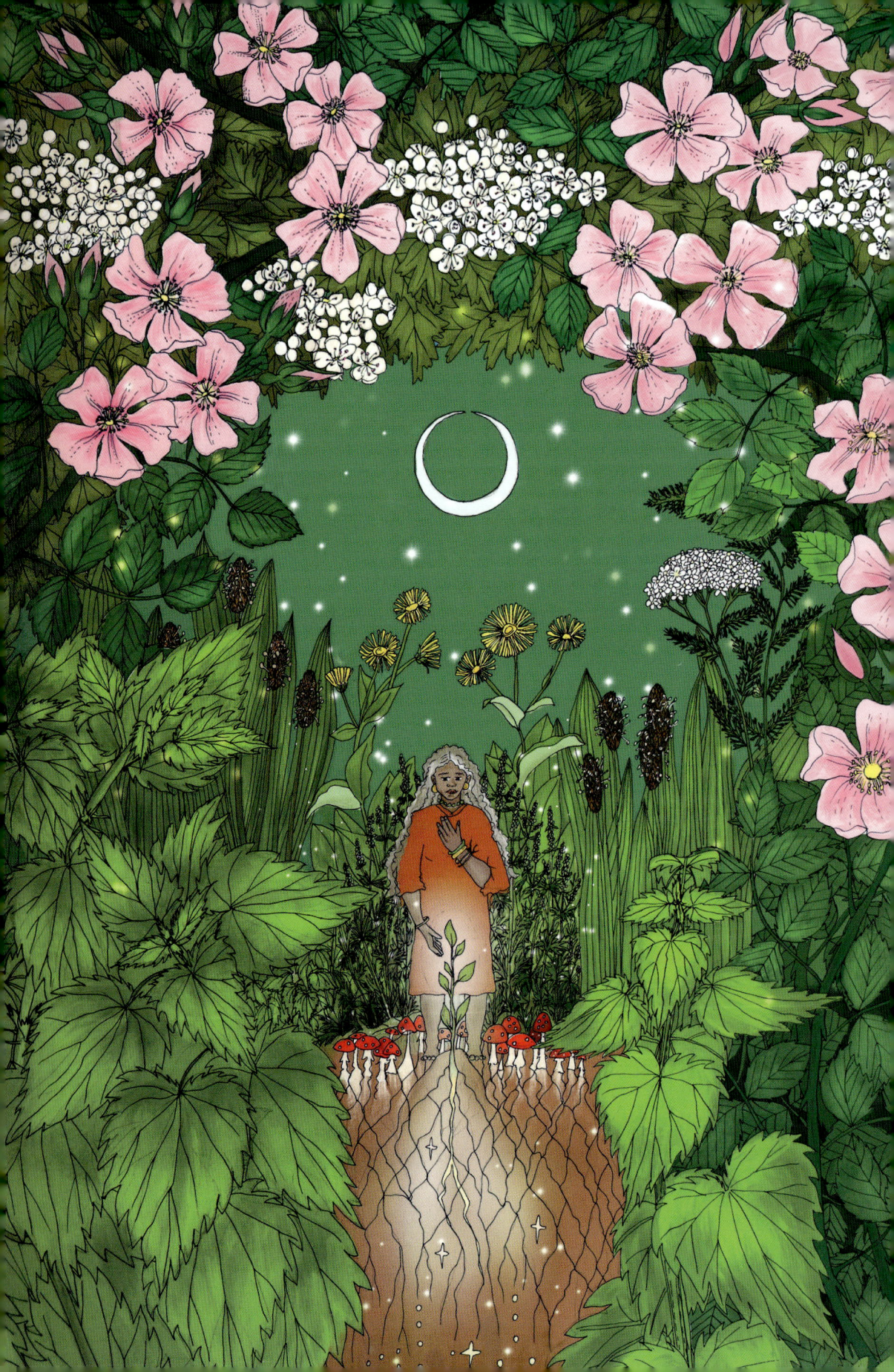

Hot flushes

The majority of women in the West experience hot flushes when going through menopause. Some are so severe that they hinder normal life and can bring about menopausal depression or low self-confidence. The lessening amount of oestrogen in the body affects our ability to regulate temperature which causes sweating in order to cool the body at times it is not normally needed. Shivering can then occur to try to warm up. It can feel very disorienting and can make a woman feel physically sick let alone cold, hot, or wet.

When this happens at night it can lead to insomnia, worry, and nightmares which are followed the next day by fatigue and frustration.

Plant allies

If the woman is a choleric or sanguine type, heat may be part of her constitution and general cooling mixes may be indicated. If she is melancholic or phlegmatic a more tonifying mix may be needed as too much cold won't necessarily suit.

An example cooling and tonifying tincture blend for hot flushes:

```
HOT FLUSH TONIC

Ashwagandha     2 parts  (eg 100ml)
Jujube date     2 parts  (eg 100ml)
Vervain         1 part   (eg 50ml)
Lavender        ½ part   (eg 25ml)
Sage            ½ part   (eg 25ml)

2.5ml with water 2-3 x daily.
```

```
COOL AND CALM TEA
Sage
Lavender
Spearmint
Applemint

Equal parts, brew 1-2 tsps of the tea blend per cup
for 5-10 mins, strain, and drink liberally through
the day.
```

```
COLD SAGE TEA
A simple infusion of sage which is left to cool can be
really helpful just before bed for night sweats.
```

```
FOR DIFFICULTY SLEEPING, A COOLING INSOMNIA MIX
OF TINCTURES CAN HELP
Wild lettuce    4 parts (eg 100ml)
Hops            1 part (eg 25ml)

5ml before bed with water and on waking if needed.
```

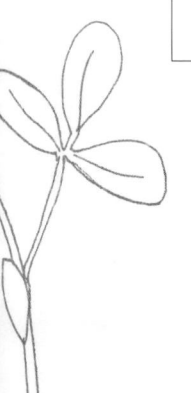

Depression and anxiety in menopause

There may be many reasons why depression occurs when women pass through menopause. The transition is a big one and the marginalisation in society of older women is evident. In healthier cultures the matriarch or older woman is celebrated, respected, and listened to, and depression is not seen in older women.

Much like depression in menopause, anxiety can manifest due to symptoms affecting a woman's life, relationship, work capability, etc. it can also be caused by the nervousness that her place has changed in society and she may not be seen anymore, or may be judged to be something she is not.

While herbs that help depression in menopause aren't specific to menopause as such, it may be that there are constitutional influences as to which herbs to choose for the individual, and also more tonic herbs might be chosen if debility or fatigue is present.

Some herbs will be helpful because they support the adrenals and increase vitality and some will calm the feelings of worthlessness or the critic inside, and others will be uplifting.

By alleviating menopausal symptoms such as hot flushes, mood usually elevates too. If depression has affected the woman prior to menopause, it may be that constitutional work, particularly for earthy temperaments, are needed or the addressing of a much more complex picture.

Plant allies

Mimosa, or Persian silk tree (Albizia julibrissin), nourishes the heart and calms the spirit and is known as "collective happiness bark" in traditional Chinese medicine! It can be used for irritability, depression, insomnia, anxiety, poor memory – many traits which can affect menopausal women. It is a wonderful uplifting herb that is well worth trying. Other herbs might include lemon balm, orange blossom, and St John's wort.

```
NO MORE ANXIETEA

Passionflower          2 parts
Lemon balm             2 parts
Jujube                 1 part
Sage                   1 part

1-2 tsps infused 5-10 mins, strain and drink 1-3
cups daily
```

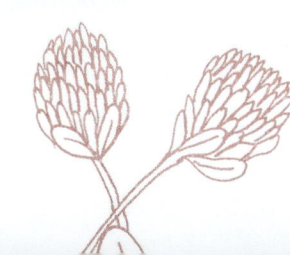

```
CRONE GODDESS DROPS

Rose

Mugwort

Lady's mantle

Sage

Rosemary

Equal parts of these tinctures. Take 5 drops when you
forget to feel like a goddess.
```

Osteoporosis

Osteoporosis is the degenerative condition most associated with, but not exclusive to, menopause; for as oestrogen levels decline so too does the protection of bones. Porous bones aren't as strong as healthy bones and increased risk of fracture is evident. This condition may present very slowly, from years or decades of slow demineralisation.

If there are deficiencies in mineral and vitamins (calcium with magnesium, phosphorus, zinc, boron, and vitamin D) they will affect the strength and vitality of the bones. The bone matrix is set by around thirty years of age – after that age, we need to maintain good levels of nutrition to keep our bones strong.

Plant allies

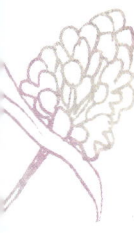

When menstruation ceases in a woman's life, reabsorption of bone minerals accelerates and loss of bone density occurs. Exercise, diet and herbs will help support retention of bone mass.

To keep bones strong, minerals and nutrients must be properly absorbed from the gut so that enough nutrients reach and are retained in the bones. Herbs to astringe and tone the gut to facilitate this include meadowsweet, agrimony, chamomile, and gentian. There are herbs which promote bone health through their nutritive effect such as milky oats, nettle, dandelion, and horsetail. Phytoestrogens are useful as they prevent the bone loss associated with low oestrogen; these include red clover and alfalfa. Preventing and managing osteoporosis is not about the cure, it is about a healthy lifestyle with lots of exercise and a nutritious diet.

```
BONEY VINEGAR
Horsetail
Rosemary
Nettle
Organic cider vinegar (preferably with the "mother")

Fill a jar up with the herbs – at a ratio you like –
equal parts is good but you might want an emphasis on
the horsetail or nettle for example. Cover with the
vinegar and seal, label, and macerate for 2-3 weeks.
Shake daily. Then strain and take 1-2 tblsp daily, as
is, on salad, in hot water, etc. This is a great way to
get the minerals from the brilliant herbs into your
body and bones.
```

Tips to maintain healthy bones

Avoid eating a lot of meat as calcium is needed to neutralise the acids.

Avoid smoking, alcohol, sugar, and caffeine as they encourage calcium loss from bones.

Eat calcium-rich foods.

Reduce consumption of spinach, chard, and chocolate as they contain oxalic acid which blocks calcium absorption.

Reduce or avoid wholegrains as the phytates interfere with calcium absorption – sprouting or soaking helps reduce phytic acid content.

Add lemon juice to your salad to increase calcium absorption.

Exercise caution with drugs that reduce calcium absorption.

Do regular weight bearing exercise.

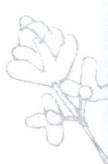

Get outside and get some sunshine on your skin to absorb vitamin D or if you can't, supplement with a few thousand iu of D3 daily.

Vaginal dryness

Vaginal dryness can be one of the most difficult conditions accompanying menopause and post-menopause as it can affect your intimate life and there aren't many people who talk about it. It is a direct consequence of declining oestrogen during menopause. Itching, dryness, irritation, and bleeding can occur in the vagina and sex can be too painful with consequent self-doubt and loss of libido also manifesting. Women are more prone to infections and are at risk of uterine prolapse. The wall of the vagina can be physically affected with tissue integrity at stake.

Plant allies

Phytoestrogens may be used for oestrogen decline along with topical or internal anti-inflammatories, anti-pruritics (anti-itching), alteratives, and demulcents to soothe the tissue.

Herbal or natural lubricants can be used during sex to allow a greater freedom and encourage intimate relationships (with oneself as well as with another).

Marigold works as a cream or salve applied directly to the vagina morning and night and can be of help where infection is present.

Alfalfa is a great phytoestrogen containing genistein which is helpful in menopause and will help with vaginal atrophy or dryness.

Hops is another useful phytoestrogenic herb that helps with vaginal dryness and atrophy as well as hot flushes, night sweats, and insomnia. It is cooling and bitter. Tea or tincture is often given but not in large quantities or for too long. Consult a herbalist.

Lavender is a great topical herb for neuralgia, pain, and soreness and can be used as a suppository or lubricant. Lovely pessaries can be made with lavender essential oils added. Douches can be done with lavender water and of course it can be taken as tea or tincture.

Shatavari works internally as a remedy for vaginal dryness. It is great taken as capsules or tincture.

Damiana is a beautiful tonic herb with a gentle aphrodisiac action, helping with libido, sexual satisfaction, and vaginal dryness.

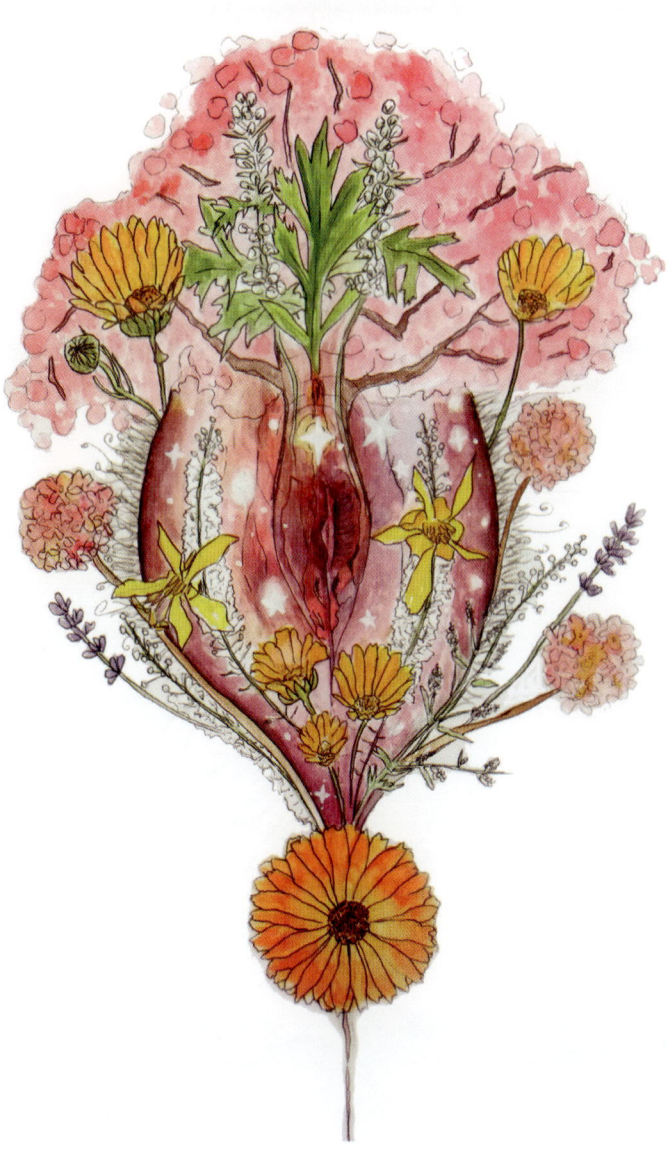

Galactic vulva and plant allies

VAGINAL PESSARIES FOR DRYNESS

Using melted cocoa butter as the carrier oil, make an infused oil of marigold and comfrey.

Infuse half a cup of melted cocoa butter with marigold, comfrey, or both, over a bain marie (water bath) for two hours (see "External remedies"; "Infused oil").

Strain and add up to 20% powdered fenugreek, marigold, or shatavari.

Pour into pessary moulds. If you don't have any, pour into a jar and leave in the fridge. Scoop half a tsp at a time and insert into vagina as high up as is comfortable for you – lying down so it doesn't melt and dribble out.

Usually pessaries are inserted at night. Of course you may choose to wear a sustainable pad if needed.

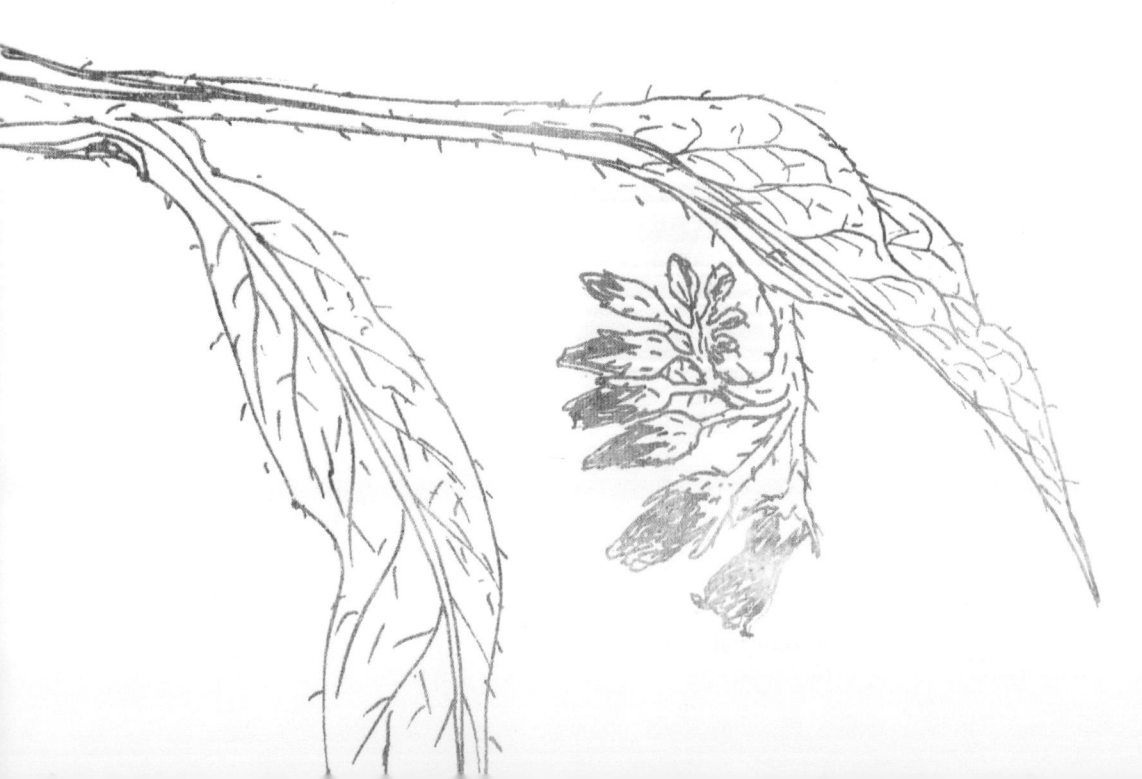

A word on phytoestrogens in menopause

It is worth noting that phytoestrogens may aggravate oestrogen dependent conditions, for example, endometriosis and breast cancer, so make sure if you are taking herbs for any hormone-responsive condition to know what your herbs do and how the condition may react to the plants or hormones in the body. Please consult a herbalist for help.

Red clover is a phytoestrogen that reduces the adverse effects of declining oestrogen.

Dong quai is used to strengthen the blood. It acts as a tonic reducing dizziness, memory loss, confusion, nervousness, and insomnia while bringing menstrual flow into balance. It can be used at any stage of menses, not just perimenopause. If you experience heavy bleeding, taking dong quai just before your moon flow can cause it to become heavier so care is needed here. Seek the support of a herbalist who can help guide you to the right herbs for you and your cycle. If your moon flow is irregular, consider using other herbs if you do experience heavy bleeding.

Sage is used as a cooling infusion for hot flushes and night sweats.

Wild yam is a phytoestrogen that reduces the adverse effects of declining oestrogen.

Jujube is used for night sweats and to promote sleep. In its native land it is commonly sucked as a fruit and used as a calming tonic.

Shatavari is an excellent herb for vaginal dryness.

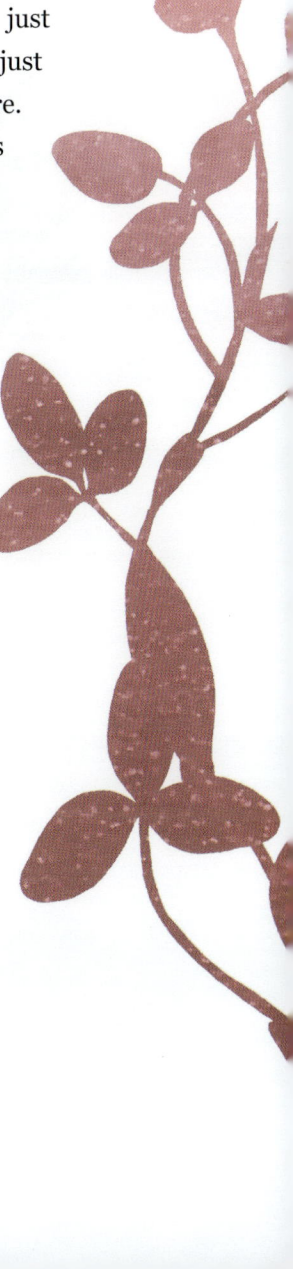
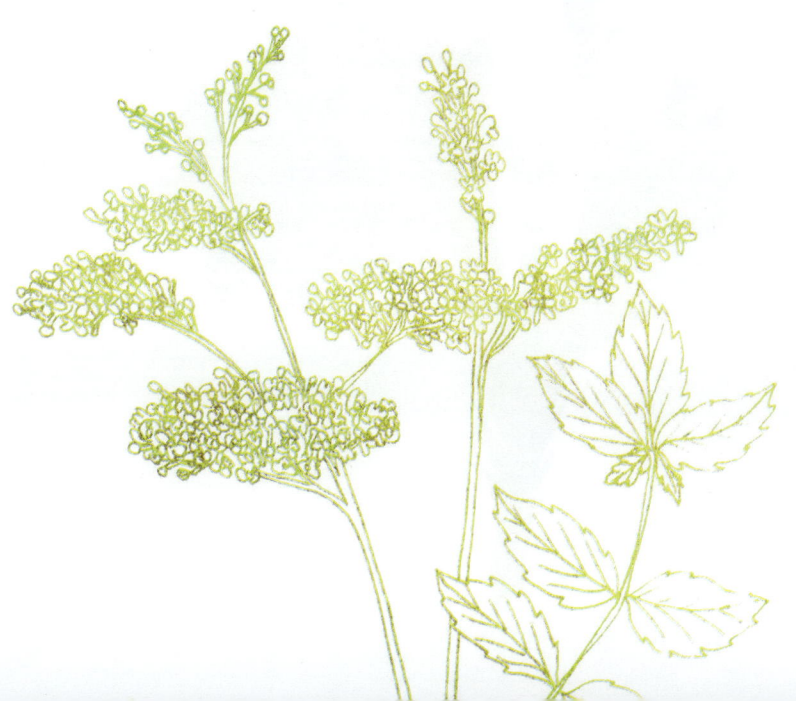

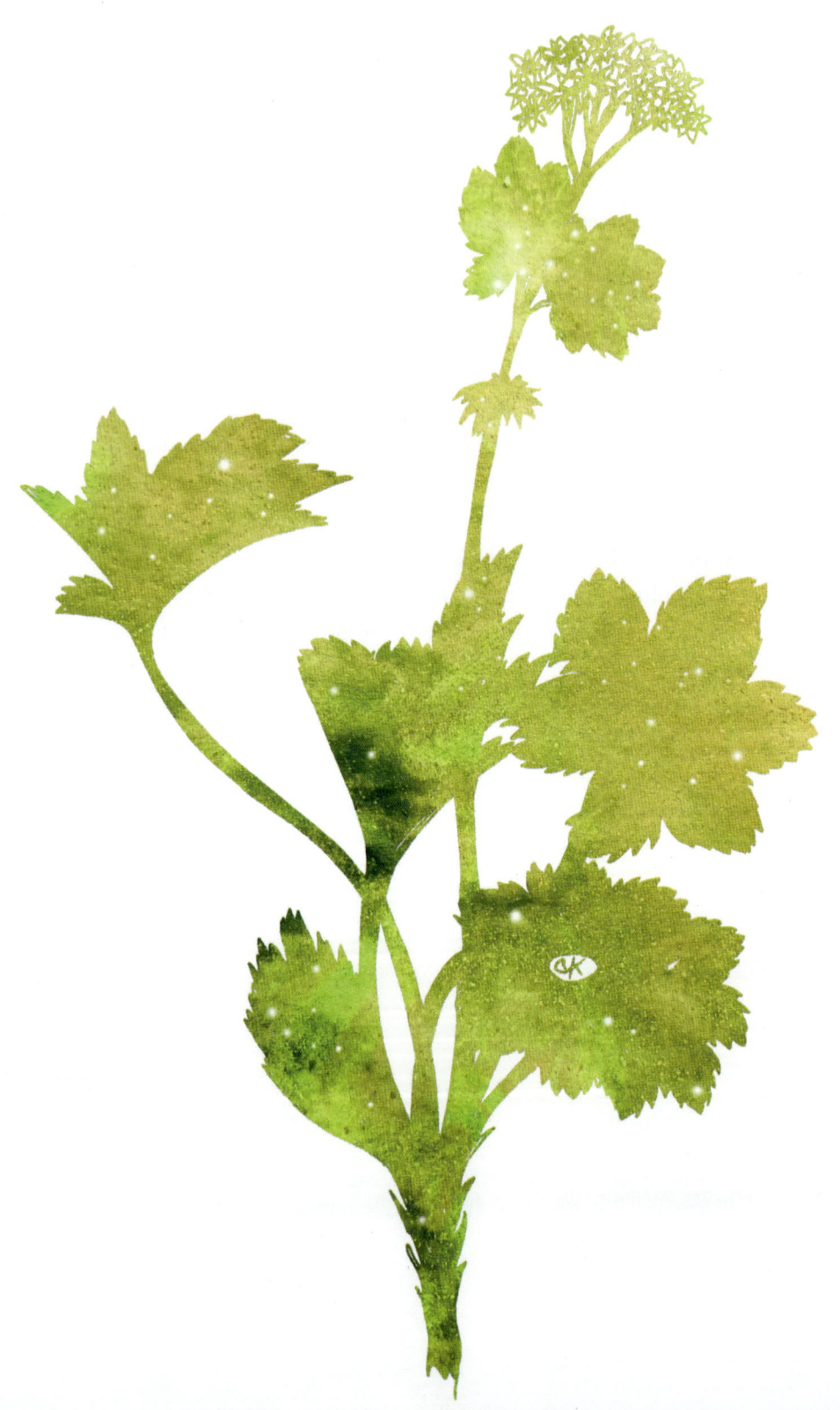

PLANT ALLIES FOR ALL WOMEN

Lady's mantle *Alchemilla vulgaris*

Nature: hot and dry

Planet: Venus

This herb is the alchemist's herb. It has a soft beautiful leaf that pushes water through it to sit in magical pools of wonder where the stem meets the leaf. It is often used for women's gynaecological conditions and is a great tonic for the uterus. In the UK it is certainly one of the foremost women's herbs but it doesn't seem to feature so highly in other parts of the world. It aids menstrual cramps, fertility challenges, menorrhagia, loss of tone in the womb, and wounds in the uterus. It is a strong astringent and can help tone uterine tissue and heal wounds resulting from birth, infection, or intrusion. It is a tonic herb for the uterus and helps rebuild physically and emotionally.

Its alchemy makes it a great herb for those in transitional times, from girl to woman, from fertile woman to crone, or in any transition. If you are melancholic and would like to step into a more spiritual life, this herb may allow the release of stuck emotions and a magical entrance closer to otherness. It is also useful for those of any temperament stuck in a pattern that you just can't shift – it will bring on the transition. So be prepared! I like tea, fresh plant tincture, and elixir of this beautiful, humble wonder.

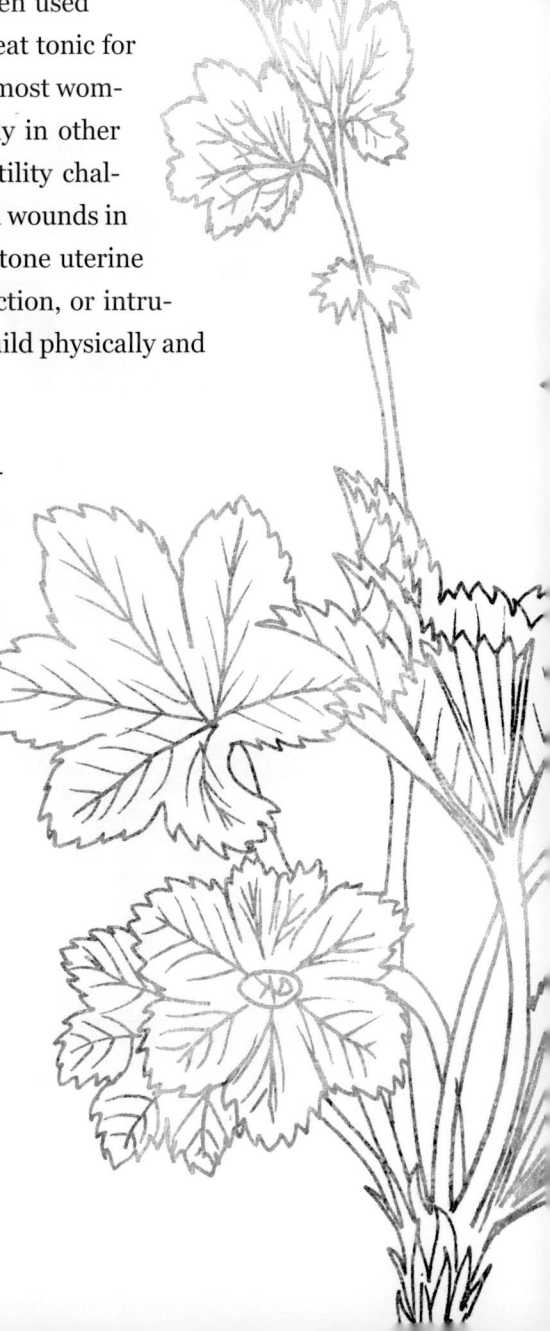

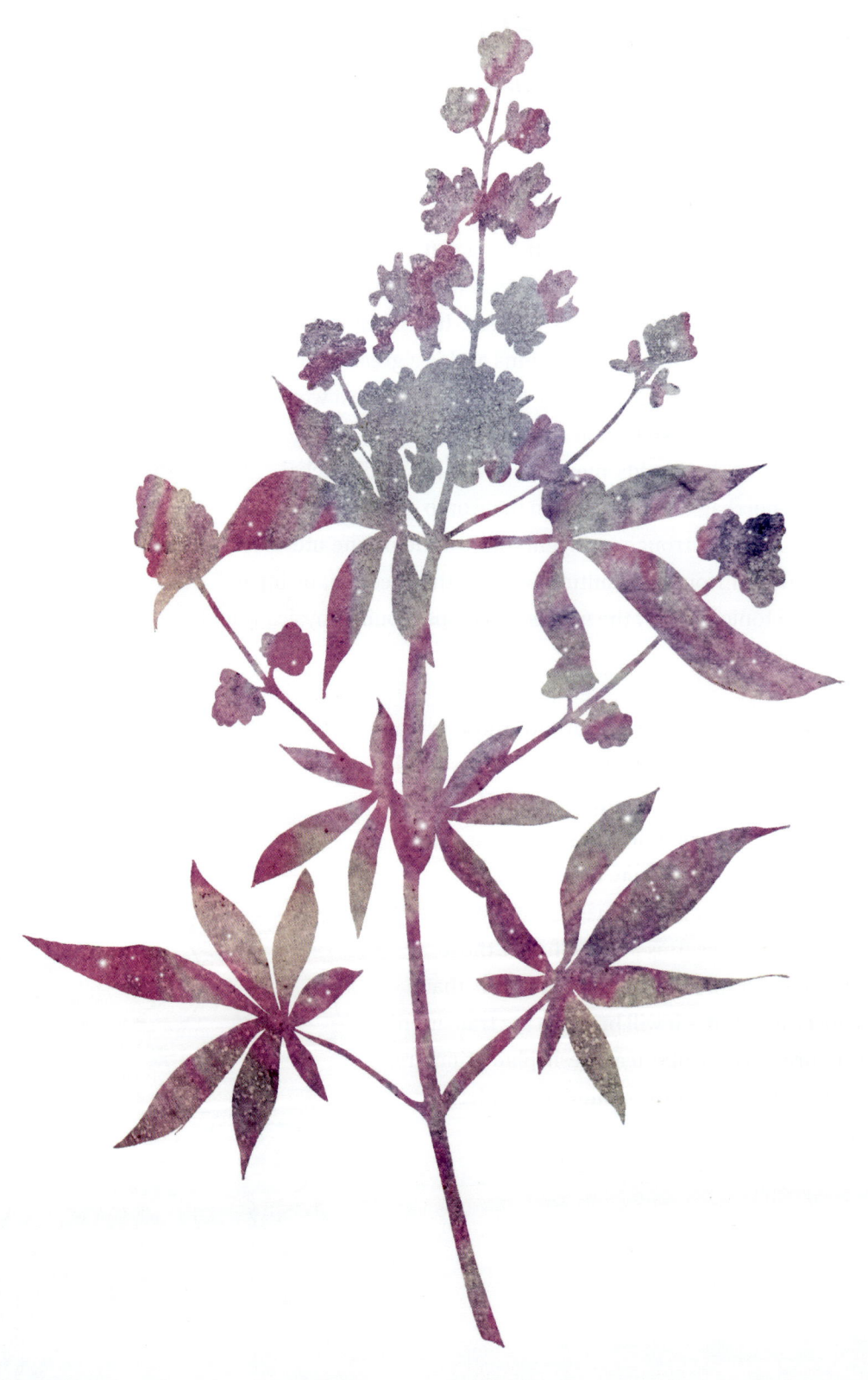

Chasteberry *Vitex agnus castus*

Nature: hot and dry

Planet: Mars (or the moon)

This wonderful tree is a beauty to behold in its flowering glory in warmer climes. It grows well here but doesn't fruit so easily. Plato (428 BCE) described chasteberry (or chastetree, vitex or agnus castus as all are commonly used) as an aphrodisiac but it is also called monk's pepper as it seems to have dose dependant paradoxical effects so it a useful to consult a herbalist for your needs.

The berries are most effective in exerting a dopaminergic action (probably the diterpenes) and inhibit prolactin secretion. High prolactin inhibits corpus luteum formation, which causes a drop in progesterone secretion in the luteal phase.

Low dose chasteberry supports a longer luteal phase, a thicker corpus luteum and promotes fertility in those with hyperprolactinaemia. This beautiful herb is also utilised for premenstrual symptoms including breast tenderness and water retention.

Chasteberry has been associated with the moon due to its silver under-leaf, its link to menstrual cycle regulation and association with water, however some say it's also a herb of Mars with its hot and dry qualities, opposing the cool, wetness of the moon. Asian and African varieties have been used for contraception and to help children sleep. The flower remedy is also very calming and nourishing.

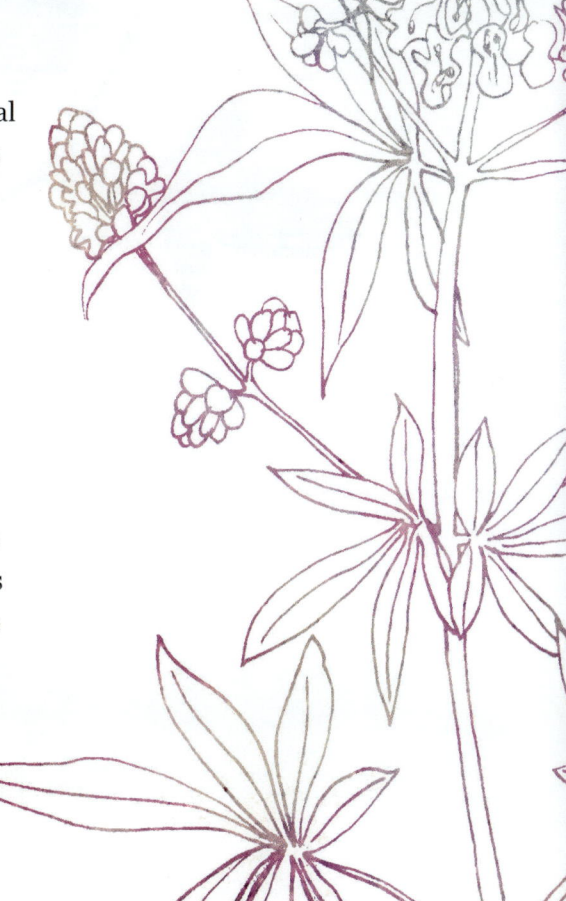

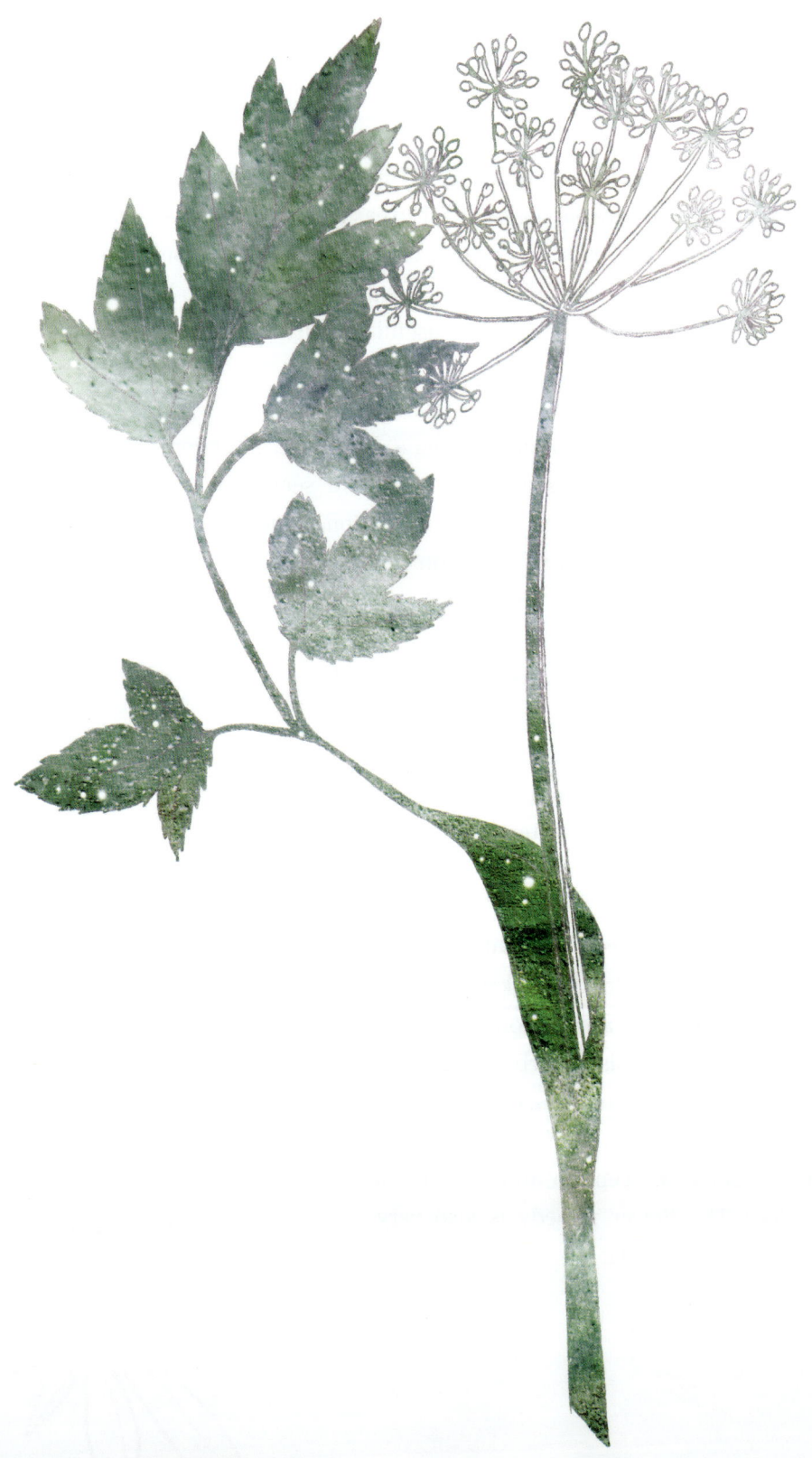

Dong quai *Angelica sinensis*

Nature: warm, moistening

Celestial body: Sun

Chinese angelica is a beautiful plant and often seen in different parts of the world as a female wonder herb. Its roots are used, like yarrow's aerial parts, to move the blood. This means these herbs are great for gynaecological issues to do with stagnancy but also throughout the body – conditions with vascular congestion will be aided, such as heart disease or dementia.

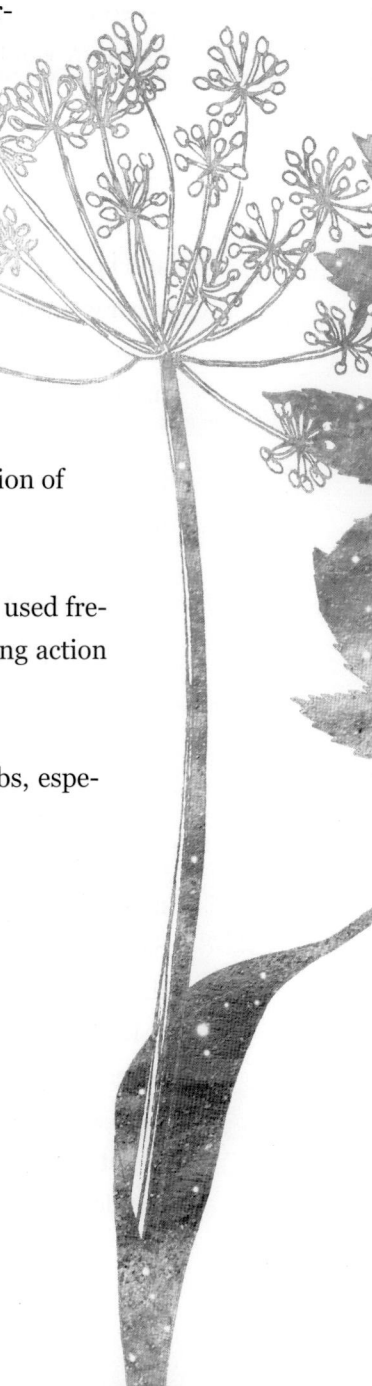

Angelica is considered a "female ginseng" – so is liquorice by some – but the attribution does seek to demonstrate the wonders of the herb. Not only will it move blood but it will feed the blood, reduce blood pressure, and regulate the heart. It also stimulates the production of white blood cells and helps our immune system and vitality.

It is a first-choice herb in endometriosis and aids fertility. It is used frequently in menopausal conditions and with its warming, moving action can soothe, nourish, and invigorate.

As dong quai can promote bleeding, consider using other herbs, especially just before your moon flow if your bleed is heavy.

The above herbs should be avoided in pregnancy.

JOURNALING

Think about how you connect with your menstrual cycle, your fertility, your lack of menses. If you don't menstruate, including because you were born a cisgender man, think about your relationship with menstruation. Even this week (February 2020), humiliation occurred for girls in India because they failed to declare their menses and were forced to have a knicker inspection so that they wouldn't "pollute" others. It is still taboo, there is still stigma. It is also amazing, life-giving, and nourishing for the earth. Do you know much about menstruation? Do you connect to it or do you have negative feelings towards it? These are things to think about.

In terms of rewilding and connection to nature, think about how we connect and how our cycles connect us. Menstruation is connected with the moon and other women – if we spend time together, often our cycles coincide. If you don't bleed, how does that make you feel? If you are using a contraceptive pill or implant, how do you feel about your cycles?

If you are menopausal or post-menopausal, think about how you feel in terms of your growth into an older woman. How does it make you feel? If you have time, think of the trees and the age of those older beauties we all stand in front of sometimes in awe. Choose a tree and reflect back to yourself how you feel about it. Describe it and how it makes you feel being near it. Then apply this description to women and yourself. See if you can absorb the beauty of the great trees and note which ones you are drawn to and why.

If you realise through your journaling that you feel negative in some way – disgust, disconnection, worry, etc., make a cuppa – preferably one with nervine herbs in and gently consider why. If you can journal this too, that would be great. If it hurts or brings up anything emotional like loneliness, disappointment, or fear please do seek support – from friends, family, professionals, the Samaritans. Try to also note down or consider what you might do to redress this imbalance.

Remember to give yourself love and care and tend yourself as you would others. Allow the earth to help if you get stuck – practise the rewilding exercises such as putting your hands on the ground and breathing in. When in doubt go for a walk in the woods. If you can't walk then go outdoors or at the very least, look outside. There is beauty everywhere. It just needs finding.

Womxn with vervain tending themselves outdoors

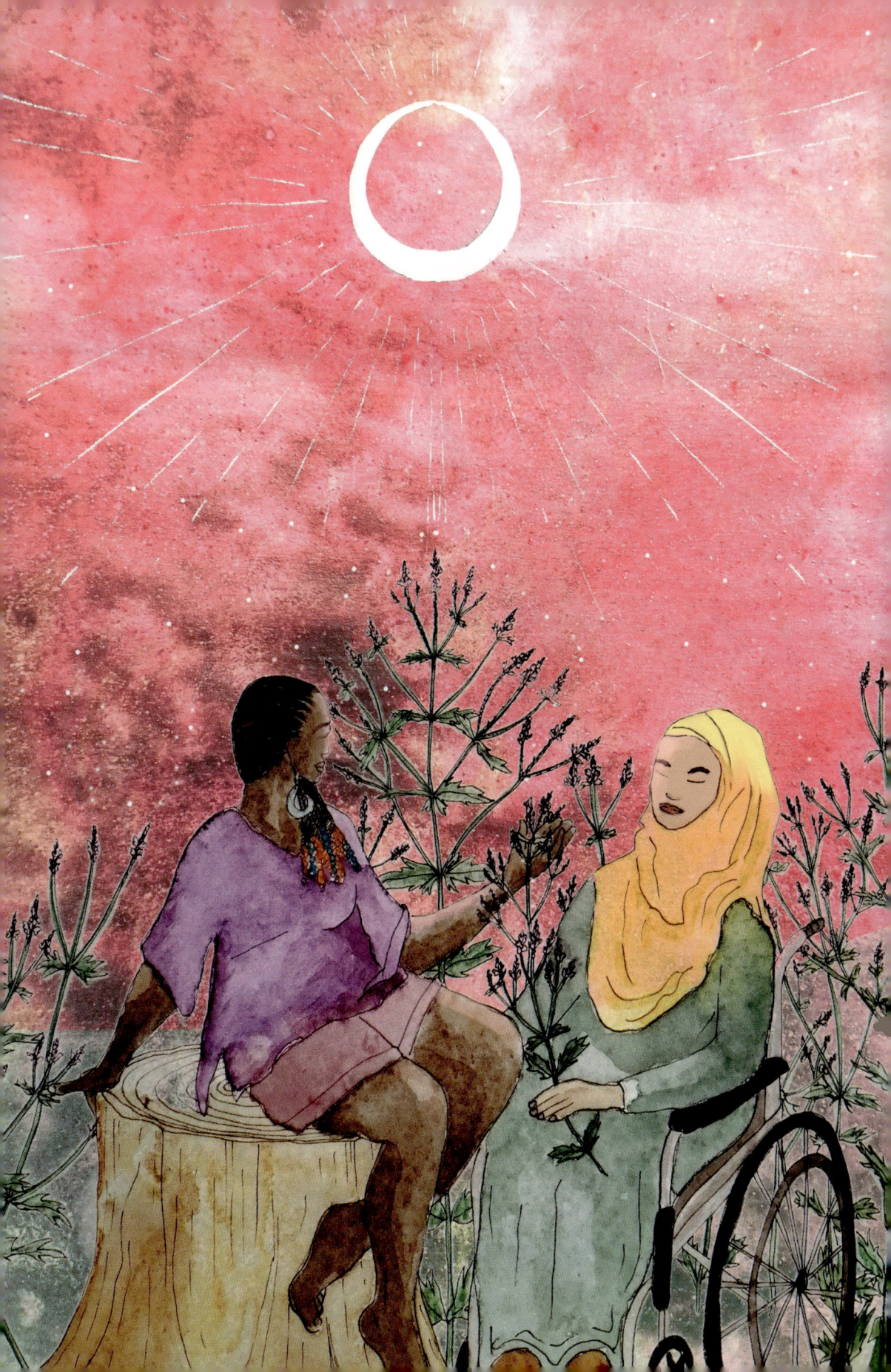

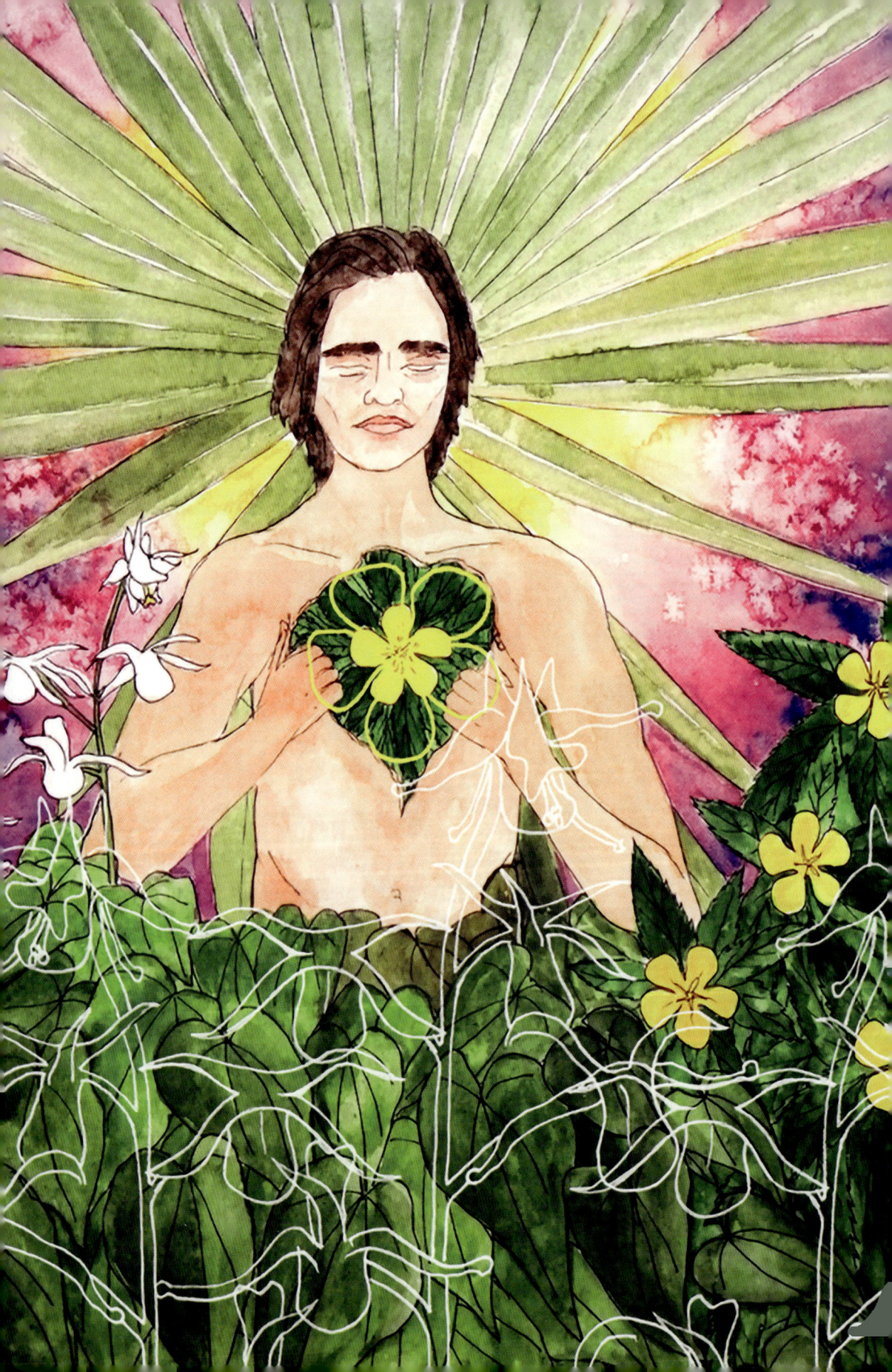

CHAPTER 8

BLOOM: MEN

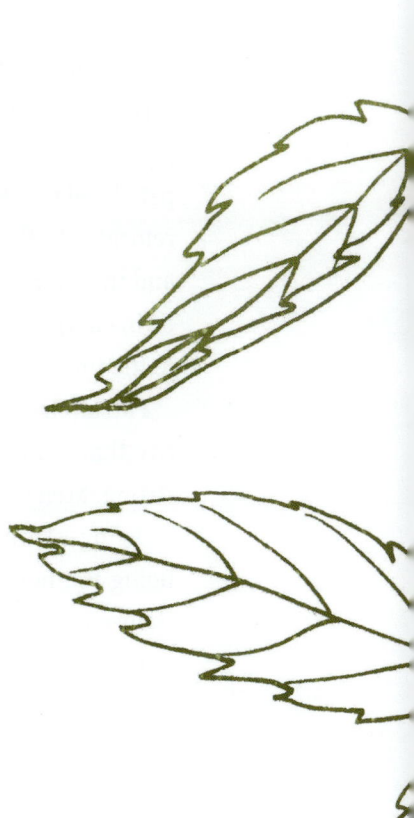

If there is a paradise on earth,
It is this, it is this, it is this.

Amir Khusrau

A man with damiana, horny goatweed and saw palmetto

ENERGETICS AND ELEMENTS

Men denied access to their own feelings are men oppressed by the system that fails us all. Failed by the system, it is sadly consequential that men "fail" others. Men commonly demonstrate anger, greed, and power as if it defines them, as if their authentic voices are denied. This is my understanding of the toxicity of patriarchal masculinity. These traits have been attributed to men in many ways – even in the attributes of plants: angry hurtful nettles are under the influence of Mars which is attributed male characteristics, for example. We are all, sadly, trapped in this system until it is broken down.

Plants actually have a lot to do with patriarchy, in a tragic sort of way. It seems that the hunter-gatherer society was fairly egalitarian and when agriculture (the growing of lots of plants to eat or as a resource) came along, patrilocalism began occurring and women began to lose their autonomy. A patrilocal residence is one where the woman leaves her own family or tribe and relocates to that of the male figure. Most families or tribes have strong bonds and the woman who has left loses that. The men, being stronger, also begin to be in charge as they defend the newly acquired resources that weren't "owned" in the time of hunting and gathering.

Patriarchy, however, doesn't benefit anyone. There is a false sense of security that comes with power and domination. Patriarchy requires men to be strong. Men then have to be strong. What happens if men aren't strong? What is being strong? Being angry? Being successful? Having kids? Leading? Being the boss? What happens if men cry? If men dance or sing sweetly or show emotion?

The adult male energetic picture is part of the turning of summer into autumn and again into winter, depending on what age you are and of course, your own constitution. In traditional Chinese medicine, the male aspect is considered yang with light, energy, heat, dryness, and the sun. It is worth remembering that relating to outside is considered a yang quality, and while subjective and open to interpretation, I think this connection for men, who are born under patriarchy, must be noted and embodied as it is a direct relationship with nature and that brings wonder.

Earth and autumn, which predominate in adult life, are calming and quiet and the male, yang, aspect may bring life, activity, and power. It may also bring domination, anger, and expectation. Patriarchal idols of maleness have dominated our understanding of men and with it comes much negativity. Through rewilding, careful tending, and sharing, the contemplative nature of autumn, and the predominance of earth energy, change may bring authentic understanding about true maleness and the essence of that meaning may rise once more.

Toxic masculinity affects everyone. To be brought up in a culture which makes boys think tenderness is shameful only ends in hurt, repression, misguided stoicism, and models we may never fulfil. While men can explore into this and find a better way by doing "the work", it is up to all of us to embrace change and challenge the system which maintains this structure. It is our job, as folk who serve, to try to bring authenticity and beauty to all and guide ourselves to a loving, caring community that will bring down the system as it stands.

Our brothers, especially young men, may be lonely, disconnected, addicted, and all too often, suicidal. Repression of feeling starts so young. "Boys don't cry" – boys are told this in the sweetest of ways as babies; "Don't cry darling," mamas and papas whisper, but at what cost? Feelings are moved into denial state and shut down.

To feel into tending of the self, listening quietly to the self while outside among trees or plants may be the first step on the long and worthwhile road to healthy masculinity.

Rewilding exercises

Unlearning in nature is a beautiful exercise. We have learned our roles, our habits, our thoughts and our behaviour. Spending time in nature unlearning is really helpful when trying to rewild ourselves, reconnect to our feelings and become more in tune with our natural habitat.

Go outside. Then just do what you normally do. After ten minutes, note what it is that you tend to do outside (if you consciously do new things, you'll probably notice that too). Next time you go on a walk, check through what it is you were doing in your notes and try to figure out why you do that. It could be touching all the plants, walking with your headphones on, humming, talking to people, not talking to people, eye contact, no eye contact, delighting in views, thinking a lot. Our actions every day give us clues as to what is going on for us inside.

The next time you go outside, see if you can allow yourself some softening – some softening of the way you move, the way you hold your body, your shoulders and jaw . . . the way you talk or think. Allow softness to reconnect you a little with the plants you can see, the air you can feel, and the soil underfoot.

At the end, wherever you end up, allow a few minute's gentle journaling or thinking through what called to you and a heart-nourishing minute of breathing quietly.

Repeat this kind of experience at least once a week if not all the time. See how it feels, see if something changes in you, see what you notice (birdsong, new plants, signs, litter, wonders . . .)

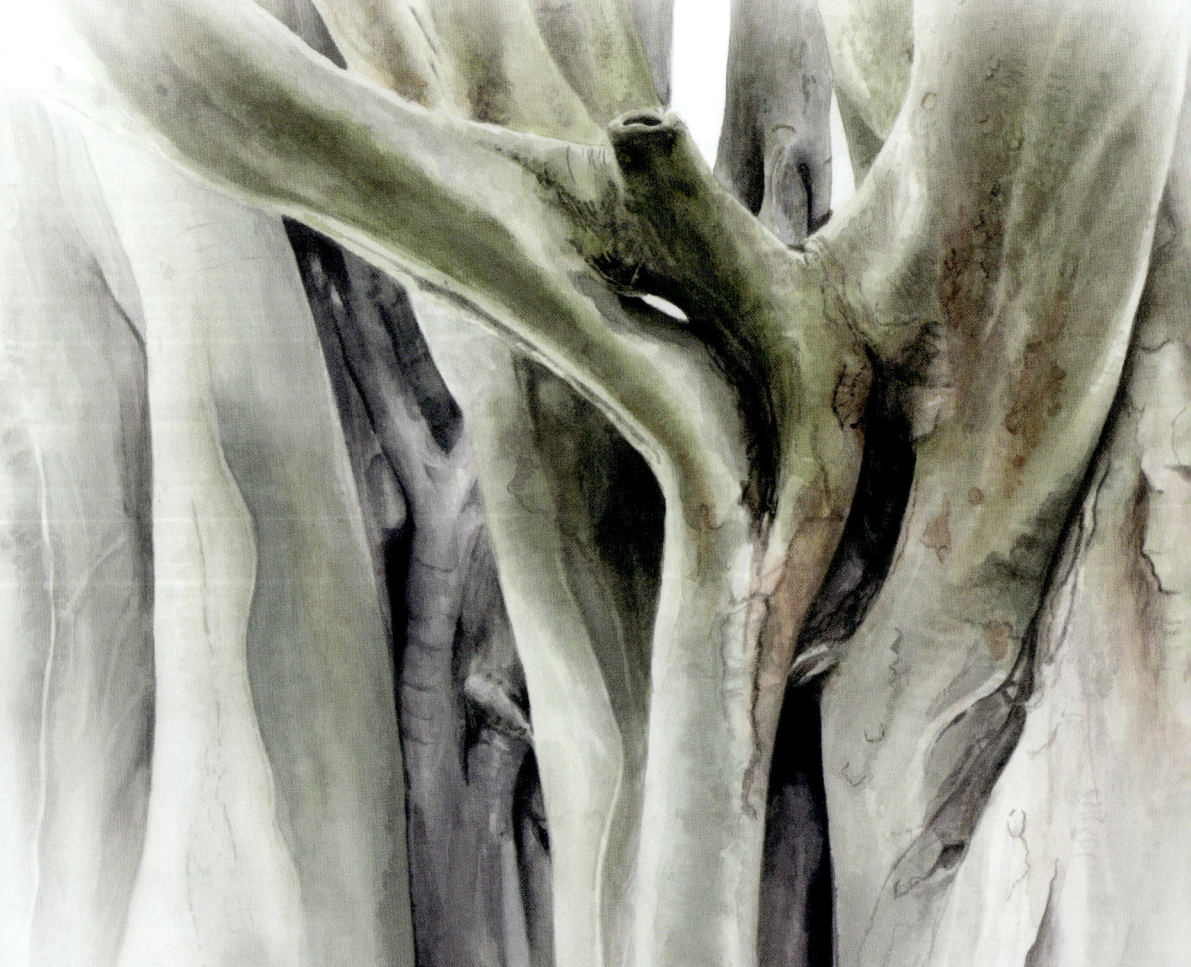

CONDITIONS

Male pattern baldness

This is characterised by a receding hair line and thinning hair which mostly affects men. The male sex hormone dihydrotestosterone (DHT) thickens the tendinous membrane at the crown of the head. This reduces blood flow to the scalp which means nutrients that usually reach the hair follicle aren't able to get there. Eventually the follicle shrinks and baldness occurs in those with the genetic trait. 90–95% of men who experience baldness have thickened membranes.

Elevated amounts of DHT are found in less hairy scalps, and the enzyme 5-α reductase which converts testosterone to DHT is found in high levels in hair follicles. When there is a lot of DHT it starts to bind with androgen receptors, thickening the scalp and eventually atrophying the hair follicles. This enzyme can actually be blocked and hence stop the path to hair follicle destruction.

Male pattern baldness is challenging for men who experience it. It can affect confidence, self-worth, and lifestyle choices so it is important that however a man's hair is growing, he tends to his heart. This is no mean feat – learning how to care for oneself and remain healthily positive in body image is hard when the ideals of success and beauty or strength are so strong in this society.

Plant allies

Herbs can help the hair follicles and hair growth by blocking 5-α reductase.

Saw palmetto is the main herb used to encourage hair growth associated with this kind of hair loss. It works by blocking the conversion of testosterone to DHT (which is similar to its role in BPH). It may also trigger the hair to regrow and allow time for the follicles to repair themselves – to what extent is dependent on the person.

Liquorice may also block the conversion to DHT and is very nourishing so will help stop the process of male pattern baldness and also aid the body in getting nutrient-rich blood to the follicles. Rosemary can act as a circulatory stimulant to the head thereby also assisting with nourishment and potential hair growth.

Benign prostastic hyperplasia (BPH)

The prostate is not a well understood gland but it is really important for folk to connect with their prostate and understand its function. The prostate is a small muscular gland, which is about 4cm wide, surrounding the urethra just below the bladder.

The main function of the prostate is to release the milky white protein liquid into the urethra when semen is released to help sperm on their journey through the vagina and womb. If male sex hormones decrease, the prostate atrophies. Even if there is no ejaculation, a little fluid is released from the prostate every day and is released through urination.

As men grow older, from around forty years old or more, testosterone declines and oestrogen and other hormones increase. This physiological phenomenon is sometimes referred to as the andropause. The prostate is oestrogen-sensitive so hyperplasia could be associated with increased levels of the unopposed hormone in later life and excessive testosterone in the prostate itself. When it is in the prostate, testosterone is converted to DHT which causes cells to multiply with eventual enlargement of the gland.

BPH is common and refers to the swelling of the prostate. When the prostate is enlarged – usually over a period of time – symptoms start to appear such as dribbling while urinating and low flow. Sexual intercourse and ejaculation can become painful and fertility challenges can arise. It is very individual – some men can have relatively huge enlargement and not notice it much, others can have a tiny amount of swelling with noticeable adverse effects.

There are three main stages of hyperplasia, the first being the thinning of the stream of urination. The second is difficulty emptying the bladder resulting in more frequent urination, and the third is bladder distension caused by the residual urine in the bladder. This can create pressure backing up to the kidneys and eventually kidney damage. Surgery is commonly recommended at this stage but lots can be done with herbs in the prior two stages.

Prostatitis is similar to BHP in that when the prostate inflames, it also enlarges so appears similar. However, in prostatitis infection can be present and inflammation can spread to the urethra and bladder. Aching is usually present as are many of the symptoms of BPH. Stress, poor dietary choices, and lack of exercise can contribute and infection can cause it.

There are quite a few lifestyle choices that can help, such as drinking lots of water, eating lightly, adding seeds into the diet, supplementing with nutrients if there are any deficiencies, hot and cold packs to the prostate area, Kegel exercises, and relaxation.

Plant allies

For prostate conditions, soothing herbs like demulcents are indicated if there is any discomfort. Anti-inflammatories and anti-infectives are needed for prostatitis, and for both BPH and prostatitis tonics, diuretics, and hormonal balancers may be indicated.

Saw palmetto berry and nettle root are often given in BPH. Saw palmetto is used with nettle root amongst other herbs to inhibit the pro-inflammatory enzyme 5-α reductase. They also inhibit the arachidonic acid pathways which are inflammatory and epithelial growth factors. The berry is anti-infective so in cases of prostatitis with infection it is a great choice. It has an antispasmodic effect and is also anti-inflammatory and acts like a lymphatic and diuretic reducing swelling.

Saw palmetto berry inhibits oestrogen so unopposed oestrogen decreases and therefore symptoms of BPH are less apparent as it improves. Nettle root and small-flowered willowherb (*Epilobium parviflorum*) also contain beta-sitosterol which reduces prostatic inflammation.

In Germany, the drug of choice for BPH is indeed nettle root while in the UK it remains relatively unknown. Lignans in nettle root attach to prostate membranes and alter the proliferation of cells causing enlargement which is excellent for reducing the swelling. Nettle roots are anti-inflammatory, anti-tumour, antiviral, and immune-modulating. The phytosterols, lignans, and polysaccharides present in the root reduce symptoms of BPH.

Nettle root helps normalise the function of T-helper lymphocytes and NKCs following stress; it also improves urinary flow. The root helps prevent aromatase to oestrogen conversion, thereby maintaining lower levels of unopposed oestrogen. The suppression of cell metabolism is encouraged through some of the constituents in nettle root and growth in the prostate is thereby inhibited. Nettle also has an inhibitory effect on the proliferation of HeLa cells and various viruses so it increases immunity.

Plant allies like cornsilk, couch grass, and dandelion leaf will help through a

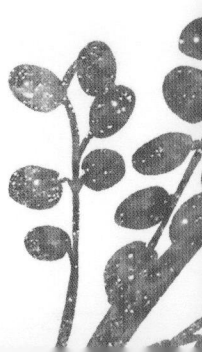

diuretic action reducing urine stagnancy and ensuing infection. Demulcents will soothe the tissue in the prostate and penis – cornsilk is an excellent choice for this.

Immune modulators include echinacea, bearberry, and oregon grape and will help support the body overall.

```
A BPH TONIC TINCTURE (SEE A HERBALIST FOR
PROPER USAGE)
Saw palmetto                    2 parts (eg 50ml)
Nettle root                     2 parts (eg 50ml)
Small flowering willow herb     2 parts (eg 50ml)
Meadowsweet                     2 parts (eg 50ml)
Cramp bark                      1 part  (eg 25ml)
Bearberry                       1 part  (eg 25ml)

Up to 5ml three times daily with water before food.
```

Orchitis

Swelling of the testicles is called orchitis. The testicles can become inflamed, painful, and feel heavy; swelling can be accompanied by fever. Symptoms may last around ten days, and it is possible for the testicles to atrophy which could lead to fertility issues but this is uncommon.

Ice packs are useful, as is treating an infection such as mumps which can cause the condition.

Plant allies

Dong quai is indicated here with its tonic effect on the reproductive organs alongside cramp bark and chamomile to relax the area.

Anti-infectives and febrifuges can also be used depending on the presentation of the illness. Yarrow, elderflower, and peppermint tea can be drunk liberally at the first sign of fever, and other anti-infectives like echinacea and boneset can be used.

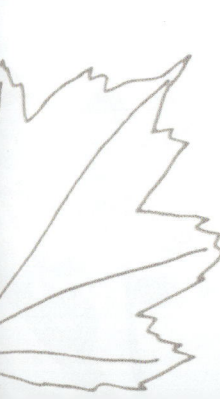

Prostate and saw palmetto

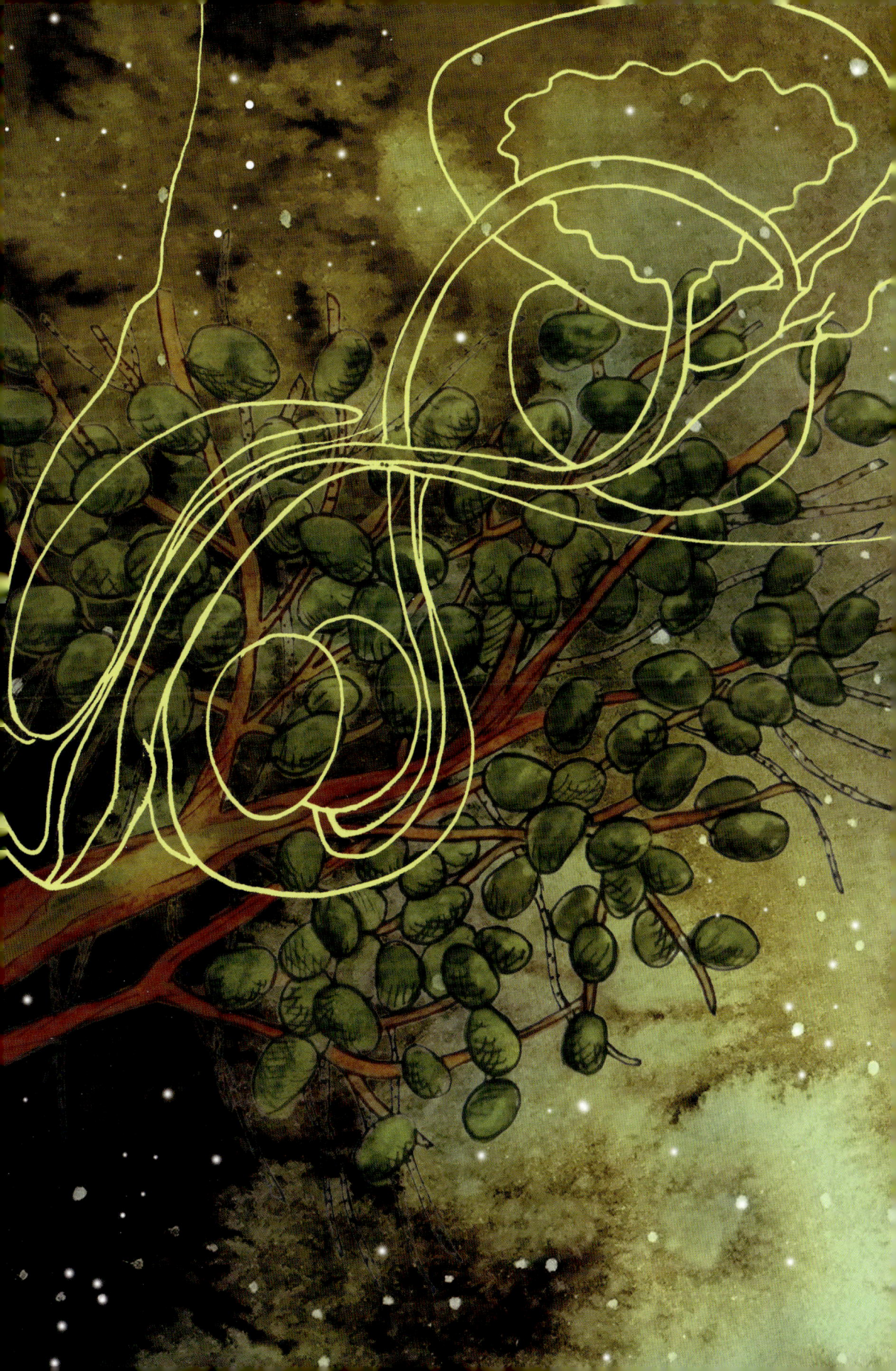

Circumcision

While this isn't a condition as such, it is a controversial procedure that affects millions of those born with male genitalia. There are a multitude of reasons given for circumcising babies, from cleanliness to fitting in, to preventing masturbation, to stopping disease spreading – though religious reasons are most commonly cited.

The penis can be affected physically following circumcision – sensation is lost, difficulty urinating or ejaculating may occur, deformation may ensue and sex can become more difficult, painful, or awkward, and emotional trauma can develop.

Furthermore, and in some ways more importantly in my opinion, when young children are cut against their will for reasons that aren't medically necessary, their sense of safety may be affected well into adulthood, or all of their life.

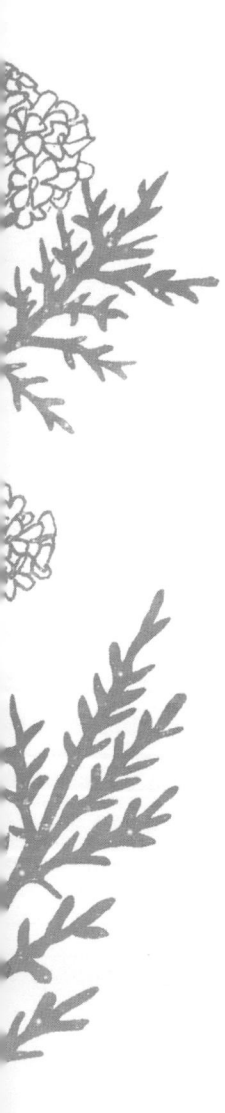

When I have talked with some men who have been circumcised and their penises affected, they carry with them sadness, hurt, anger, resentment, and bewilderment. Let alone shame at being different, deformed, or less sensitive, these are not emotions that anyone needs to feel and they stem from this culture of circumcision which is absolutely unnecessary, unless for medical reasons. One in five boys around the world has experienced circumcision.

"I feel anger rising – anger at the system that intimidated my parents to proceed with this senseless and risky mutilation. I feel indignant displeasure . . . at the collusion of the physicians and my trusting ill-informed parents who made that decision for me, abusing my rights and destroying my birth right with irreversible genital surgery," explains James Green in his book *The Male Herbal*.

In the UK there is a much lower incidence of circumcision than in, for example, North America – fewer than 10% of men are circumcised. In the USA it is more like 60% of men. In Judaism and Islam, babies are circumcised as dictated by their Holy word, male babies are circumcised as an initiation rite and a sign of their loyalty to the faith. While I would never want to offend anyone who is circumcised or their faith, I feel circumcised men often don't know who to talk to or how to share their pain.

There are complications each year – it is estimated that just under 0.5% of circumcisions result in some kind of impairment after the procedure (El Bcheraoui *et al.*, 2014). There are an estimated 2.6 million babies circumcised each year in the United States – it's possible that around 104,000 of them will suffer some form of impairment afterwards. That's a huge amount. Sadly folk will suffer from circumcision like any other invasive procedure. While being part of a faith, community, religion, or culture is really important and often the most beautiful experience, if there are problems such as complications from circumcision, tending to our folk is of utmost importance and care must be acknowledged in that community or religion and given to all.

Reference: Rates of adverse events associated with male circumcision in U.S. medical settings 2001-2010. El Bcheraoui et al., 2014.

Plant allies

While there is nothing herbalism can do to reverse the procedure, there are herbs which can help physiologically by soothing tissue and helping stretch the skin should that be required through softening and strengthening. There are herbs which can help with any infections following the procedure and of course there are plant allies which tune in to the pain and suffering that men have undergone or are experiencing at any time of life.

Self-care cream could include lavender, marigold, rose, and rosehip as a gentle moisturising cream that can be used if stretching the skin is needed.

If there is shame or lack of self-confidence associated with circumcision, herbs like damiana, rose, ginseng, and liquorice may well bring healing and vitality. See "Erectile 'dysfunction'" for further information.

The key here is to accept yourself in your form and go gently with care, tending to your whole self.

Rewilding visualisation

If you feel shame or embarrassment around your penis or perhaps pride in your penis, it is worth trying to find an authentic healthy relationship with this part of your body for it is you. One way to do this is to imagine yourself as a child and wrap your arms around you as a little child and tend your younger self, you are so worthwhile and beautiful. That child doesn't deserve shame, or the loss of ego or pride, detracting from your wonder. Feel into that hug you give yourself and your child self. When ready, release your child and come back into your present being.

Imagine your own body, above the earth with roots going deep into new earth, a place of wonder and dreams, full of plants and birdsong and magic. What do you see? How do you feel? Seek out that which makes you feel nourished and good – is it green? Is it wild? Can you feel yourself in your wholeness? Allow the plants to nurture you, hold you. Is there shame in this beautiful world? Can you release any shame and watch it transform into butterflies or beauty? Allow yourself to know your worth and your beauty.

When ready, gently come back to your body, bring your roots up inside and know that they are always there ready to connect with the best of Mother Earth. When you feel strong or ready, come back into the present space in which you are, and rest a while with a good view or a cuppa.

Erectile "dysfunction"

This is a huge, emotionally charged condition and can affect an adult at any time. It is far more common, though, in later life and is commonly referred to as impotency which may cause feelings of unworthiness or a loss of self-confidence. Low self-esteem, feelings of inadequacy, and relationship to self must all be taken into account and tended when erectile "dysfunction" is present. Difficult relationships with a partner may also affect erection or ejaculation (often premature or absent).

Nerves and the state of the nervous system can have an effect on the ability of a man to produce a satisfactory erection. Stress can be a major player in erectile dysfunction and sympathetic dominance can have an effect on the whole body and affect erection. If adrenaline is relied upon too much because of chronic stress in all its positive and negative forms (anger, too much work, excitement, partying), no replenishment of the nervous system cycles occur and a state of chronic adrenal exhaustion or insufficiency occurs affecting vitality and life force.

Vitality within is needed to achieve erection and ejaculation. Lifestyle, emotional health, and worries or anxieties must be taken into account. There may be impotence in relationships (to other or self) or there may be other health issues that don't seem apparent at first. I don't like to use the term impotence as it implies a weakening, a loss of power, a losing of something, a lack of potency.

This is a physiological and/or emotional condition and even "dysfunction" doesn't hold enough positive imagery. There are causes of softening of the penis and that is really what we are looking to help the individual work with.

It's important to check liver function and circulation when any softening or loss of vitality is present. By aiding the liver and lessening hepatic congestion, the body is supported in doing all the clearance work it may be struggling with in cases of hormonal excess.

By increasing circulation, more blood can flood into the penis and erectile tissue when needed and help initiate and maintain erection. In fact, if it is a physical issue (as opposed to emotional block), it is most likely to be a circulatory issue in those over forty (ish) years and herbs that encourage blood flow and health are indicated.

Sexual stimulation is a complex process. When aroused, a message is sent to the brain by way of the central nervous system to the nonadrenergic and noncholanergic nerve cells in the penis. Nitric oxide is released from these cells near the blood vessels there and, along with the contractions of the veins and the relaxation (dilation) of the arterioles in the penis, increased blood pressure occurs which pools in the sinuses and creates the erection.

If the arteries aren't relaxed enough or relax slowly, the erection will not manifest properly. The erection begins to soften when the chemicals used to create the signals to stimulate erection start to break down, spurring new signalling. Herbs can prevent that breakdown of chemicals (cGMP) so that signalling for the softening of the erection does not occur so quickly. This is indeed how Viagra works (and that was a side effect of the drug which was first trialled for angina).

Plant allies

Damiana is a fantastic aphrodisiac with tonic and uplifting effects. Whilst it lifts low mood (due to feeling inadequate or similar) it is also a circulatory stimulant and may also mimic anabolism.

Ashwagandha has traditionally been used as an aphrodisiac and tonic herb increasing low vitality and life force. It strengthens the body and helps restore fertility and sexual health.

Ginkgo has a circulatory stimulant action on the body and supports peripheral vasodilation, thereby helping blood reach erectile tissue. Ginkgo

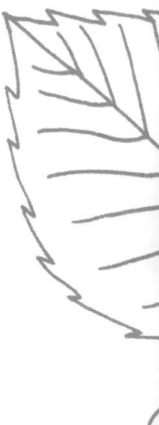

improves the nitric oxide pathway so blood can start to flood into the penis more easily.

Ginseng (Ren Shen) boosts energy and stamina and is traditionally an aphrodisiac and tonic herb. Ginsenosides support sexual function though kidney nourishment and, similarly to ginkgo, ginseng increases the levels of nitric oxide in the blood and also circulation. It strengthens the body and calms the spirit (shen).

Horny goat weed (*Epimedium brevicornum*) is a herb which exerts moderate androgenic effect on the testes and prostate and has been used traditionally to improve libido. It increases sperm production and stimulates sensory nerves. One of its flavonoids, like Viagra, inhibits the breakdown of cGMP thereby helping to maintain erection.

Milky oats and oat straw can be used to nourish the nervous system, especially if the impotence is accompanied by depression, anxiety, or low feelings.

Fertility

Fertility complications affect both men and women and are challenging for all involved. Around 20% of people experiencing difficulty with fertility are men. In terms of spermatogenesis, various factors can affect production and efficacy of spermatozoa, including low sperm count or maturation deficiency possibly caused by insufficient activity in the testes (hypogonadism) or low pituitary activity.

Low percentage of motile sperm or short-lived motility of sperm and low percentage of healthy sperm must also be evaluated. There may be obstruction causing difficulty in conception and other illnesses or conditions such as hypothyroidism, stress, anxiety, or low immunity can affect fertility. Temperature is also important – keeping the testes cool and avoiding tight, sweaty clothing and hot tubs may help.

Plant allies

Horny goat weed is a traditional herb for erectile dysfunction and helps increase sperm count, motility, and endurance as well as testosterone and sensory nerve sensitivity.

Ginseng (Ren Shen) – see "Erectile 'dysfunction'" above.

Saw palmetto is used in impotence and has tonic value. It is a strengthening herb which can nurture the reproductive system in both men and women.

Adaptogens including schisandra, ginseng, liquorice, sarsaparilla, and ashwagandha can all be beneficial for increasing vitality. This is key in erectile dysfunction.

Liver herbs such as mugwort, gentian, and yarrow are all bitters which have an affinity for the reproductive organs of both men and women. Liver herbs are needed to process hormones and toxins and to imbue the body with vital force. Stagnation can be cleared but it will always go through the liver at some point, so a healthy liver is vital.

Fleeceflower (He Shou Wu, or Fo-Ti) supports the kidneys and liver and increases sperm count and motility.

Schisandra has bitter elements which support the liver and balance hormones. It is also traditionally used for enhancing sperm production.

Maca is well-researched as a herb to increase sperm count and motility.

Hawthorn, ginger, and ginkgo will support the cardiovascular system.

A tonic with some of the above herbs may be the right herbs for a man but a consultation with a herbalist may be much more beneficial as the tonic can be tailored to suit each individual. Herbs that boost vitality, encourage blood flow, and ease anxiety are most needed.

TONIC FOR MEN (TINCTURE)

Saw palmetto	1 part	(eg 50ml)
Horny goat weed	1 part	(eg 50ml)
Ginkgo	1 part	(eg 50ml)
Ginseng	½ part	(eg 25ml)
Orange blossom	½ part	(eg 25ml)
Orange peel	½ part	(eg 25ml)
Prickly ash	½ part	(eg 25ml)
Cinnamon	½ part	(eg 25ml)
Rosemary	½ part	(eg 25ml)

5ml twice daily with water.

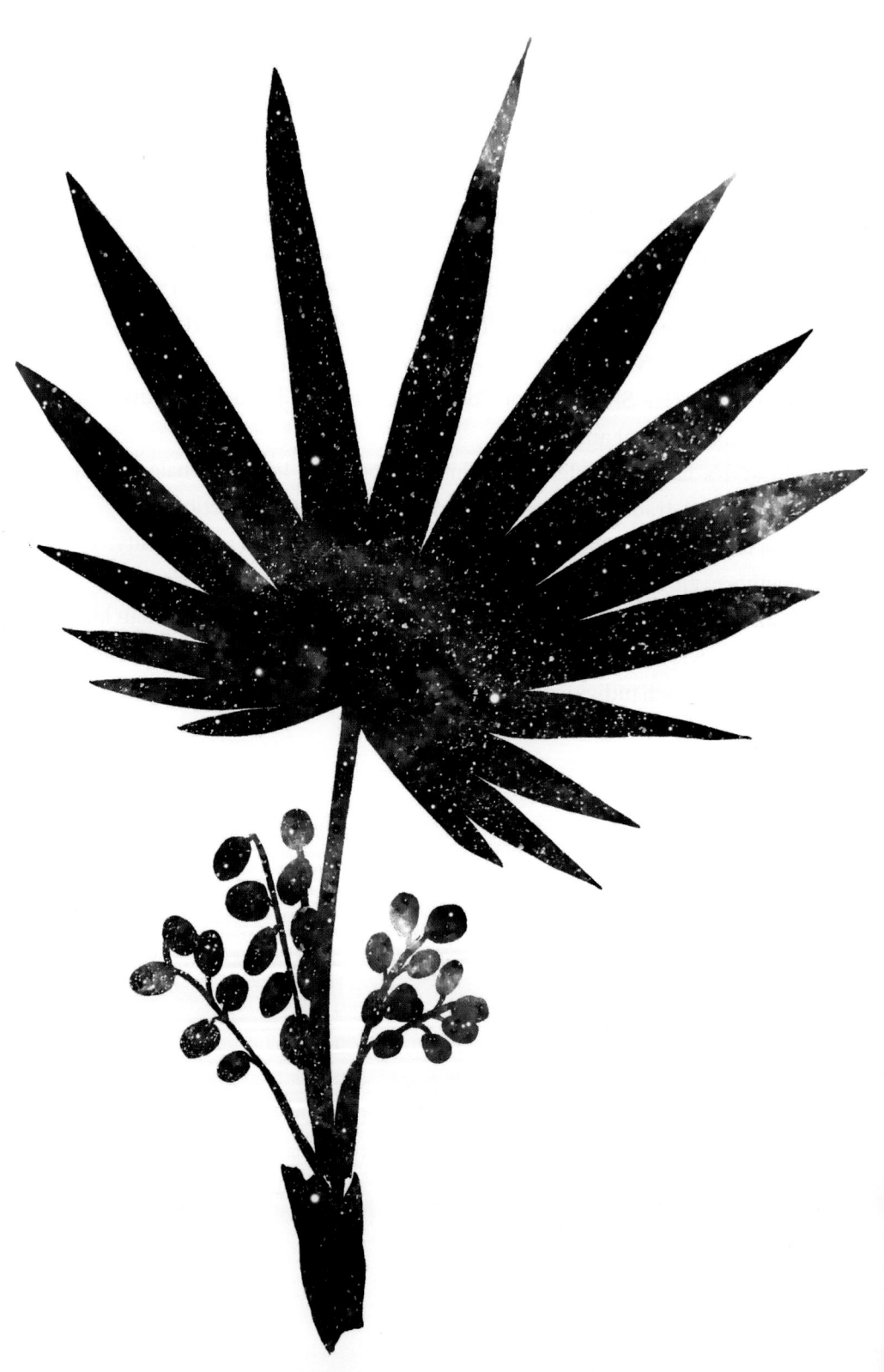

PLANT ALLIES FOR ALL MEN

Saw palmetto *Serenoa repens*

Nature: pungent, sweet, sour

Planet: Mercury

Saw palmetto is a nourishing tonic. It is sour in taste and pretty soapy but so important. The berry can be drunk as a tea or decoction and I often give it as tincture to those (men and women) with hair loss or perceived thinning and as a tonic, nutritive, and hormone influencer when needed.

It is often used for low libido, low sperm count, and, as described above, erectile dysfunction, and as a tonic for the reproductive system. It is used alongside nettle root for BPH and relieves pain or aching, improves the flow of urine (which becomes dribbly or intermittent), and has a direct effect on the size of the prostate. Along with nettle root it inhibits 5-α reductase, inflammatory arachidonic acid metabolites, and epithelial growth factors.

It is a great herb for genital and urinary infections and can be combined with herbs like bearberry and cornsilk.

It is not just a male herb but can be used in men and women alike for cystic acne and delayed puberty.

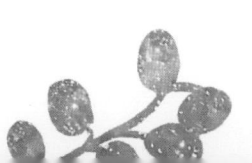

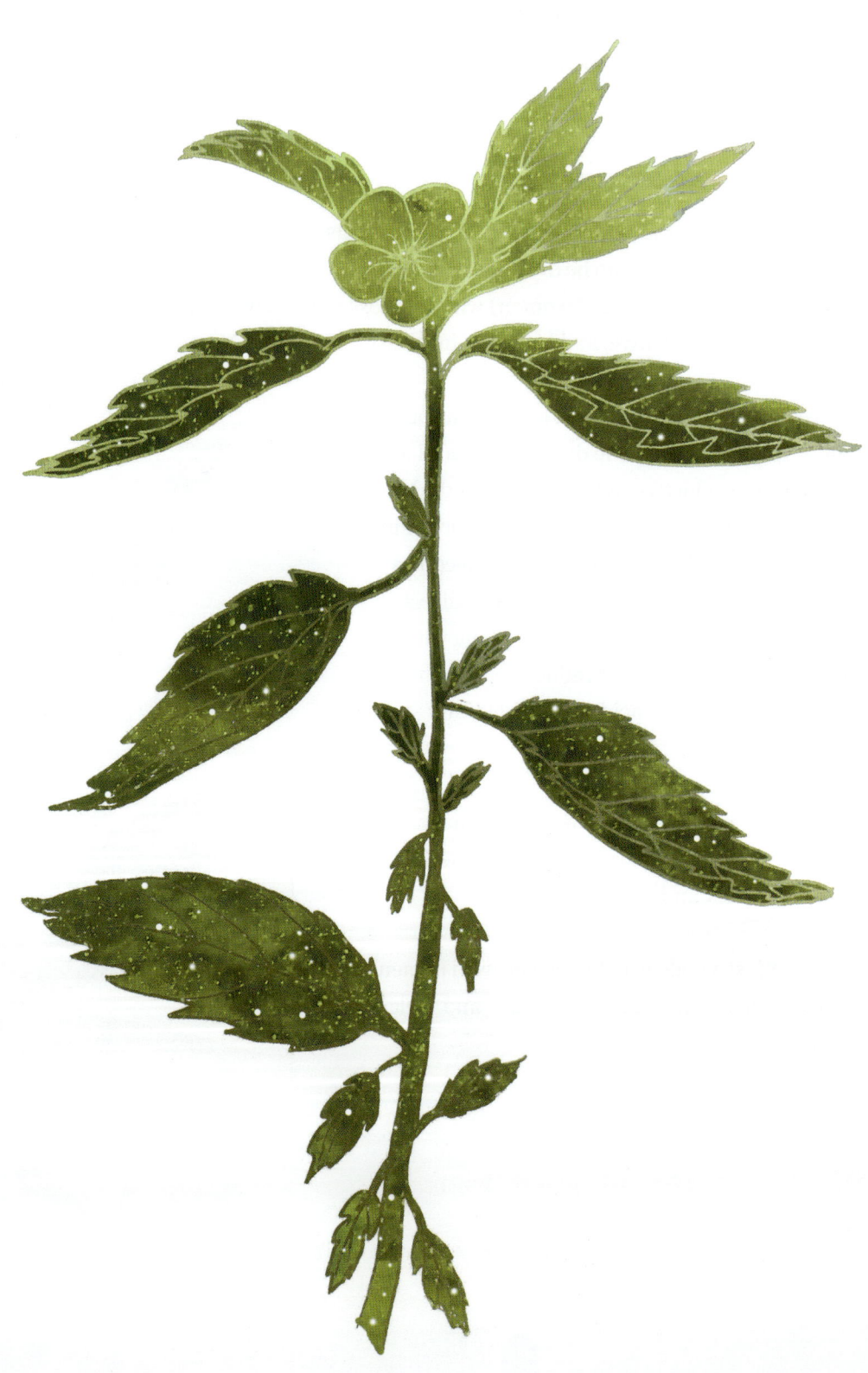

Damiana *Turnera diffusa*

Nature: warm, aromatic, dry

Planet: Venus

This herb has a fantastic reputation as an aphrodisiac. It is an incredibly aromatic plant, the aerial parts being used for medicine and is great as tea or tincture. It is a sexy tonic herb that seems to dance its way into aiding any difficulty in having or maintaining erection, to break through what might be affecting the man, or anyone experiencing low libido or self-doubt in their sexuality.

For men it is useful in orchitis, erectile dysfunction, lack of orgasms, and tension. It is a wonderful nervous tonic, relaxes physical and emotional tension, and alleviates spasm. It is useful in genito-urinary disorders as it soothes the urinary tract and works as a diuretic. It will also help with bed-wetting as it strengthens musculature.

For women, damiana is also used in menstrual and menopausal conditions and in conditions where fertility is challenged.

As a relaxant, it is helpful in respiratory conditions, drying excess phlegm, soothing coughs, and aiding asthma.

As a nourishing tonic herb, damiana is very uplifting and is used for anxiety and depression. This kind of action is really helpful in challenging conditions that affect our confidence and vitality.

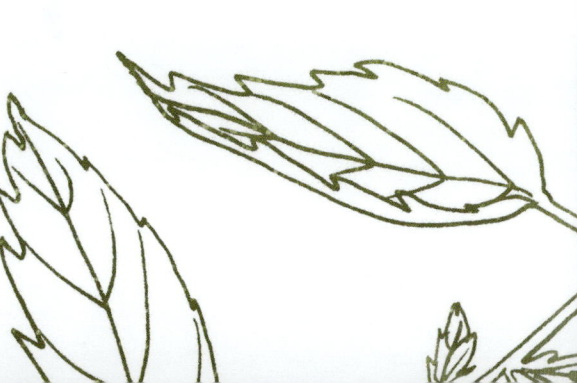

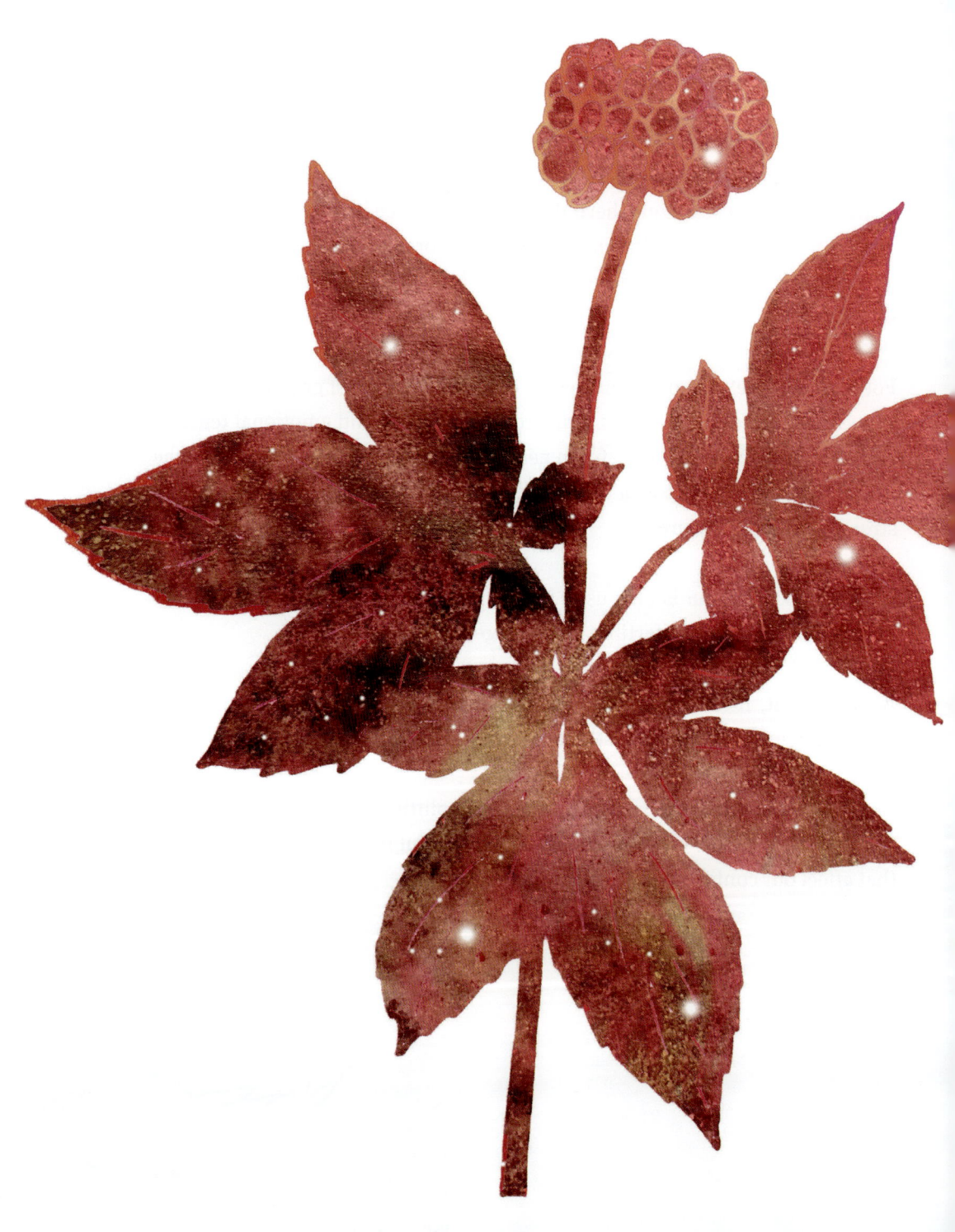

Ginseng Ren Shen *Panax Ginseng*

Nature: slightly cooling, sweet

Planet: Jupiter

Ginseng is warming, sweet and a little bitter, it is famed throughout the world for its tonic effect, bringing up vitality and life force. As an adaptogen it is beneficial for the adrenals and hormonal balance within the body.

If the body is cold, deficient, sluggish or tired, ginseng in small doses is a wonderful herb as it stimulates the cardiovascular system and increases corticosterone in the blood. In China, it is used in trauma to bring a patient's pulses up, usually alongside herbs like schisandra. It is used for convalescence and also helps protect the liver which is very much needed where fatigue is present. Ginseng aids and strengthens the heart, lowers hypertension and improves intramuscular oxygen use which reduces muscle fatigue. Its help in erectility is thought to be due to its influence on lowering higher levels of prolactin, this also means it is also helpful for menstrual imbalances.

It is a fantastic immune booster, helping the body remain resilient when challenged. As an immunomodulator it stimulates the activity and production of T-lymphocytes and interferon. Ginseng helps mental acuity and focus through its effect on cognitive function. It is lovely for pulling the self together, choosing what to focus on for nourishing yourself and softening the worries of spirit. It allows wisdom to come to he who seeks it. It is, however, used so much that ethical supplies must be found.

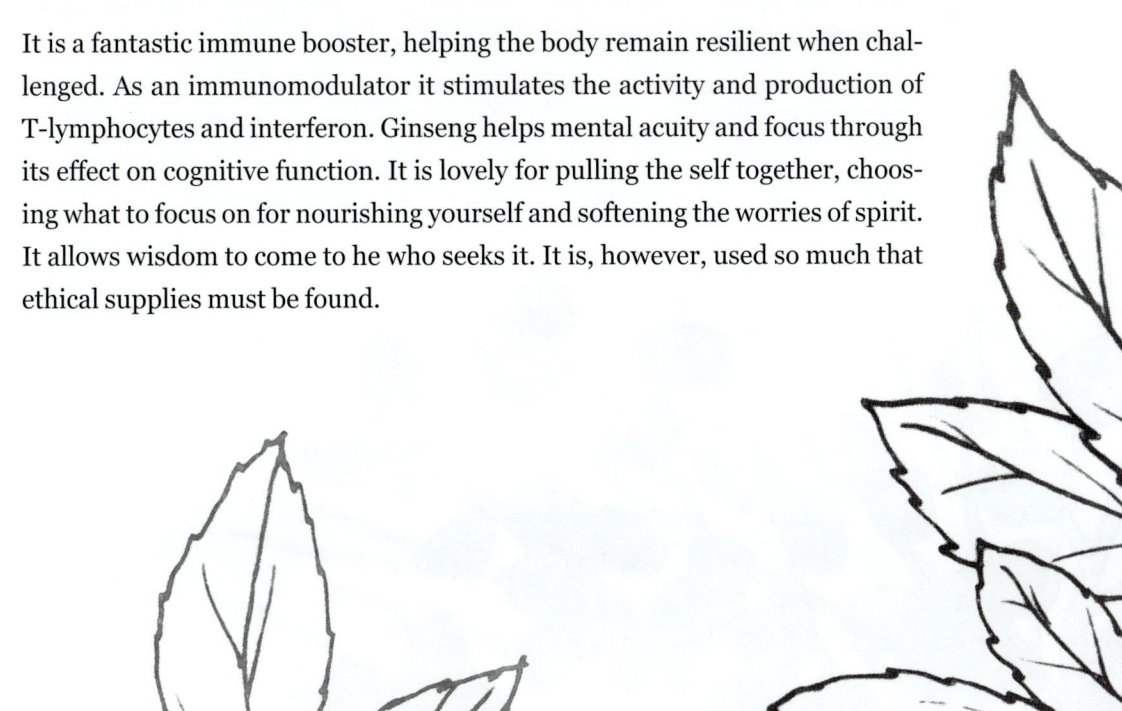

JOURNALING

In addition to journaling your unlearning experiences, take some time to write about new plants you see – note down where they are and if you don't know what they are, write notes to describe them. It is really nice after you have built up a relationship with them to find out what they are, but not before! For example, I might note down three plants in the cracks of the walls between my house and the local shop. I might stay a while with the first, make notes, draw it, and generally listen to anything that comes to mind when I am near this plant.

Once I have a body of work about this plant, I may notice characteristics which tell me it's a mint family or umbel and I may have seen its growth cycle. On identifying it I may learn new things or I may realise that I knew quite a lot about the plant. Keep plant notes as you discover more plants or learn more about the ones you already know.

Another aspect of journaling may be to do with your own role in life and how you feel about the life you find yourself living. As you start to spend more time being mindful in nature, notice how it changes you. Journal after plant communication or walks or time spent outside. See how it makes you feel. Notice what comes up and what doesn't – whether you feel negative or positive, grief or joy. If we notice what nourishes us, we can make changes that enable us to live life in a more nurturing and fulfilled way.

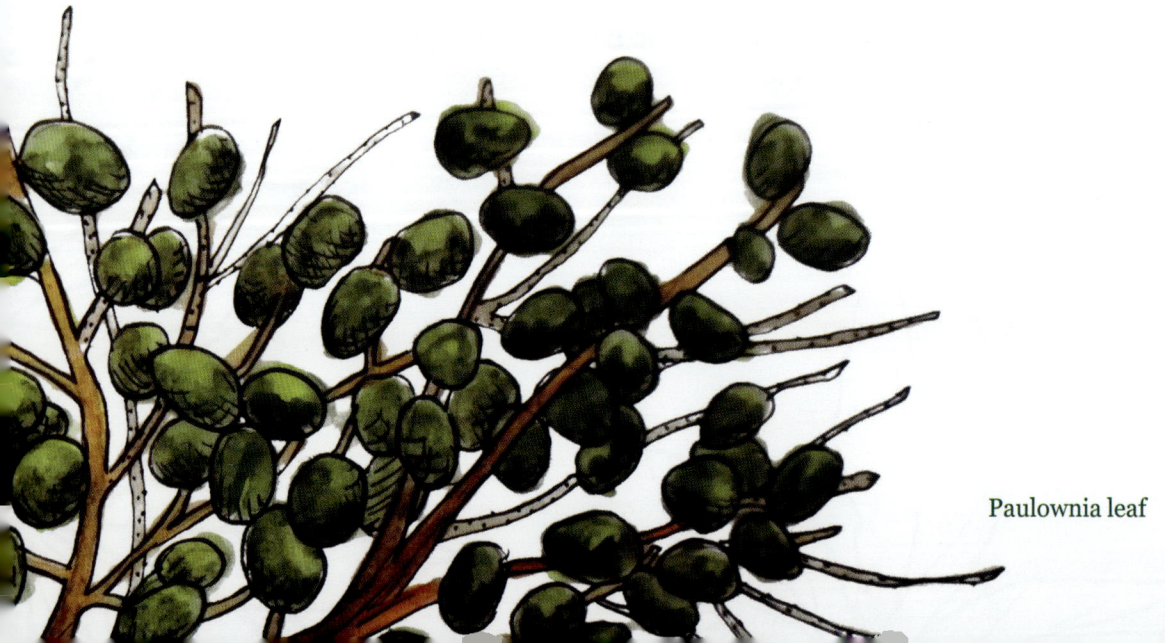

Paulownia leaf

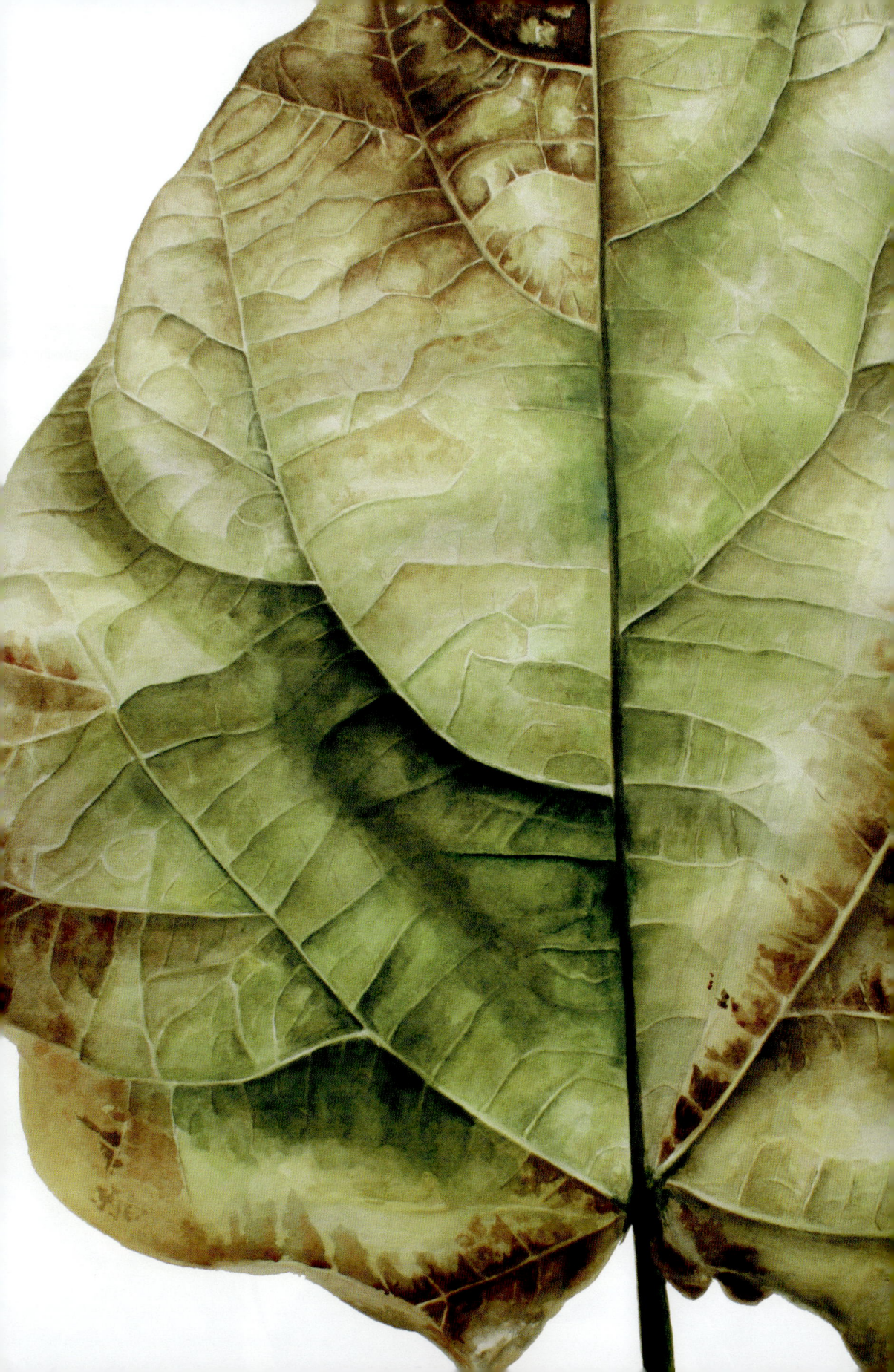

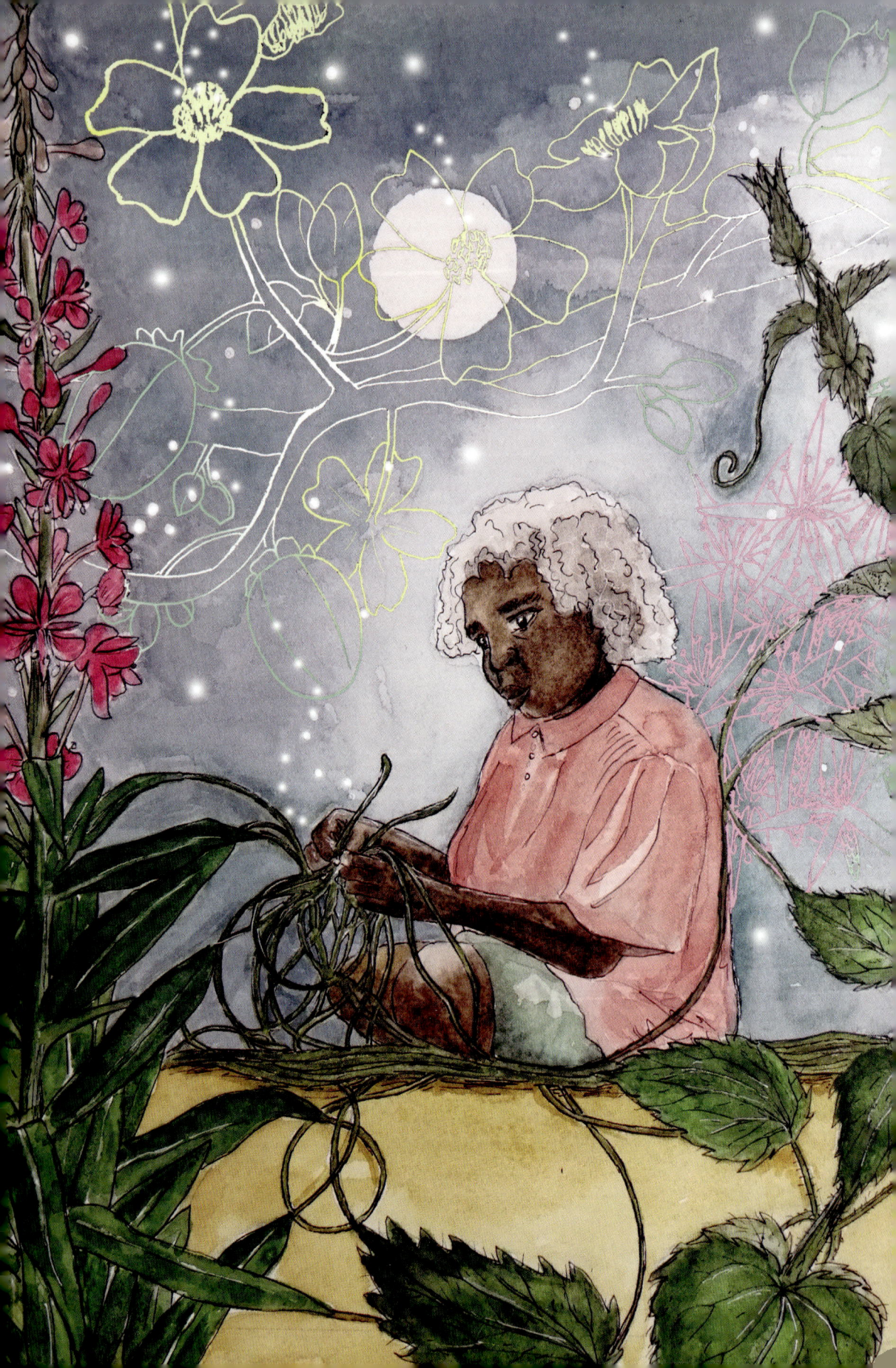

CHAPTER 9

PLANT KIN: WISDOM OF ELDERS

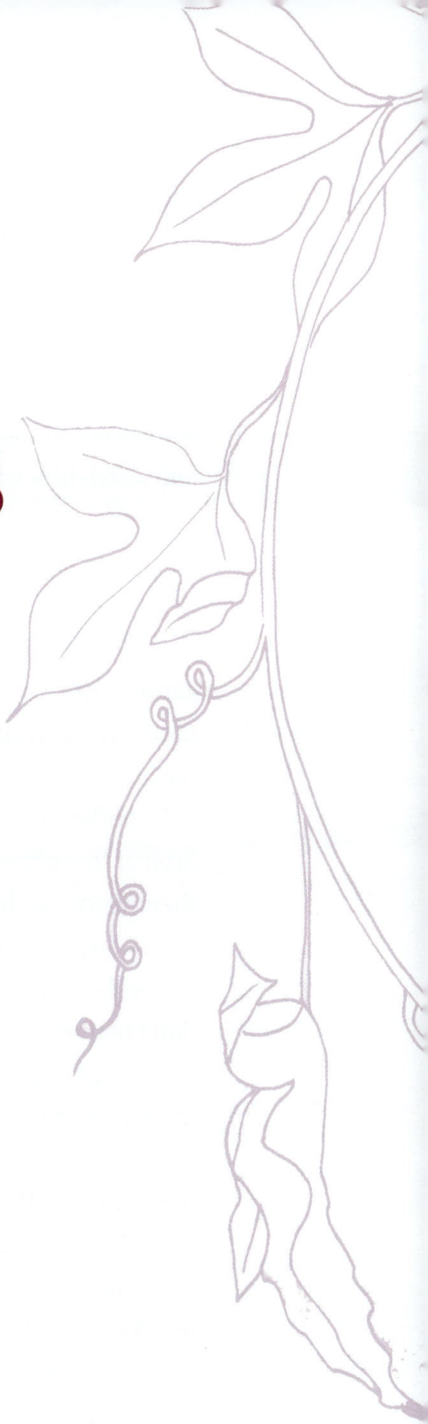

And don't think the garden loses its ectasy in winter
It's quiet, but the roots are down there riotous.

Rumi

An elder weaving plant allies and surrounded by kapok and turkeybush. Inspired by elders in the Kakadu lands. Nettle and rosebay willowherb are local to me and form the foreground. They are often made into fibre.

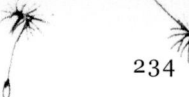

In so many cultures our elders are revered, cared for, and respected. Elders are folk with experience, wisdom, and wonder. All too often in our modern culture we push folk with these gems of life to the edges of society while we revere the youth and accomplished adult.

When I was a child, I would wander down my lane in the hope of being able to see old Tom who lived on the main road and had a little bench he would sometimes sit on. Once or twice I was lucky enough to join him on his bench and watch him whittle a stick and listen to him telling stories. One of his fingers was missing and would tell me how he used to bite his nails. He said that one day, he went too far and bit his whole finger off before he noticed and that his mother gave him a great telling off for it.

I believed that story for many years and cherished sitting out with him in the garden with my legs swinging from the bench. It was only years later that I figured out this couldn't be the case and he probably couldn't bring himself to tell me how it had really happened.

I wonder now, as I grow older, how much wisdom I could impart to my children or those around me, how many stories I could tell, and how I could protect them from the horrors of war or the goriness of accidents. I wonder who is able, now, to impart wisdom to me. I wonder who are my elders? I see the way we treat older women, and men to some extent, as if they don't exist, as if they don't matter.

I also see a generation of elders who haven't been guided in their growing up, in their growing wise, in their growing into leadership because the leadership role has been moved to the younger generation of successful adults. Those who have reached the pinnacle of individual success and have got the job, house, car, and kids. It makes me sad that the aspirations of youth in this culture stop in adulthood. I never once heard "I want to be a wise old woman when I grow up." Yet wise elders are precious beyond belief and are so very needed.

Elders in other societies have *become* an elder, they haven't grown old with a quiet life in mind. They have practised their roles and been guided by others so that they can step into a place of mentorship and responsibility. They have not, as we often witness in the West, been in isolation, unable to grow into this role. Community holds dear all those in it. Elders need us and we need them. So how do we look after our elders so they can look after us and guide us and we reciprocate care and respect? In terms of rewilding, many elders will know much more than I do, but I will share what I do know in fearlessness as this is something I am cultivating as I journey through adulthood.

ENERGETICS AND ELEMENTS
PHLEGMATIC TIME OF LIFE: WINTER

As we age, we enter the winter of our lives. We have passed through the spring of childhood, the fiery summer of youth, and the hard work of autumn adulthood and now seek to restore and nourish ourselves gently in the winter.

Burning of the oil, a metaphor for the body

My teacher used to say we can think of the body as an oil lamp. It begins by burning gently (childhood) and then brightly (youth and adulthood) but the flame starts to dim as the oil runs out and eventually extinguishes (elderhood and eventual death).

The body, like the lamp, becomes drier as we age and we need to keep this in mind as we nourish ourselves at different stages of life. Elders are generally a little drier or weaker – this is noticeable in the skin, the bones, the joints, the muscles, the digestive fire, and the spirit. Softening, calming, grounding are all traits of elderhood and winter.

Elders generally need building up and strengthening as the body slows and the pace of life changes for many. Vitality begins to reduce and healing capability slows down. Care and tending take a different role as gentle nourishing becomes key rather than the high activity of younger years.

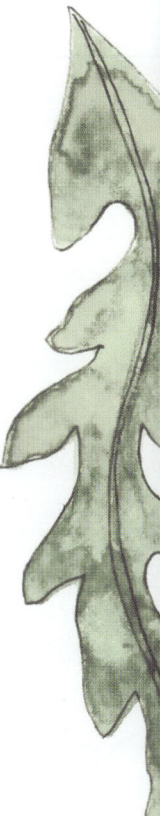

> ### Rewilding exercise
>
> Rewilding exercises for the elderly include a range of gentle activities. As the body is slowing down so the level of understanding and wisdom deepens for many. There are many exercises that can help elders connect or reconnect with the wild.

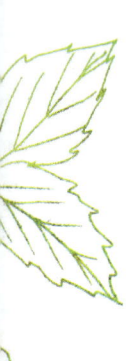

Exercise: a sensory walk

Take the time for a walk on three different mornings at around the same time of day. These walks could be as long or as short as you like but around five minutes to twenty minutes might be a good start. On all of the walks try to empty your mind of anything from your daily life and focus on your walk.

For the first of the three walks try concentrating only on your sight (vision). See the plants, gates, clumps, horizon. Notice what you are seeing and what you are drawn to. Take note of the shapes created by the positive matter (eg. a branch) and the negative (eg. the shape created between a few branches). Try to use only your sight to interpret what is around you.

At the end of the walk, see what feelings come up for you as you notice and observe what is in your path. Notice anything that you were interested in or anything new that you might not have taken note of before. Or journal any experiences you felt.

For the second walk, repeat how you approached the first one but instead of using sight, try to focus on listening. Tune into your hearing. You may need to close your eyes for parts of the walk just to minimise the sensory overload that can come through our sight.

After your walk make notes of what you heard, how it felt, and what it may or may not have brought up for you.

On the third walk, use your sense of touch to feel your way through the walk. Touching with your hands but also with your feet, skin, and body. Try to notice the tactile sensory input as you walk along. Slow down, speed up, see how this changes your understanding of the landscape through touch.

Once again, at the end of the walk note down any feelings that were elicited and how you found the experience.

At the end of the three days, you might choose to do another walk using your sense of smell. You can smell the earth, the leaves, the bark, the air

PLANT KIN: WISDOM OF ELDERS

from afar or close up. Again notice what happens to you, how you feel afterwards and the experience as a whole.

Then take a little time to think about the three (or four) walks – see what you enjoyed, what you noticed about the walk each time or overall, how you feel now compared with then, whether you want to do more of the same, whether you were able to focus or not.

Often doing exercises like this a few times, or many times, enables a gradual build-up of understanding of the land on which you walk.

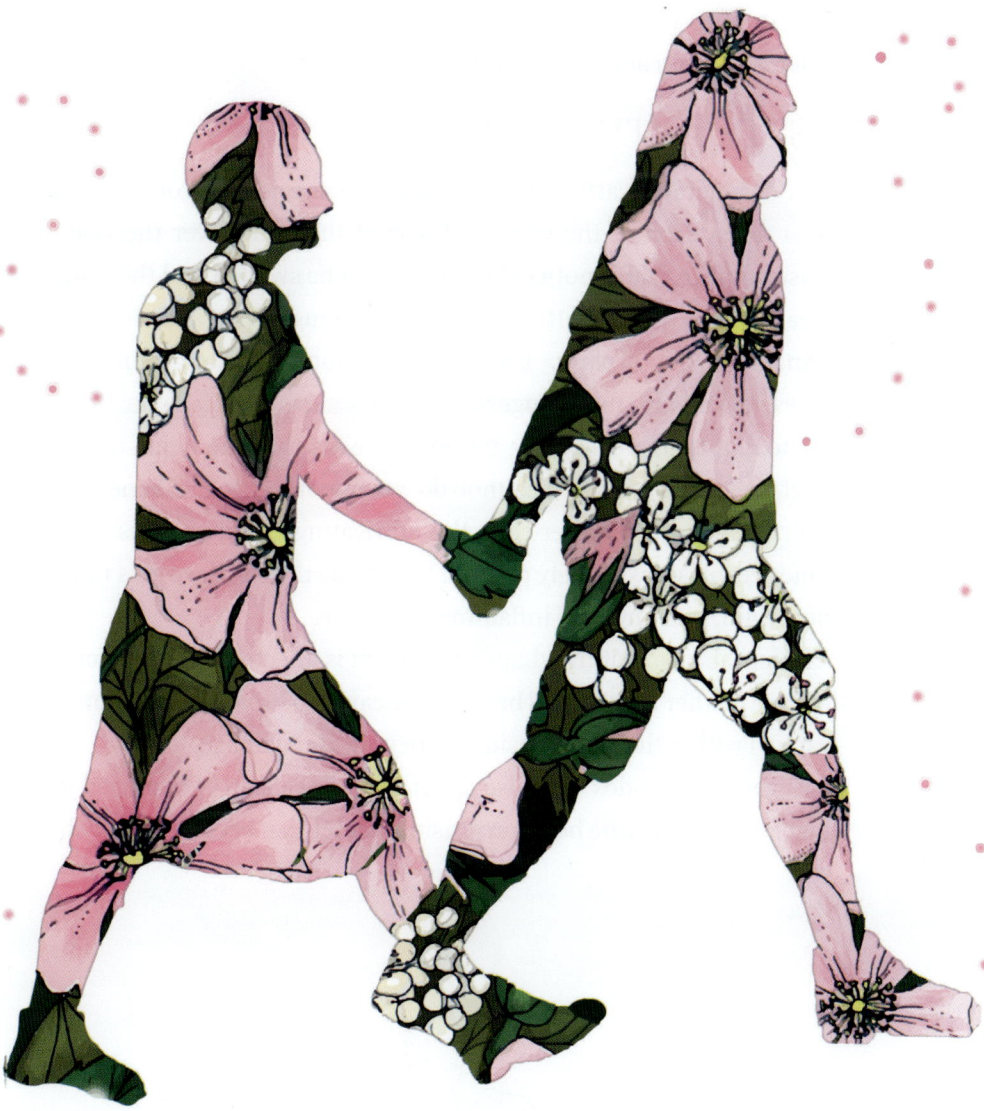

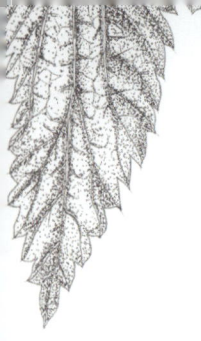

CONDITIONS

ARTHRITIS

There are many different conditions which fall under the term arthritis. Arthritis actually means inflammation in a joint. Generally, when elderly folk refer to their arthritis they are talking about rheumatism or osteoarthritis. Either way there will be pain, stiffness, and swelling in the joints, muscles, or tendons around the articulations.

Rheum is the watery liquid that drips from the eyes and nose; it is an old word for phlegm and rheumatism is a classic phlegmatic condition, thought by many to be caused by an excess of secretions in the body, leading to a damp constitution. Rheumatic conditions are considered a connective tissue disorder which can also be autoimmune in nature.

OSTEOARTHRITIS

This degenerative arthropathy (disease of the joints) commonly affects the older generation as the wear and tear of the joints over the years begins to cause damage that is noticeable. Joints can be swollen and there may be a loss of cartilage in the joint. It may also affect younger men and older women more than their counterparts. The most commonly affected joints are the hips, knees, lower back, neck, fingers.

The damaged cartilage in the joint means that the bones which normally meet and glide together cannot do so smoothly as the bones begin to rub against each other rather than the lubricating cartilage. This may be almost unnoticeable or extremely painful. With time the cartilage gets more worn and more pain, swelling, and inflammation occur.

It may also be that the shape of the joint is affected as bony spurs grow. This leads to further pain. Small bits of bone can also break off the joints and remain trapped within the joint causing more pain and damage.

Herberden's nodes may also appear and are a sign of damaged joints in the fingers. They are little bony protrusions which can become noticeable.

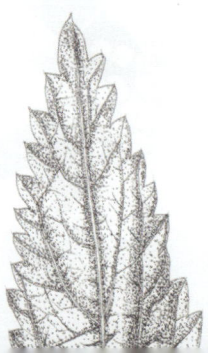

DIET AND LIFESTYLE

As in any inflammatory condition it is important to minimise inflammatory foods which can exacerbate the condition. Oily foods are great not only for arthritis but for elders, and in fact everyone. Tins of sardines (not in sunflower oil) can be really useful as they are high in fatty acids, especially Omega-3, and can be stored easily.

Gentle exercise keeps the circulation and lymph flowing which helps ease swelling and encourages the removal of toxins. Swimming or very gentle seated yoga or Pilates may be tolerated by those with pain.

Nature-bathing can be very beneficial. Gentle walks or even sitting on a bench among trees can encourage positive feelings and well-being. Mental and emotional health always needs tending where there is pain or chronic illness and time in nature is a good strategy to maintain well-being in this respect.

Hydrotherapy – using hot and cold water treatment can be useful in cases of inflammation, fatigue, and muscular soreness. A simple version of hydrotherapy involves having a hot shower followed by a cold one – particularly on the crown, spine, underarms, and chest. Try it and see how you feel.

Anti-inflammatory bath

Bathing in herbs is a lovely way to get them into the body. You can literally pop the herbs in the water – the only issue is catching the herb when the bath plug is pulled. I like to make a really strong brew – either an overnight infusion or just a good strong tea and pour a teapot of it into the bath just before getting in.

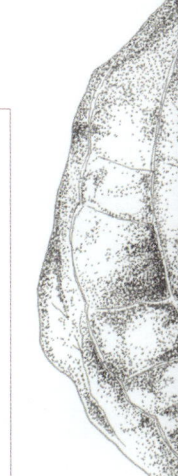

```
AN EXAMPLE OF AN ANTI-INFLAMMATORY BATH
Plantain
Nettle
Calendula
Meadowsweet

In equal parts. Brew a strong pot of these dried or
fresh plant allies and add to bath.
```

Herbs for arthritis and rheumatism

We commonly use anti-inflammatories, alteratives, antispasmodics, and circulatory stimulants.

Anti-inflammatories can halt the pathway of destruction to some extent and lessen the inflammation and pain. Salicylate-containing herbs reduce inflammation and are commonly used. Plant allies – nettle, comfrey, meadowsweet, willow.

Alteratives are useful because they tend to the eliminative organs which maintain healthy blood and act on a cellular level restoring balance in the cell. Plant allies: dandelion, nettle, and burdock can be given for long periods – useful in chronic illness.

Antispasmodic herbs allow the muscles around the arthropathy to relax and take pressure off the inflamed area. Plant allies: black cohosh (see a herbalist), valerian, guelder rose.

Circulatory stimulants keep the blood moving, bring fresh nutrients to the joints, and aid lymphatic flow which removes toxins. They encourage heat to the affected area – useful for those who are cold in constitution or in those whose arthritis gets better in hotter climes. Plant allies: yarrow, ginger, cayenne, nettle, comfrey.

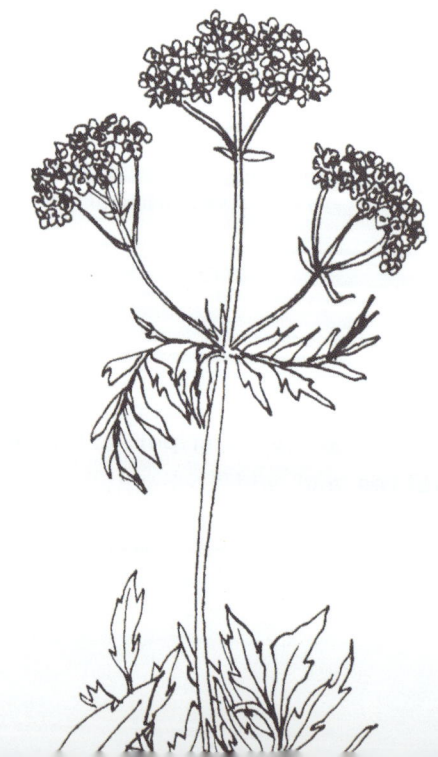

Recipes

```
RHEUMA TEA

Nettle          1 part
Marigold        1 part
Angelica        1 part
Ginger          ¼ part
Cardamom        ¼ part
Cinnamon        ⅛ part

Infuse 1-2 tsps of the herb in boiled water.
```

Comfrey leaf is an excellent anti-inflammatory. It is not used internally for chronic conditions by most herbalists anymore due to its pyrrolizidine alkaloid content which is higher in fast-growing parts of the plant.

An external preparation can still be made, especially of the root or older leaves which are slower growing. These can be foot soaks, creams or ointments (balms), or poultices. A "hot" comfrey balm is very comforting – made with cayenne, ginger, or pepper as potential additions.

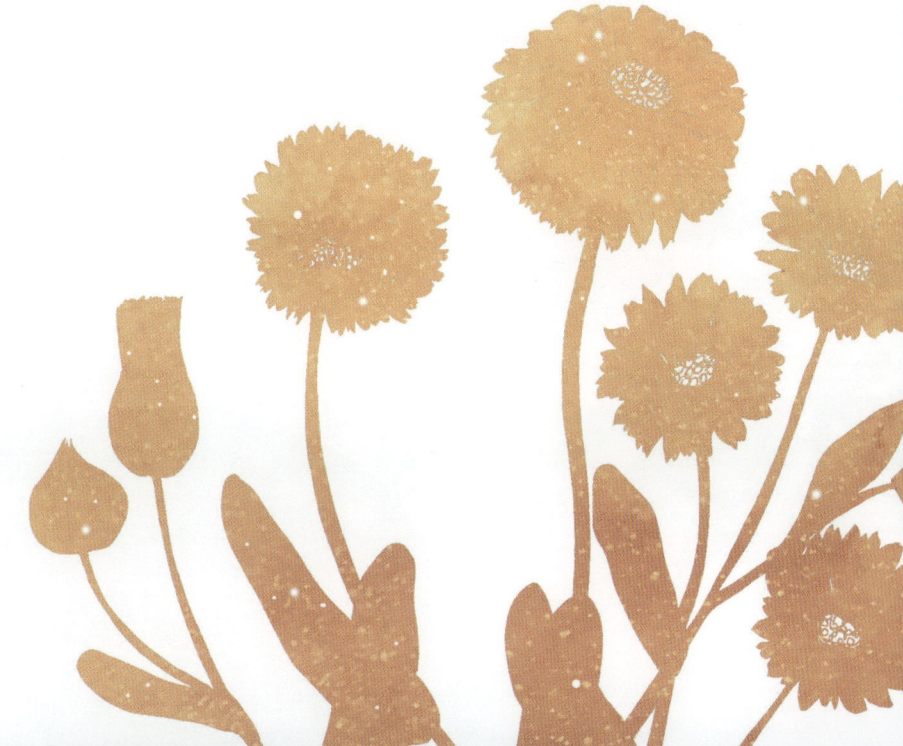

HOT COMFREY BALM

Make an ointment with comfrey infused olive oil (see Chapter 2). Just before you add the beeswax add 5 drops of each of these essential oils:

Wintergreen, ginger, clove, turmeric, black pepper, yarrow.

Stir in then add wax and pour into individual jars.

Leave to set.

Apply to aching joints or tender muscles daily.

To add cayenne to the balm you can infuse chillies (*Capsicum annuum* is the one commonly used) with the comfrey leaves, or you can mix a powder into the balm if absolutely dry. I often add tincture of cayenne (which is very strong!) by bubbling it gently through the oil or making a very similar cream of comfrey, cayenne, and the essential oils.

Do wash hands after use!

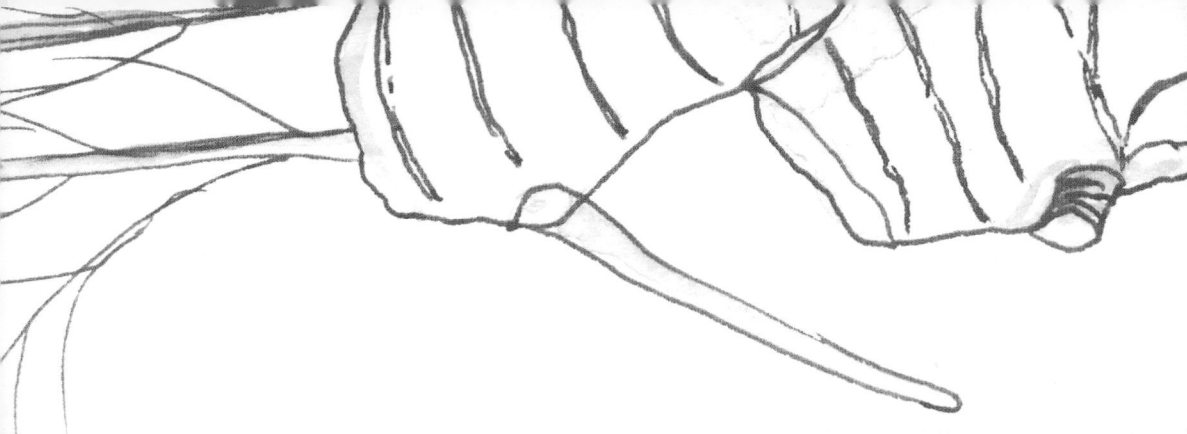

WILD HEAT BATH SALTS

Bath salts are wonderful in arthritis as the magnesium content helps the muscles relax and regain free movement. Dried herb or essential oils can be added to the salt and stored in an airtight container.

Take a half-litre jar of rock salt and a few drops of the essential oils of:

Wintergreen

Ginger

Clove

Juniper – the dried berries also make a great infusion which you can add to the bath

Cedar.

Add a couple of teaspoons to the bath. You can add also add more salt without the added essential oils (up to 1 teacup) for a good magnesium soak. You can use Epsom salts as the base if you prefer. Nettle stings – lots of people still swear by flagellation of nettle leaves and stems. It is difficult to brave but worth trying if you have stiff aching joints. They are heating and anti-inflammatory and aid nervous regeneration in conditions such as carpal tunnel and some nervous or muscular damage.

> ### Rewilding exercise: nettle stings
>
> If you've never been stung by a nettle other than by accident, this may take some bravery.
>
> Approach a clean patch of young vibrant dry green nettles. Spend a few minutes just relaxing with the plants.
>
> Then when ready, having asked the nettles if you may make medicine with them, firmly grip a stem with your thumb and finger and pluck the top of the plant. Or just pick one leaf. You most likely won't get stung by the nettle that you pick but perhaps by a neighbouring nettle leaf that blows towards you or is pulled in your direction.
>
> Once picked, roll the nettle leaf in your hands – quite briskly if you don't want to be stung - and then eat it. When you break the needles, the sting is lost, just as blanching the leaves in hot water breaks down the needles.
>
> See how you feel when eating freshly picked nettle – notice if there is any difference this way in contrast to picking it with gloves on.
>
> Note: I have picked and eaten it without rolling it properly and it will sting in the mouth so just take care to roll it well until you get the feel for it.

PNEUMONIA OR BRONCHITIS

Conditions of the lungs are more common in elders as phlegmatic build-up increases and immunity decreases. Infections in weaker folk are more common due to susceptibility.

Pneumonia may be caused by a virus, mould, inhalation of foreign objects, or, more commonly in the elderly, bacterial infection. The cough, shortness of breath or difficulty breathing, fever, racing heart, and malaise all need attention.

Medical help must be sought with this condition. Herbs can be given alongside orthodox care and generally strengthening the constitution of the elder is key.

Bronchitis is the inflammation of the bronchioles and commonly affects older folk. It can be acute or chronic. If chronic it may be part of a more complex picture of chronic obstructive pulmonary disorder (COPD) where emphysema may present.

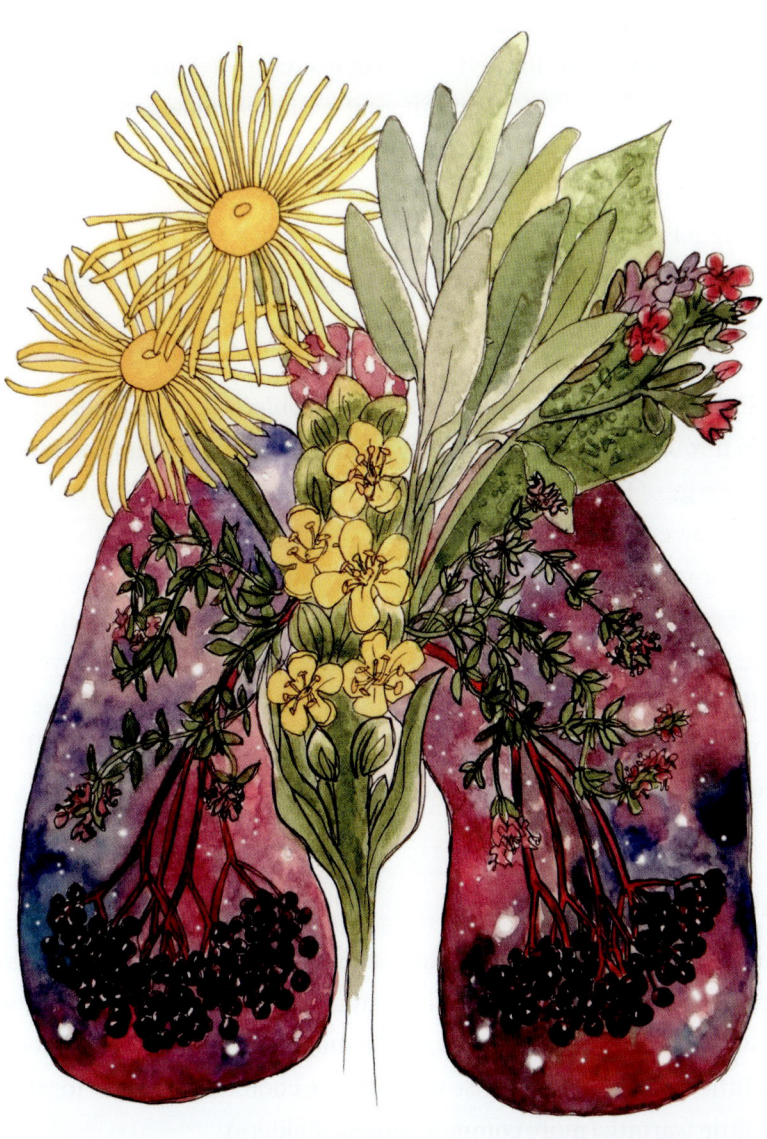

Galactic lungs and plant allies

Rewilding exercise: deep breath of winter

Breathing is a fundamental part of life but we don't always do it well. Tuning in to our breath if we are struggling to breathe is a must.

Find a comfortable spot where you can see something natural – a tree, field, river, part of your garden, a plant. Choose something that you find makes you feel good. That in itself is a great exercise – taking the time to feel how you are when you look at different natural wonders. Some folk feel great looking at trees, or being surrounded by them, others are mesmerised by flowing water.

Definitely get comfy.

As you settle your body and lengthen your spine, feel out your lungs and chest – do they feel open, closed, relaxed, or tense? Notice and try to relax as best you can.

Focusing on the beautiful natural scene or object you have chosen, breathe in through your nose, all the way to the base of your lungs. Imagine the good energy of that plant (or river) entering your lungs and sharing it with them, the energy dissipating all over the body. As you breathe out through your mouth or nose – whichever you find more soothing – gently exhale the air, energy, and a little wisdom to give back to the earth, or water, etc. Continue this for at least five minutes. When you are ready to finish, allow yourself a minute of normal breathing and gather together your thoughts or feelings of how the object of your vision made you feel. Relax, release, and move on gently with your day.

Plant allies

As stressed, with elders, the key is to nourish and strengthen. Sage is a fantastic herb for this as it does both while also battling any infections. A couple of leaves a day would be great as an infusion. Thyme and liquorice are also lovely teas with a little mint added for those who like the coolness or ginger for those who seek a little warmth (more common amongst elders).

There are many other useful herbs – to treat fully and properly, please contact your herbalist.

```
DEEP BREATHE TEA

Sage            2 parts  (eg 100ml)
Thyme           2 parts  (eg 100ml)
Applemint       1 part   (eg 50ml)
Liquorice       ½ part   (eg 25ml)
Ginger (dried)  ½ part   (eg 25ml)

Infuse 2 tsp. for 5-10 minutes and sup daily. If hyper-
tension is present, monitor the blood pressure as
liquorice taken over time may increase it.
```

HYPERTENSION

High blood pressure is not something to be taken lightly as care of the heart is paramount for good health. When systolic or diastolic blood pressure rises above what is considered to be safe, hypertension is diagnosed. Hypertension can be primary (unknown cause) or secondary (known pathological cause, eg. kidney disease). Blood pressure is the measurement of the force of blood pushing against the wall of the arteries as it circulates around the body.

Resting heartbeat is generally 60–70 beats per minute, every heartbeat being a single pump of the heart squeezing oxygenated blood into the arteries. Systolic pressure is created from the contraction of the heart to pump, and diastolic when it relaxes between pumps, hence the lower reading of pressure.

Hypertension can be symptomless or can produce complications such as dizziness, flushing, headaches (red flag if no history of headaches or any changes), fatigue, nosebleeds, and anxiety.

Blood pressure varies from individual to individual so not one measurement fits all, but generally high blood pressure is thought of as 150/90mmHg (systolic/diastolic) for a period of time in the elderly.

Hypertension must be taken seriously as it can lead to arteriosclerosis, myocardial infarction, cardiac hypertrophy, kidney disease/damage, or stroke, amongst other conditions.

Please seek professional help with hypertension. There is a lot you can do to support your health with herbs, diet and lifestyle changes while receiving professional care.

DIET AND LIFESTYLE

It is really important to eat well with any serious heart condition. Plenty of fresh vegetables and less inflammatory and stimulating foods like coffee and sugar. There are various supplements and specific foods you can take or eat to encourage a healthy heart. Ask your herbalist or nutritionist.

Stress is a major cause of hypertension and using techniques that help maintain or encourage emotional health and well-being such as meditation, walking outside, exercise, good food, and good company is crucial. Slow exhalations can bring blood pressure down so it's well worth bringing breath work into your life.

As we try to rewild ourselves and connect to our natural habitats, we must also remember that it has been demonstrated that the most important thing we need to feel happy is human interaction. This may be the essence of community – meeting the milkperson or postie, chatting, even briefly, to other parents or workers or folk on the bus. Of course, this may not be possible for some, due to community breakdown, personal trauma, or modern day isolation – we drive cars to work, we use our laptops or phones to communicate. Connection = happiness.

Rewilding exercise

Each morning when you get out of bed, take a few moments to stand, or sit if standing is hard, with a view to a tree, or hill, or the sea, river, or canal. Put your left hand over your heart and right hand over your belly. Breathe into your belly and relax the body so you feel comfortable and safe. Allow the power of yourself and the tree or river (etc.) to nourish you. Gently focus on your heart, calming and nourishing the body with blood. Maintain this practice for a few minutes every day.

Rose within the Ash

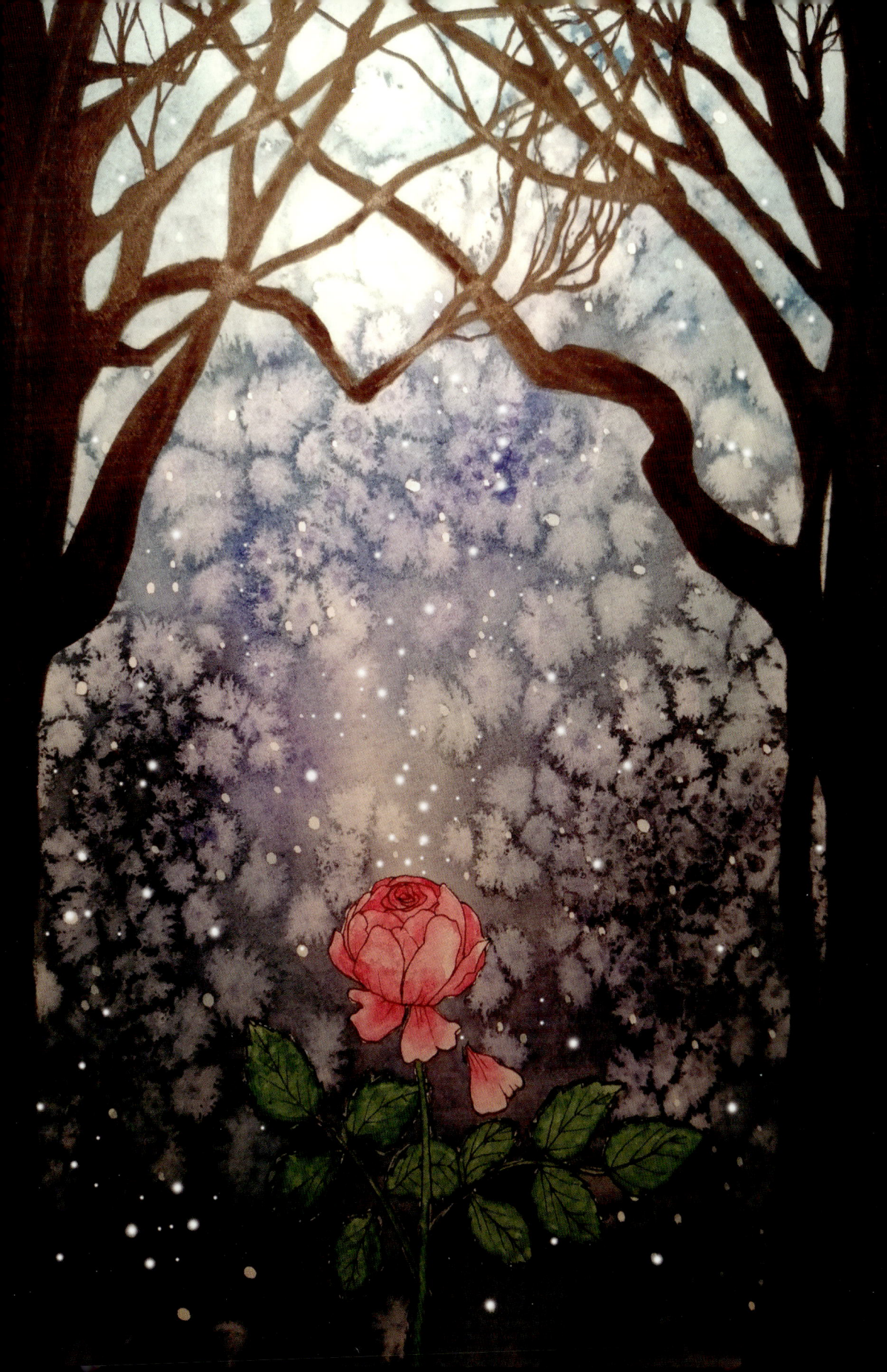

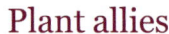

Plant allies

Actions for plants that may be helpful in hypertension include: hypertensive, cardiotonic, diuretic, antispasmodic, and astringent.

Hawthorn is the number one heart herb. It is a cardiotonic and helps make the cardiac muscle work more efficiently. It is also a hypertensive and diuretic so aids the heart in high blood pressure in different ways.

Motherwort is excellent for spasm in the heart causing palpitations and tachycardia (racing heart). Its Latin name is lion heart (*Leonurus cardiaca*) and it is indeed such a fantastic plant ally for the heart.

HEARTEASE TEA

Hawthorn flowers	1 part
Motherwort	1 part
Linden	1 part
Heartsease	¼ part
Skullcap	¼ part
Oat straw	¼ part
Yarrow	¼ part
Dandelion leaves	¼ part
Valerian flowers	⅛ part

1-2 tsp of the tea blend brewed for 5-10 minutes. Strain and enjoy 2-3 cups daily.

This tea may also be used as part of a plan for atherosclerosis which can be lethal and is one of the most common cardiovascular diseases. The inconsistent thickening of the arteries is attributed to fatty deposits called plaques which block, and can sometimes completely occlude, the arteries. This can lead to heart attacks if occlusion occurs in the arteries, or strokes if a piece breaks off and makes its way to the brain. In the Western world, blockage in the coronary (heart) arteries is the leading cause of death due to ischaemia.

Cardiotonics and vascular tonics such as hawthorn, guelder rose, linden, and garlic are useful along with peripheral vasodilators and hypotensives which bring down blood pressure and increase flow in the vessels. Nervines are also a great addition to a blend.

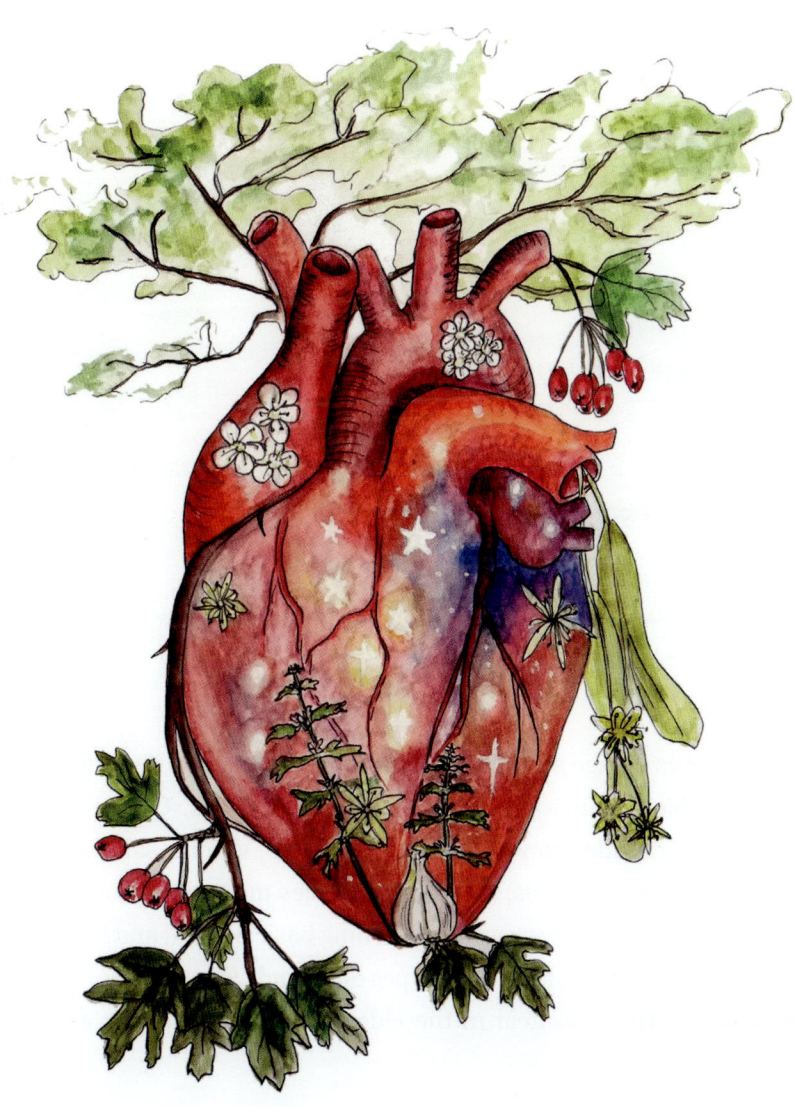

Galactic heart and plant allies

HAWTHORN HEART BRANDY

Pick as many hawthorn berries as you need to fill a jar. Once packed, add brandy and fill to the top. Leave for a few weeks to macerate – shake gently each day. You can also add cinnamon, cardamom, orange peel, cloves, garlic, and honey should you choose to. Strain and use as an evening tipple that happens to be excellent for the heart.

HEART PROTECT CHAI

Rooibos tea	100g
Ginger powder	1 tsp
Cardamom	10 pods
Cloves	5 buds
Cinnamon	1 stick crushed
Black pepper	2-4 peppercorns

Simmer 2 tsps of the blend per cup for 5 minutes and leave to infuse for another 10 minutes. Strain and add 2-5 drops of cayenne tincture and ½ tsp of honey if desired.

ULCERS

Skin gets drier as we age and it is important to look after it. If we don't, we are more susceptible to cuts, infections, and complications. Cuts, bruises, and grazes must be attended to with care. Compresses, lotions, salves, liniments, glycerites, powders, tinctures, teas, and poultices may all be used depending on how the wound or injury presents. Learning basic first aid and how different forms of medicine work for different types of wounds is really helpful.

Ulcers can be tricky to heal in the elderly as they can fester and remain unhealed in a worrying, oozing wound. Some say it's best to heal them under damp conditions and others in dry conditions as humidity can keep cuts and ulcers from resolving. I have found that dry conditions work well with anti-infective and resinous herbs.

Varicose ulcers can present as many small ulcers and if untreated may worsen. Ulcers should be checked by professionals but a simple guide to care is as follows:

Remove any debris from the wound then disinfect it – you can use a spray of myrrh tincture, goldenseal (sustainably sourced), or gotu kola tincture.

Gently rub marigold cream around the wound (not in the wound).

Pack the wound – fill the hole with aloe gel, or honey, or leave as is if you can't get these. Make sure if you do pack the wound that the honey or aloe is clean (not from your kitchen cupboard with butter in it . . . you know who you are!)

Dress the wound with a non-stick dressing over the wound – first a mesh layer, then a pad, then a bandage, and finally a tubigrip or stocking or similar if not painful. Or if you have a proper single dressing that might be fine too. The large Mefix ones or similar are good.

If in any doubt whatsoever, call your GP, nurse, or herbalist who can help.

Plant allies

Myrrh (tincture or powder-based preparation) is really useful here as it is easier to get than goldenseal and extremely anti-infective. As it is resinous, it sticks to the wound, healing it. Goldenseal, if you can find it grown ethically, is excellent as powder but I rarely use it. Sometimes I mix it with myrrh powder to give a wider anti-infective dry medicine.

Marigold will heal the tissue around the wound and encourage healing of the wound itself, so make sure the wound is clean as otherwise it will try to heal with debris or infection in it and it will fester.

DEMENTIA/ALZHEIMER'S

Alzheimer's was once described to me as a fog-like state which suddenly clears, leaving the person standing on the edge of a cliff feeling disorientated and scared. It can be deeply disturbing to experience for the individual and for

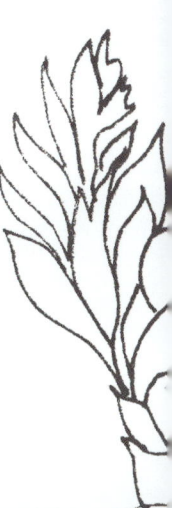

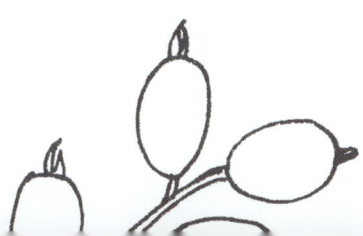

those around the affected person. As with all serious illnesses it is best to see a professional but there are lots of things you can do to ease suffering, improve memory, and calm anxiety.

Dusk and dementia

There are different forms of behaviour that can arise in people who are experiencing dementia, such as sun-downing. At dusk, elders may feel agitated and want to "go home". Dusk is a bit of an edgy time of day and to me it's no wonder that anxiety or aggravation occurs at this time. It was the same with my babies. At dusk they would become unsettled until night had fallen, then they settled into sleep. Birds are finding their way home, the level of noise one perceives from outside changes, vision is impaired. It is a difficult time of day. It is, in fact, dusk as I write this and the blackbirds and robins are still singing as the pale orange horizon gives way to indigo blue starlit skies.

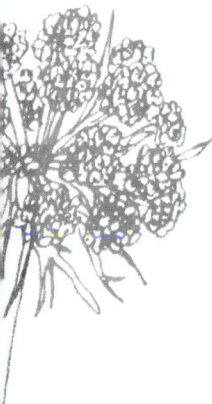

Memory

My teacher once said of elders, "They don't know what they do know." I always remembered this because as we age we accumulate so much knowledge, yet as our memories fade and we adapt to a changing body, we forget the vastness of what we know.

We know music, scent, and touch evoke much that the cerebral thought process cannot. We must find ways to connect and maintain relationship as best we can if what we know starts to become lost in the huge landscape of forgotten memories.

Plant allies

Antioxidants – you just can't get enough of them in a state of failing memory or mind. Increase all the coloured fresh foods like bilberries, carrots, beets, rocket, and broccoli. Or make smoothies with antioxidant-rich herbs.

Cerebral circulatory stimulants will encourage blood flow to the brain and aid memory. Rosemary is easy to grow and harvest and is an excellent memory herb. It is very recognisable too and smell is such a powerful sense to remind folk of memories old and new. Ginkgo is both an antioxidant and cerebral circulatory stimulant (gets blood to the brain) so a great addition as tea or tincture.

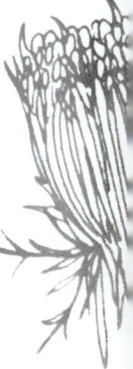

Medicinal mushrooms are fantastic and in particular, lion's mane. Check with a local herbalist about any contraindications.

```
RECIPE: MEMORY BOOSTING SMOOTHIE

1 cup organic almond (or similar) milk
½ avocado
1 handful blueberries
1 handful bilberries
1 handful hawthorn berries (without pips)
1 handful rocket
1 handful lettuce
2 inches cucumber
¼ celery stick
1 tsp cacao
1 tsp rosemary (powdered leaves are good or rosemary-
infused hemp oil)
1 tsp ginkgo leaves (powdered)

Blitz in a nutribullet or similar and drink – other
things to add could be a little ginger, or half a
banana if sweetness will bring about compliancy.
Enjoy!
```

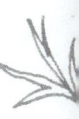

Omega-3 fats are also very beneficial. Avoid refined sugars which are inflammatory.

INCONTINENCE

Urinary incontinence can range from a weak bladder to total loss of control and is a commonly seen ailment in the elderly. It can be managed and aided with herbs but it is something that holds much stigma for many of us. Losing control is one thing, soiling yourself is another very emotional occurrence. Incontinence is seen more in the elderly because of a range of illnesses that affect our ability to control our urination. It isn't necessarily a symptom of ageing per se.

Identifying the cause of incontinence is key. In children it can often be stress or anxiety which leads to bed-wetting or soiling themselves in the day. This isn't the same as what we call stress incontinence.

Stress incontinence is commonly seen as we age, particularly after pregnancy, and is the presentation of urine leakage when the bladder has pressure pushing on it – for example when you cough or laugh a lot. "I laughed so much I almost wet my pants," is a classic stress incontinence example. Stress incontinence may be caused by damage to or the weakening of the muscles which help hold urine; these are the levator ani and the coccygeus muscles, otherwise known as the pelvic floor.

Urge incontinence is when a little leakage occurs and an urgency to urinate accompanies it. It may be caused by too much activity in the detrusor muscles.

Overflow incontinence is a form of retention of the urine, where you can't fully empty your bladder and leakage occurs. Sometimes there is an obstruction or a blockage causing retention.

Total incontinence is when you can't hold any urine in the bladder and so urinate constantly or experience frequent leakage. There is a wide variety of causes for this, including congenital bladder ailments, injury, or fistula.

Lifestyle

Pelvic floor exercises are indicated here, or core muscle work. Certain yoga and Pilates practices can also be just as beneficial or more so overall.

Plant allies

Similarly for bed-wetting in children, St John's Wort, agrimony, and crampbark may be useful, depending on which kind of incontinence is presenting.

Soothing herbs like horsetail, cornsilk, and marshmallow are also indicated.

Diuretic herbs aid the body in urinating efficiently and many have volatile oils that will help with any infections that are causing or adding to incontinence.

Make sure you have fully investigated why the incontinence is happening and try to support the elder with as much respect and care as possible. If dementia or Alzheimer's is present then gently remind the elder why you are, for example, changing their pad or washing them when they forget why they have no trousers on while you are changing them. When a person starts to lose autonomy due to illness, it is important to be respectful and to try to re-engage that individual with their own power.

CONSTIPATION

If constipation is a recent development in older age and no other causes are found, then we look to constitution. Has the elder become too dry? Think of their health picture and what they are eating, how they are moving, and their environment. Dryness can mean stagnancy or lack of movement. It is really important to regain good digestive health so no further problems arise. Stress, diet, dehydration, prescribed drugs, and other conditions can all contribute to a tendency towards constipation.

Plant allies

As elders are cooler and drier than their younger counterparts, it is important to remember warming remedies and states. Digestion and brain function take up much body heat so keeping warming infusions, cosy fires, and blankets to hand is a good idea.

If constipation is more than a mild bout, think about the following laxative stages:

Bulk laxatives – these bulk out the stools and draw water to them to encourage passing through. Examples include psyllium husks, ethically sourced slippery elm, or soluble fibres.

Bitters encourage the liver and gall bladder and there are different levels of bitters:

Gentle bitters are the first port of call – dandelion is a great one to try first. Soothing and healing, it works as a cholagogue and choleretic encouraging bile release which aids digestion.

Anthraquinone-containing bitters are a bit more pushy and include dock, senna, and aloe (notice the yellow just below the green when you cut a leaf open). Aloe is good because it is also demulcent in hot water, so a warm infusion of aloe will soothe and heal as well as encourage the liver and gall bladder.

Irritant purgatives are strong and most likely won't need to be used or will need to be used under the guidance of your herbalist. They include squirting cucumber (*Ecballium elaterium*), though I haven't used this yet, rhubarb, and senna.

Apple cider vinegar (ACV) use may also be encouraged. Along with bitters, sour tastes also aid the liver. ACV is cooling and supportive for the liver and may be taken with a little honey (or vegan alternative). As things start to slow down in the elderly supporting the liver and other organs is good general practice.

Simple dietary changes can bring about movement and good peristalsis, digestion, and comfort. Osmotic laxatives from fruit sugar (eg. soaked prunes in porridge) are a food to store in the cupboard and use if needed. Try a few prunes or prune juice for a few days and see what the results are. A beetroot every day can be really useful and essential for some.

DAILY BEETROOT

500g raw beetroot

400ml (or enough to cover) organic cider vinegar

1 bay leaf

1 crushed cinnamon stick

1 star anise pod

2 allspice berries

5 black peppercorns

1 small dried cayenne pepper if desired

2 cloves

1 tsp coarse salt

Wash the beetroot, cut into smaller pieces unless they are baby beetroots.

Put all the other ingredients except the vinegar into a heavy based stainless steel pan and heat gently so the aroma of the spice mix is apparent; you can do this in a tsp of oil or dissolved sugar, both of which will hold the aroma.

> Add beetroots and enough water to cover and simmer
> until tender. You can simmer in the vinegar with sugar
> syrup (dissolved in the pan before adding the beet-
> root) if you prefer. I like to pour the uncooked
> vinegar over the spiced beetroots in the jars and seal
> shut. Keep in fridge once opened.
>
> Alternatively, simply simmer the beets until tender
> and then add an oxymel or herbal vinegar to cover. An
> example would be all of the above spices macerated in
> the vinegar for a week or two and then poured over the
> tender beets once in the jar (having been strained).
>
> Have a few slices every day.

Plant allies for elders

Plant allies for the elderly can be different from those for younger adults. We are often looking for strengthening (tonic) herbs and remedies which can be easily tolerated if weakness has set in.

Note: some tonic herbs can be processed or raw and it is important to know the difference in effect of each preparation. Such herbs include liquorice, rehmannia, and fleeceflower. When these herbs are processed (usually cooking including baking) they are nourishing in action and when in their raw state (they might be softened for a day but are uncooked) they are more active. These three are commonly used herbs in traditional Chinese medicine but you may not find them growing in the UK unless you try growing them yourself. Which is fun! They are excellent herbs in many ways for our elders. Some have contraindications so check with your herbalist first.

In terms of the actual remedy, vinegars are great for the elderly because they are what my mentor called "thinning". This is the language of humoral medicine and it's easy to imagine what it means visually. It is to say that vinegars in general are helpful with the thickening of the fluids that build in old age. Phlegmatic build-up is a may present as rheumatic joints, clogged arteries, and phlegmy lungs. Stiffness and aching can often be attributed to phlegmatic excess.

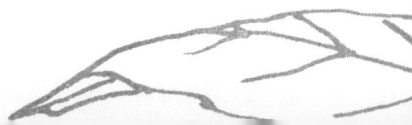

Building and strengthening herbs are often best taken as decoctions. These are pleasing to make as they involve the patient but if the individual has difficulty making them, community is needed!

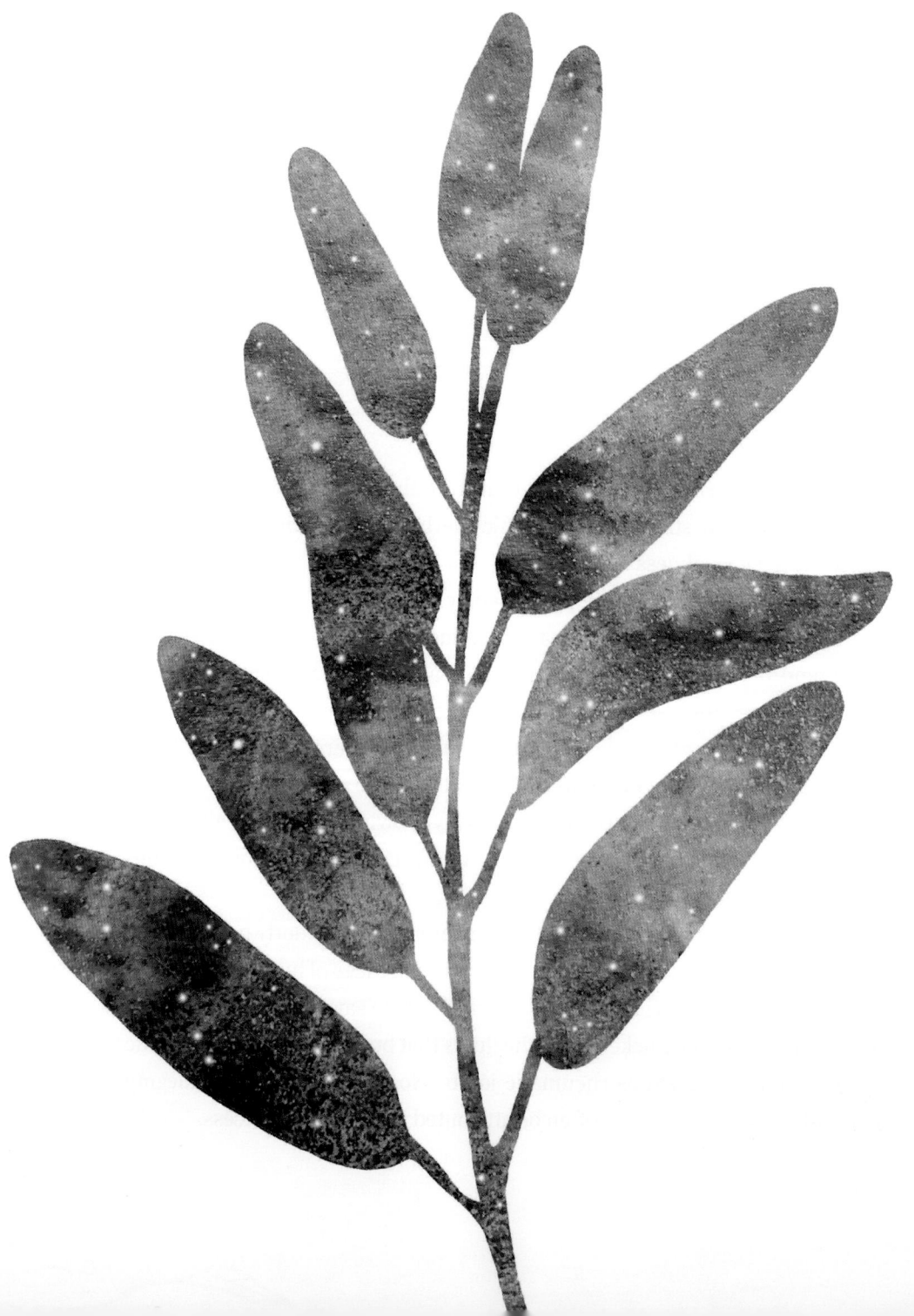

SOME USEFUL HERBS FOR OUR ELDERS

Sage *Salvia officinalis*

Nature: hot and dry

Planet: Jupiter

There is a saying that if you infuse or eat two leaves of sage every day you'll live forever (see why it's helpful in bronchitis?) The same is also said about lemon balm – both are excellent and well tolerated by elders.

Sage is a very strengthening herb and like nettle will reduce phlegmatic excess through its drying, heating, and expelling action. It is a tonic herb but as it is drying, take care to add marshmallow or another soothing moistening herb.

As sage can regulate blood sugar, care must be taken with diabetes where insulin is used to regulate blood levels.

Sage is an anti-infective and clearing herb so very useful for many stagnant phlegmatic conditions. As a diuretic it will support the kidneys and help reduce the retention of water causing swelling and aching. It will also aid sluggish digestion and cold conditions of the digestive tract where warmth is needed to invigorate.

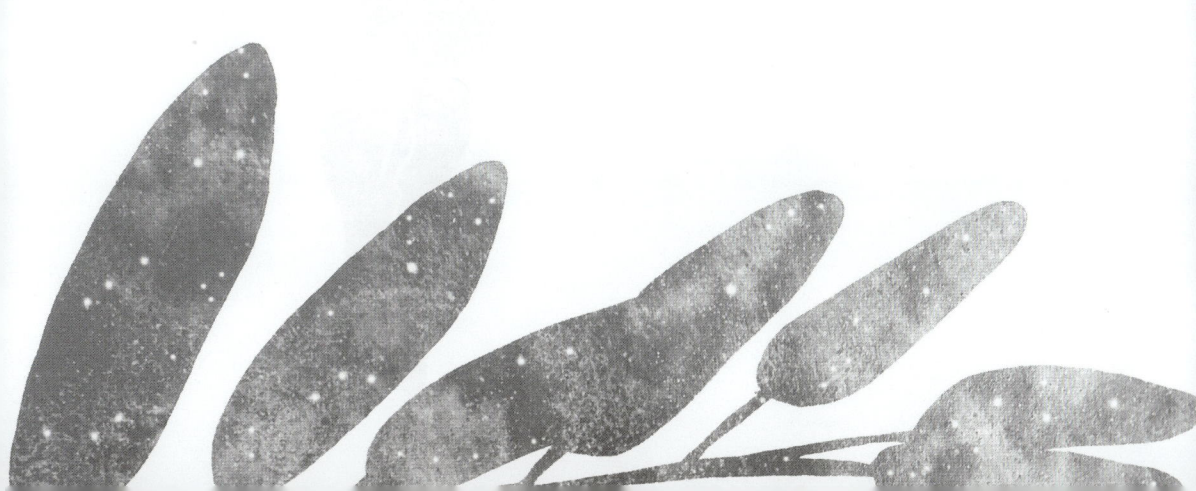

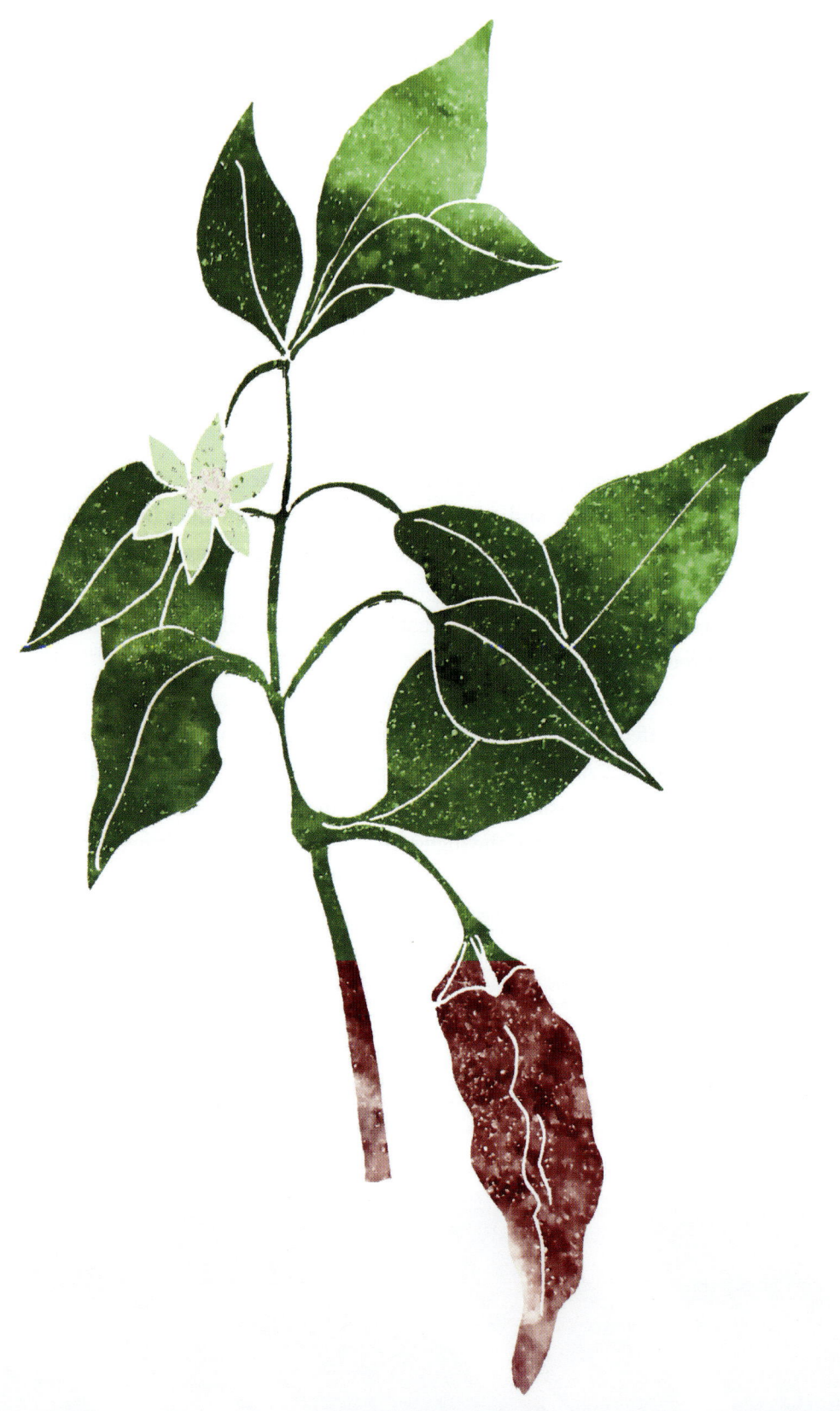

Cayenne *Capsicum annuum*

Nature: hot and dry

Celestial body: Sun

This herb is invaluable as cold and slowing metabolism in our elders become apparent. A few drops of cayenne tincture in hot drinks every day (like a chai) can restore health.

Keeping cayenne powder or tincture handy is a good idea as its use in heart attacks and intermittent claudication could be life-saving.

This herb is used in traditional Chinese medicine, and around the world including in humoral medicine, for cold and deficient states. This becomes clear when you taste it – it is hot hot hot and invigorating. If you are already hot and dry, it may feel irritating so use when indicated. Eclectic practitioners used it for both excess and stagnant fluids, including blood which was considered the "chief" fluid. Either excess or stagnant fluid may indicate a phlegmatic or melancholic excess. As neither is generally useful (except as protection in acute conditions) warming stimulating herbs are a go to for an elder's apothecary.

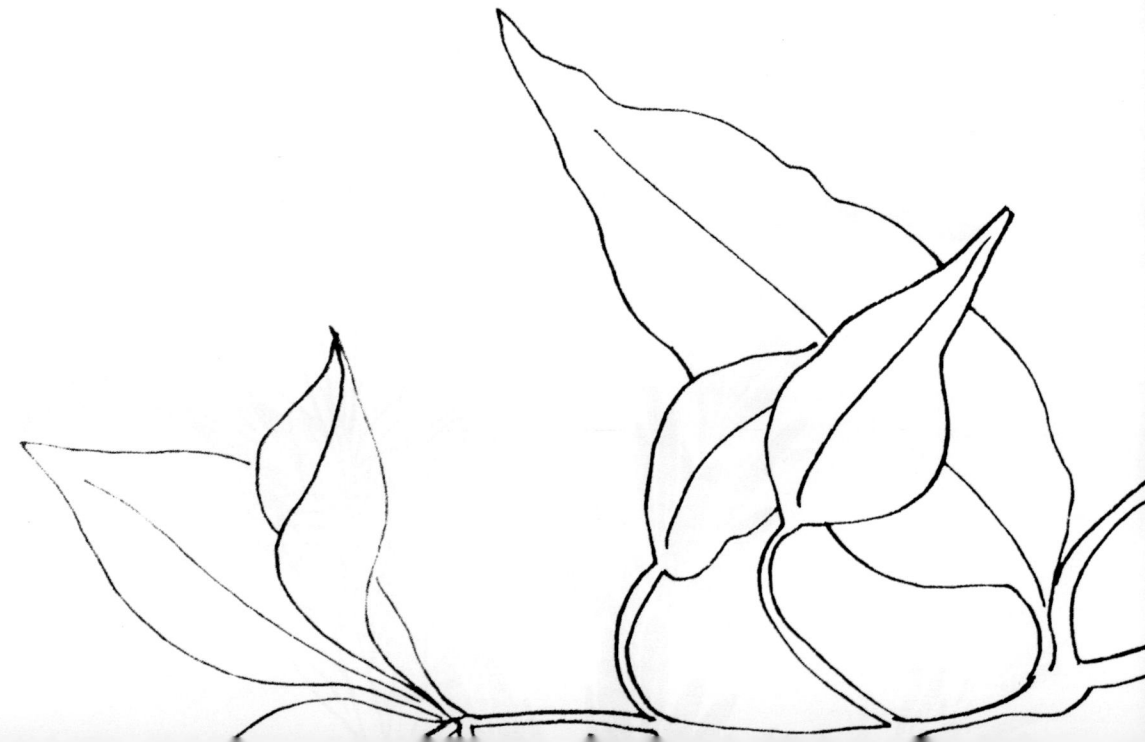

Rosemary *Salvia rosmarinus*

Nature: hot and dry

Celestial body: Sun

Wonderful rosemary is so easy to grow and useful as a hot and dry herb, because elders are often cold and damp in this country. Rosemary will aid circulation starting with supporting the heart and warming from the heart outwardly. As a tincture with alcohol it will be diffusively warming and as a hot infusion it will warm the core, so another herb like cayenne, ginger, or prickly ash may be needed to get heat to the limbs. It will warm up a cold constitution and get rid of phlegmatic build-up. It is a cerebral circulatory stimulant so will aid blood flow to the head and is often used instead of coffee for a caffeine-free morning drink.

Elders tend to remember the good old days, as do those of a melancholic disposition. Rosemary will aid memory and introversive reckoning which is a great thing. It is natural to comb through one's life as one ages and see the joy, sadness, wisdom, and wonder; and helping elders remember these experiences means they might share them with you. This is a treasure. If, however, repetition is a factor in an elder's sharing, then look to help as anxiety, confusion, or mental health conditions may be indicated.

I love Elisabeth Brooke's reminder that Greek students used to entwine twigs of rosemary in their hair when they were studying to improve memory. Have a go! Get touchy with rosemary. It is vibrant all year round and smells beautiful. It can aid focus and elicit emotion. It is a wonderful herb.

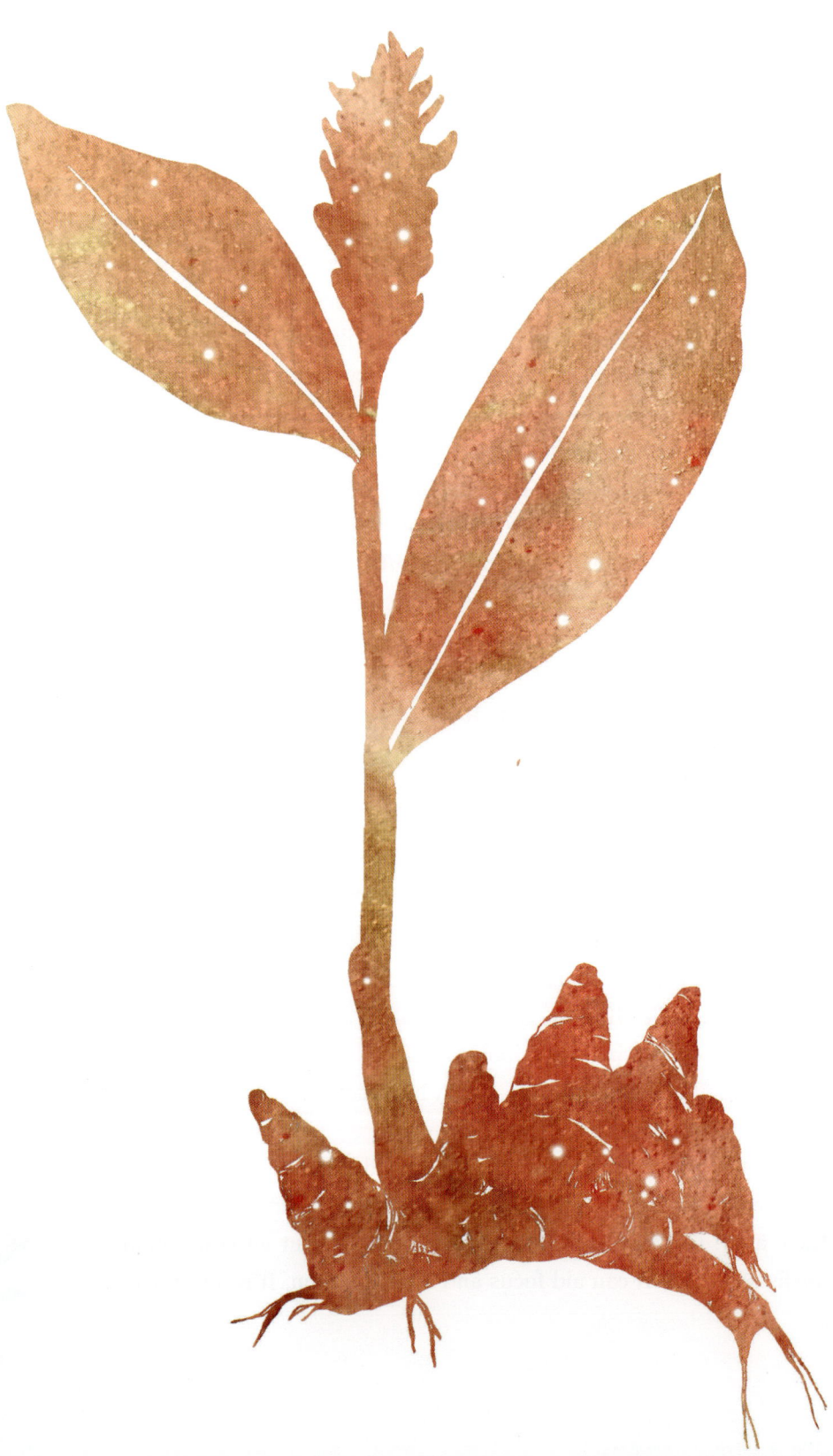

Turmeric *Curcuma longa*

Nature: warm and dry

Planet: Jupiter

A great herb which is commonly used as a nutritive in many cultures. Turmeric can be drunk or eaten as a daily tonic. Traditionally a teaspoon is taken with a little black pepper in honey or in a milk of some kind.

Turmeric is full of antioxidants and this is demonstrated in its vibrant yellow you will, no doubt, be familiar with. If not, get familiar! Be warned it does stain though – we have made great tie-dye T-shirts with it.

Christopher Hedley used to love it when we students would talk about colour, and as a visual person I would often speak of colour when thinking of herbs and feelings so I resonated well with this. When teaching us about turmeric once, he said it was like internal colour therapy. Yellow, the colour of happiness, light-heartedness, warmth, fun, and focus. It is an energising colour and turmeric indeed is an invigorating herb.

Turmeric is a food and long-term medicine is best as food if you can find what you need from your food. Turmeric builds and restores – it is a replenishing herb so deficient states, often present in the elderly and in those stressed from modern life, could do well with this herb.

If cholesterol is high, as is often the case for elders, a mix of turmeric and artichoke can bring levels down sufficiently. See a herbalist about this.

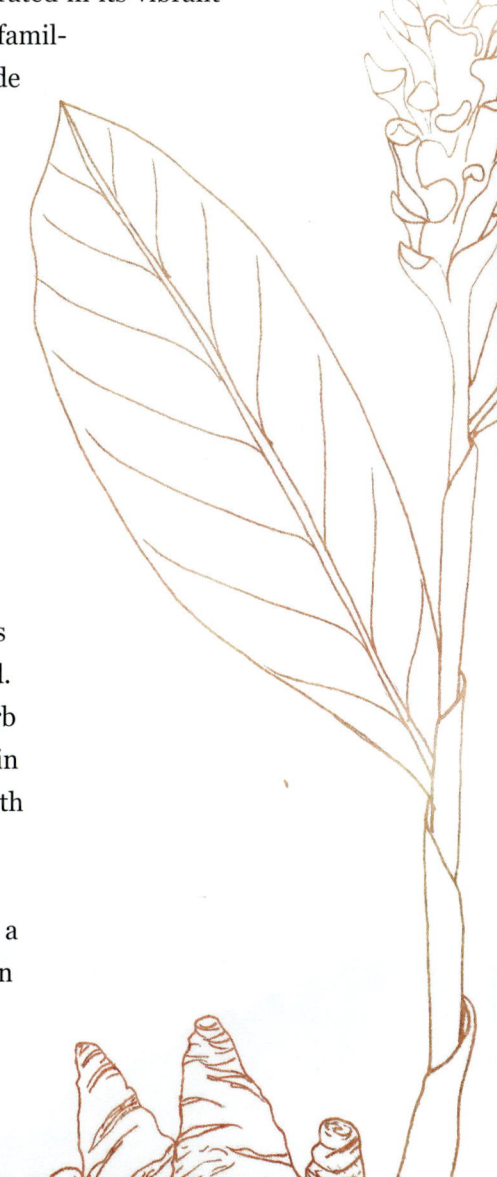

RECIPE: TURMERIC LATTE (HALDI DOODH)

You can use fresh or dried powdered turmeric – you'll experience them slightly differently and can choose how to make your own smoothies or lattes. I prefer fresh turmeric.

Fresh turmeric root – 1½ inch piece (this could equate to ½–1 tsp of powdered turmeric)

Black pepper – a pinch is fine as it is used to aid the efficacy of turmeric

Fresh ginger (this is also different in nature to dried ginger) – a 1x1 inch piece

A teaspoon of honey – or vegan alternative

Milk – organic, nut-based, or coconut, it needs to be fatty (so not oat milk or rice milk) – a cup of your preferred milk.

POSSIBLE ADDITIONS

1 tsp of a nut butter – you can use water instead of milk if you have the nut butter as it is a fat)

Cinnamon	½ tsp
Vanilla	½ capful or infused pod
Cardamom	3 pods
Cayenne tincture	2 drops
Salt	a pinch if preferred

Blend together and heat gently. Sup and enjoy.

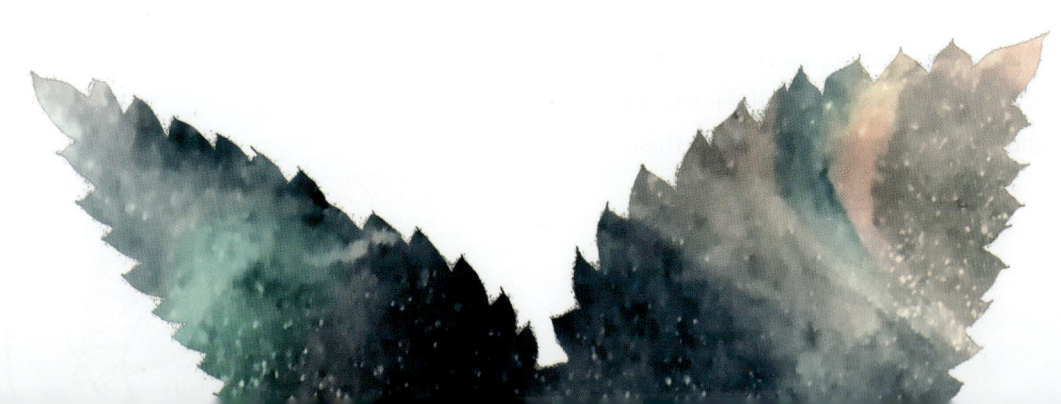

Nettle *Urtica dioica*

Nature: hot and dry

Planet: Mars

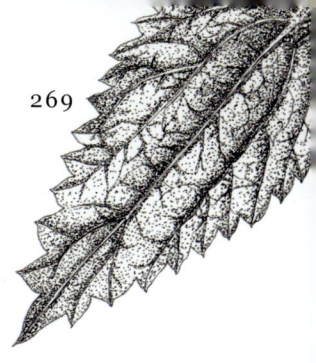

Nettle is hot and drying and therefore useful in old age where phlegmatic excess may be seen. The cold of winter, and of old age, sees a build-up of phlegm – nettle cuts through this and helps clear the stagnant accumulations. In this respect it can be seen as a spring tonic, especially as it starts growing in spring, but in fact it can be used all year in teas and tinctures, frozen soups and juices as needed.

Nettle is useful for anyone who is a little stuck, energetically or emotionally. You might imagine the sting pushing you into action but it is the whole leaf and not just the sting that stimulates action.

Nettle is warming and drying and can aid the damp cold arthritic presentations. It is an anti-inflammatory and can be taken internally as a tea or tincture.

It can also be applied to the joints as a fresh preparation – the stings are highly beneficial to cold, stiff, achy joints.

Nettle is renowned in herbal folklore and modern scientific trials have been done on it. In a Plymouth University study, out of eighteen people who used nettle therapy for their painful joints, only one said it did not help.

Nettle beer is still something you occasionally come across. I love to see it! It was brewed for rheumatism. Romans would flagellate themselves with the fresh herb to stay warm and nimble in cold damp Britain as they travelled to conquer. In this form it may also help sleep – nettle is nourishing and will aid vitality in the day so that rest will come at night. In old age rest and rhythms are really important as we replenish our energy nightly.

As it is also a urinary tonic, nettle is especially helpful as it clears the blood of urates and toxins through the stimulation of the kidney and its alterative effect.

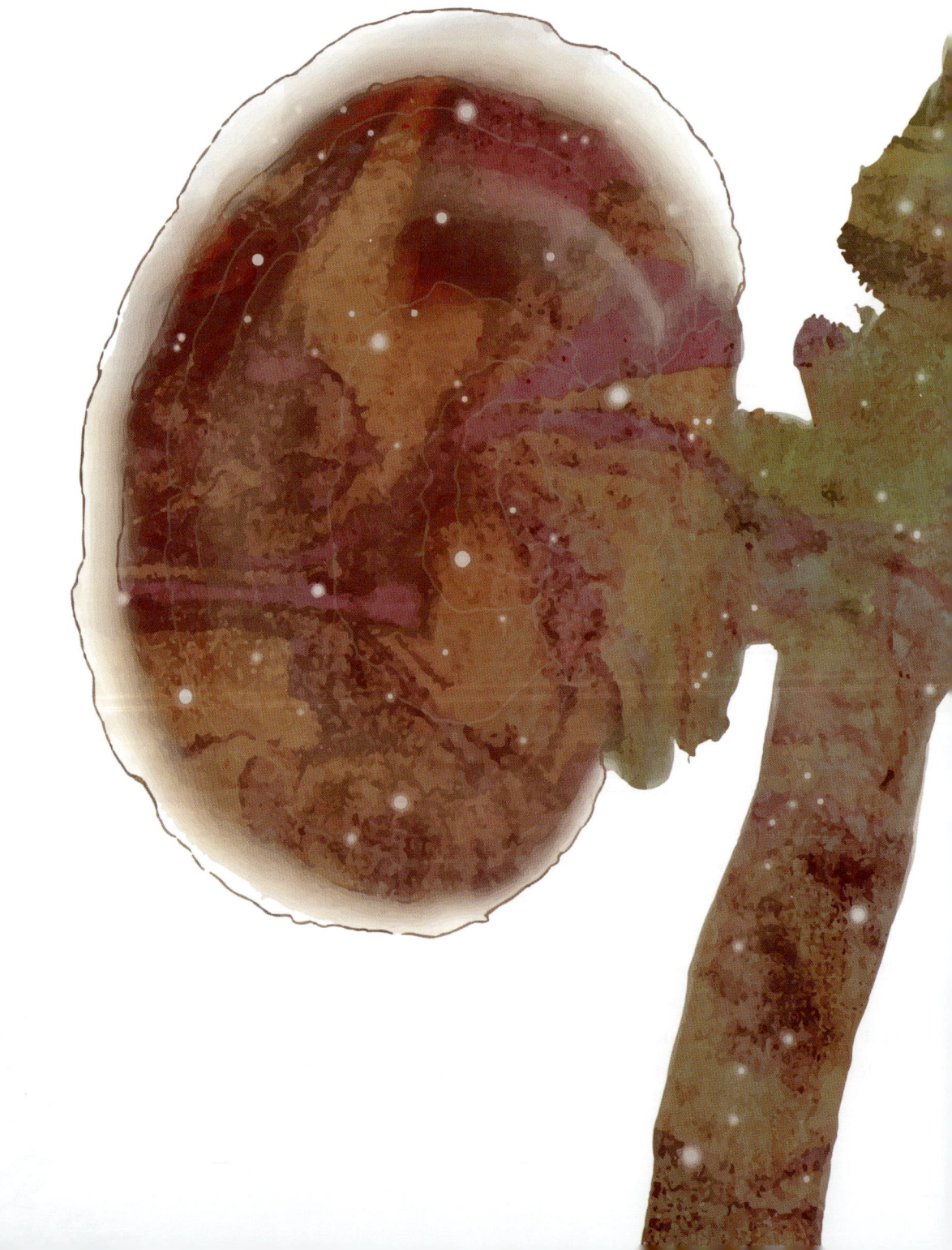

Medicinal mushrooms

While certainly not just for elders, medicinal mushrooms are a powerhouse of wonder for us humans. They work on a deep immune level and most are anti-inflammatory, anti-oxidant and anti-viral. They are magical wonders of the woodlands and fields.

I love all the mushrooms but the ones I use most in clinic include reishi, turkey tail, birch polypore, lion's mane, and chaga. The ones you can find in abundance in the UK include turkey tail, birch polypore, artist's conk, and chaga if you're based in the north. I don't use medicinal mushrooms lightly as they are a deep medicine and not everyone needs them but as they are a food as well, I love to encourage many people I work with to incorporate mushrooms into their diet.

A few mushrooms for you:

Lion's mane (*Hericium erinaceus*) is well known and a nootropic. It helps with nervous tissue growth and also acts as an anxiolytic and uplifting medicine. It is full of vitamins and minerals and is a known antibiotic, anti-inflammatory, anti-tumour, and hypoglycaemic medicine. It is protective against stomach ulcers and is used as a tonic as we grow older.

Lion's Mane has been shown to improve brain function and therefore is useful for cerebral conditions such as dementia.

Reishi (*Ganoderma lucidum*) or Ling zhi is a beautiful bracket mushroom and a cousin of artist's conk (*Ganoderma applanatum*). It is anti-inflammatory and works on cerebral potency and mental acuity. It is known as the "king of mushrooms". Not that I think it's gendered. It is, however, associated with longevity, is used as an adaptogen, and is highly nutritious.

As an immune-modulator, reishi works to aid our immune system in both under and overstimulating immune conditions. It is a balancer and harmoniser.

Turkey tail (*Trametes versicolor*) I adore turkey tail – its presence on logs in local woods makes me happy and this is perhaps medicine enough on some days!

In 1987 Japan spent a quarter of its anti-cancer agent budget on PSK (polysaccharide-Kureha and polysaccharide-Krestin, the two immunologically active constituents in turkey tail).

It is incredibly potent and so humble. There have been various studies done to suggest that PSK could be the fraction responsible for sarcoma-inhibition that turkey tail holds. There is an action that appears to be caused by PSK which activates natural killer cells and battles cytomegalovirus infection.

I could list more medicinal mushrooms but I just don't have the space in this one book! Do keep fungi allies in mind when you are thinking of local medicine. Before harvesting any mushrooms, triple cross-check your identification.

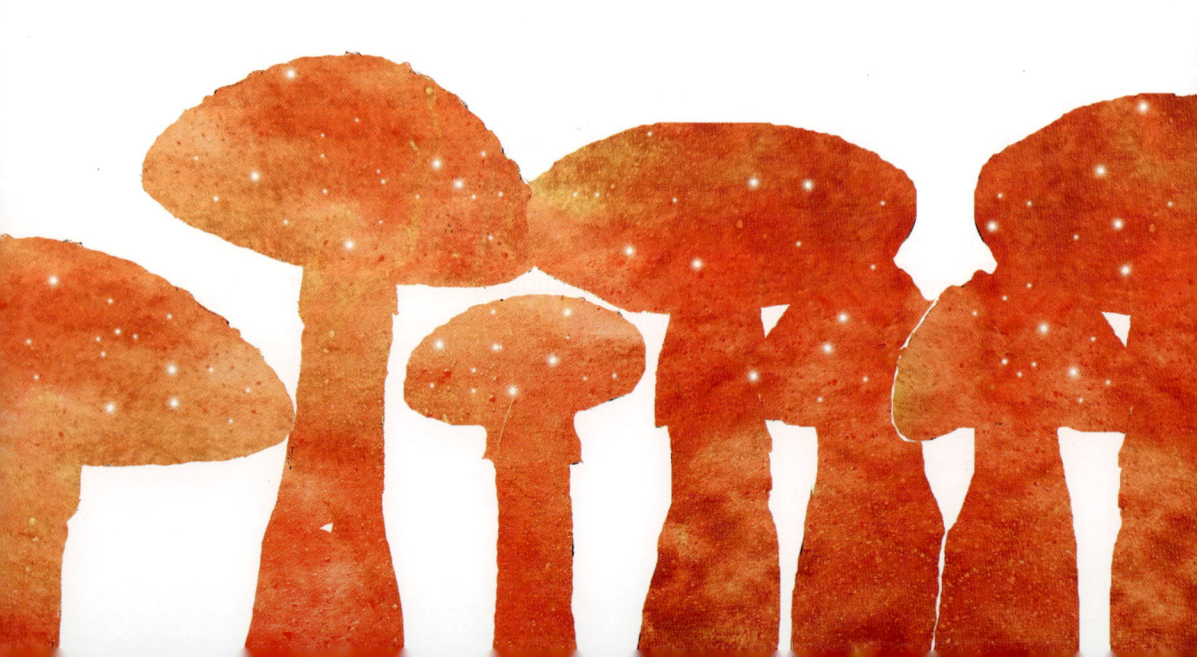

JOURNALING

As elderhood is the time of winter, a lovely rewilding exercise for your journals is to consider how you feel in winter. What does this part of the cycle mean to you and how do you experience wintriness? Writing about what you hear, see, smell, and feel is indeed a wonderful activity on a cold wintry day. What do these elements evoke for you? How do you handle the season as a whole? Can you associate this to your temperament? Choleric people might want winter done with so they can "get on"; melancholic folk might struggle through winter but actually be very creative. You might love the freshness of the crisp wintry air and long nights when you can practise your best Hygge. You might yearn for play outside on spring days! See what winter means for you.

Then, go outside and see what plants are around you. You can always count on the evergreens. Pine and other conifers always offer medicine while nettles, marigolds, and daisies might thrive all year round. Notice and write about the plants. If you can, take the time to listen to them as some learning will always happen. Though not always in ways we expect.

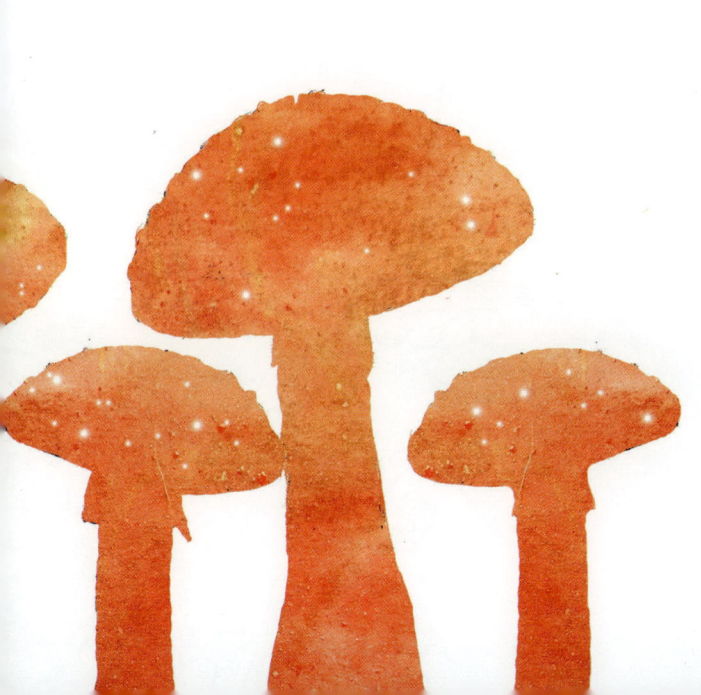

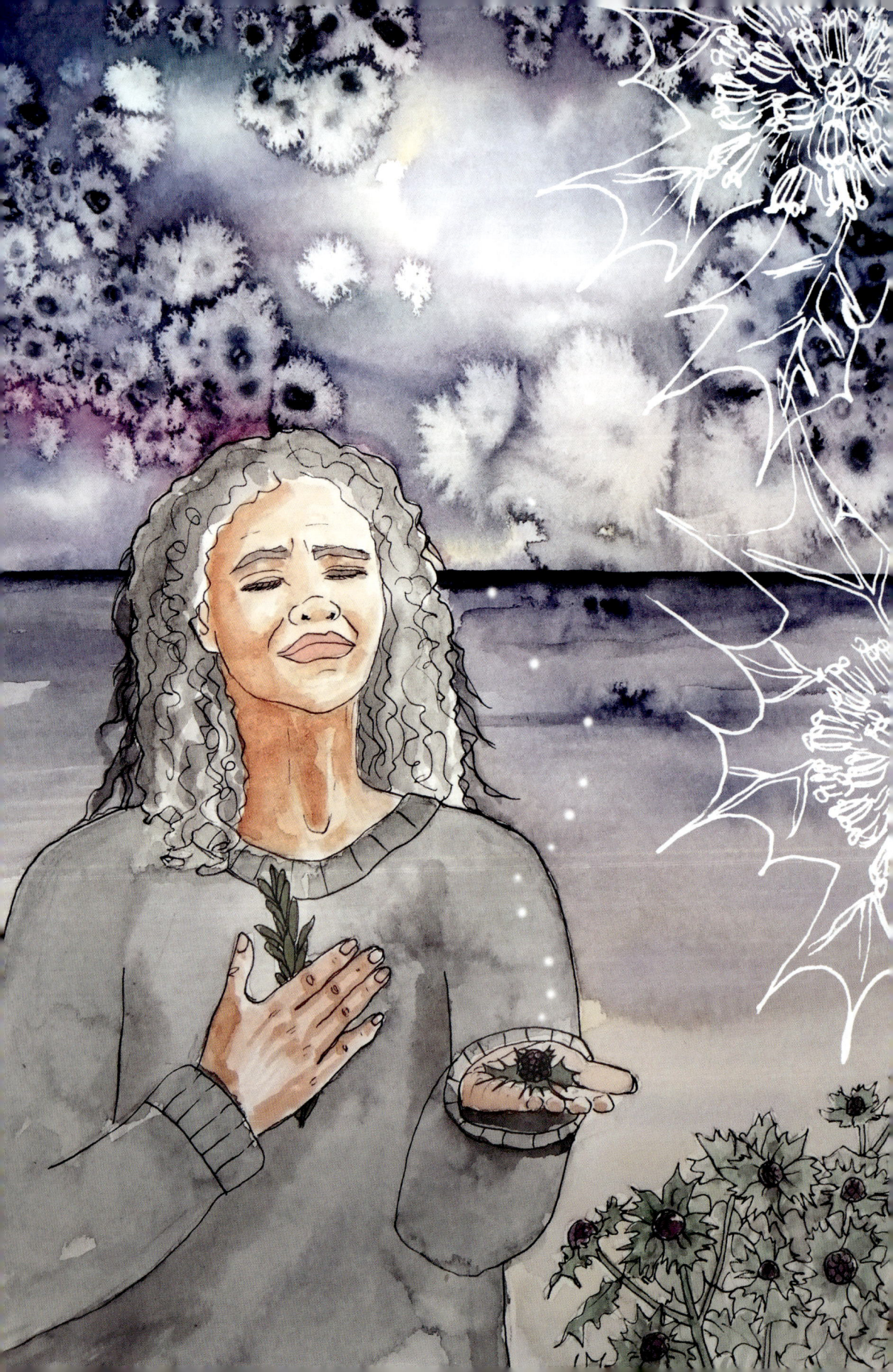

CHAPTER 10

BACK TO THE ROOTS: GRIEF

My dear child do not worry about me, Water.
I recover quickly with the song of our birds, the love of trees, with movement, moments of rest and the prayers moving around our Earth.

Message from the Water to Azul Valerie Thomé

Womxn by the sea with sea holly and rosemary

ENERGETICS – GRIEF AND THE CYCLES OF LETTING GO

What is grief and what are the energetics of grief? How does it manifest and how can we understand it?

When the oil lamp burns out, death will come. We all shine so brightly and if a natural lifetime is lived, we die old and satisfied. Hopefully we love and share and care. Hopefully we were tended and heard and found joy. Dying well is as much a journey as living well.

Embracing and accepting the inevitable allows us to let go a little more easily. I find this greatly aided by time outside. By listening to trees, lying by rivers, and walking up hills. By watching the orders of nature and glimpsing the magic. By seeing creation and witnessing destruction. By bringing all of the elements into my being and feeling the everything that this ignites.

Then trying to find ways to deal with loss, change, transition, hurt, and the wounds we all carry. The energetics of all the seasons and my whole constitution seem to suddenly sit in starkness – "Here we are!!", they call to me. "Why did you ignore us?" Time to learn them and tend them and understand them. Time to tend our hearts and all the little cracks that now hurt and stop us living well.

Grief has been taught to me in different ways. It was not something I was told much about. It was not something I knew much about first-hand as a child. And yet. And yet I learned to grieve so early, not just for life but for injustices, tragedies (that were not mine), animals, trees . . . a little empathy went a long way in my melancholic demeanour. Our way of being will certainly impact how we grieve. Our perception of the self will impact how we grieve.

I have always been quiet, not making much noise at all. Others will wail and scream and shout. Others will release by doing and moving. Others will hold and not release at all.

However you hold and process grief, it is very worthwhile tuning into your process. I often wonder why I am not making more noise – is it my temperament, my fear, my way or have I been taught that way so as not to be seen or so as to keep from upsetting anyone?

My path is to figure this out and gently take myself deeper into self-knowledge, letting go and grieving that which does not serve me, which does not nourish

Plant allies for grief

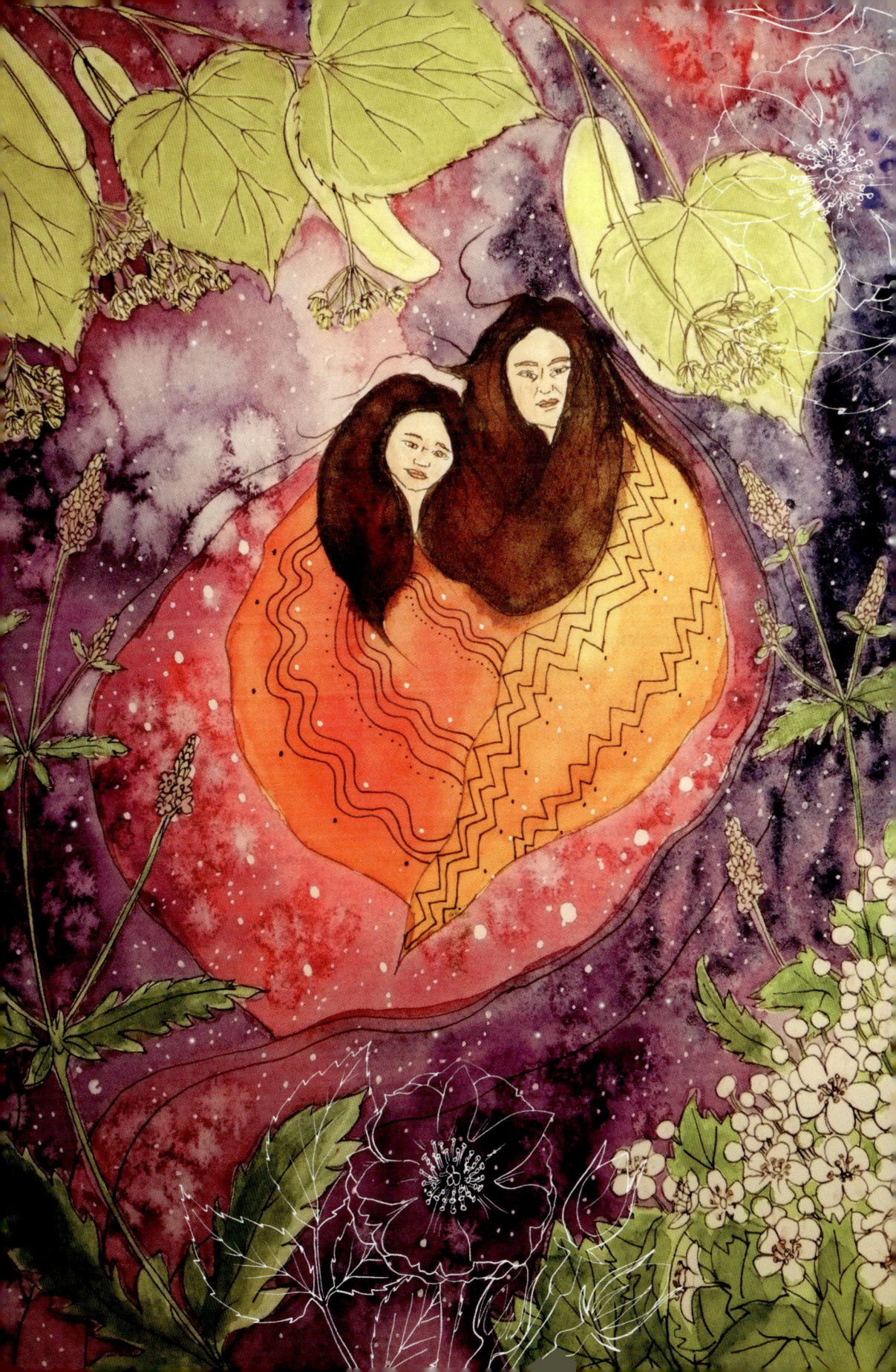

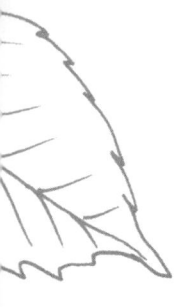

me. It is a long path and through ceremony, sharing, and tending we start to move through it, and as Brené Brown and her teacher say, "The thing in the way becomes the way."

When we look at the way grief is welcomed throughout the world, our British understanding of grief leaves much to be desired. Let us look to indigenous folk to help with ceremony, understanding, and healing. Let us look to those who have searched for sorrow and its place in the world and learn. Let us look to each other to be seen, heard, and accepted.

If you can, find a local grief circle, grief-composting ceremony or death café. At the time of writing, in my town there is a fantastic death café that welcomes anyone and brings together folk who are grieving, who have sorrow, or who are supporting others. There is cake and tea and there are guided exercises and sharing without it being therapy. It is a fantastic community resource.

We also have grief circles where we can share our grievances, sorrow, and sadness – aloud, to ourselves, with the earth, water, fire, or air. Bringing the elements into the ceremony is really helpful as we try to release some of the grief or ask for help.

If you don't have a local circle, start small with your own. You could choose a natural object to share your grief with. Once shared, you could return the object to the earth, gift it to the fire, or give it to the water.

If you are overwhelmed with grief, see if you can work with one of the five gates of grief. I came across this in the work of Francis Weller and my own friend and teacher Azul Valerie Thome. I find the gates really help me to focus on what I need to release as it can be too much to deal with all of our accumulated unattended sorrow.

The Five Gates of Grief

    The 1st Gate: Everything We Love We Will Lose
    The 2nd Gate: The Places That Have Not Known Love
    The 3rd Gate: The Sorrows of the World
    The 4th Gate: What We Expected and Did Not Receive
    The 5th Gate: Ancestral Grief

If one or two resonate more strongly for you, spend some time considering what your grief in these realms is. For example, a grief that overwhelms me and

THE ROOTS: GRIEF

those close to me is climate change and the destruction of the planet. I need to spend some time releasing the stuck emotions of this grief while concentrating on the gate of The Sorrows of the World.

Find out more about these gates and what they mean to you and other grief tending if you can from Francis Weller, Azul Valerie Thomé, or Malidoma Somé who taught both Francis and Azul, along with his late wife Sobonfu, and may still offer traditional indigenous Dagara grief tending to those who seek it.

> ### Rewilding exercise: incorporating elements into grief tending
>
> I like water for grief as it flows and moves, runs deep and clear, and reflects my tears. I like earth as it holds my most stuck feelings when I release them, and slowly composts them. I like fire when I blow out my frustration onto a stick or a strand made from wool, nettle, or cotton. I allow the fire to burn it and watch as the smoke rises and disperses while the heat and beauty warms me. I like wind to take away my unsettled feelings and refresh me.
>
> Choose an element that resonates with you and slowly, gently, deeply try to share your grief and then let it go. This isn't a cathartic experience, though it might be for some, and may require you to do it frequently. Slowly and surely you will start to see change.
>
> When you do these exercises, remember to breathe, feel it out, go with good intention, and focus well.

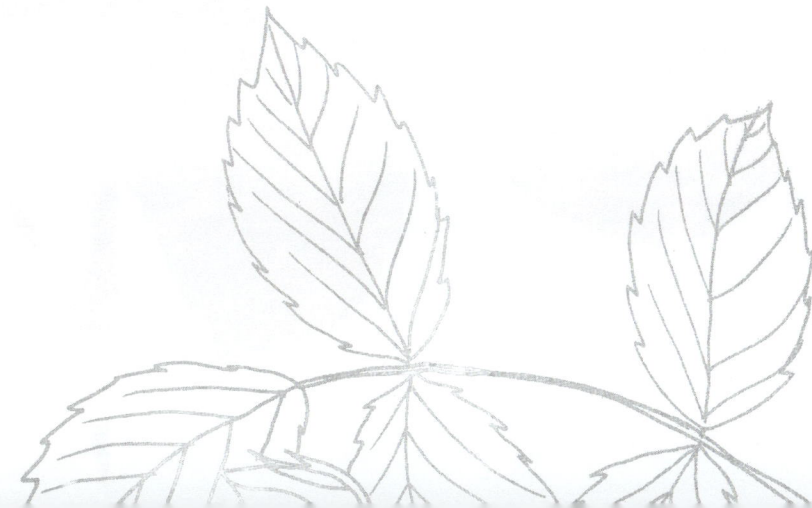

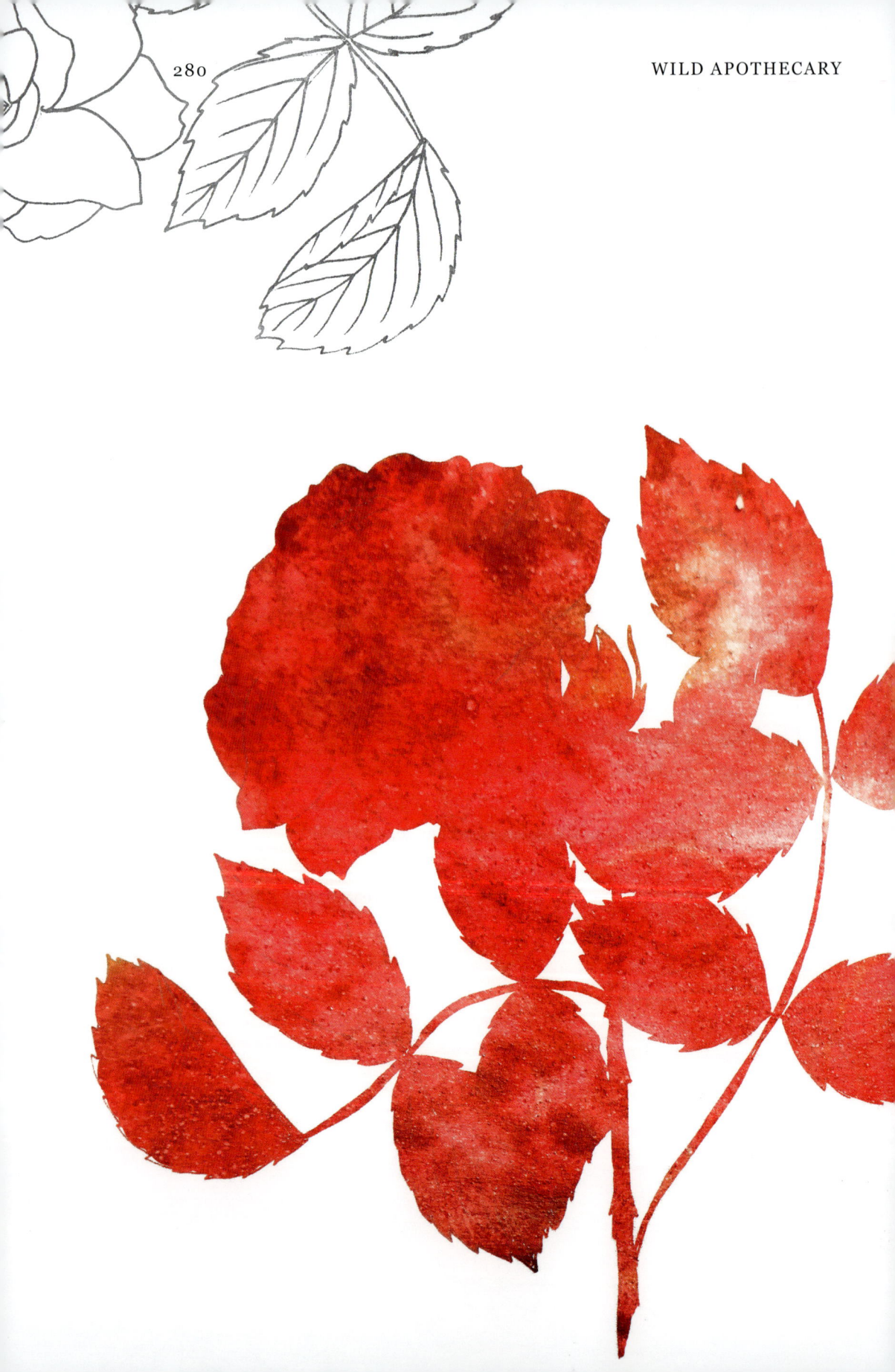

THE ROOTS: GRIEF

PLANT ALLIES

Rose *Rosa damascena*

Nature: cooling and dry

Planet: Venus

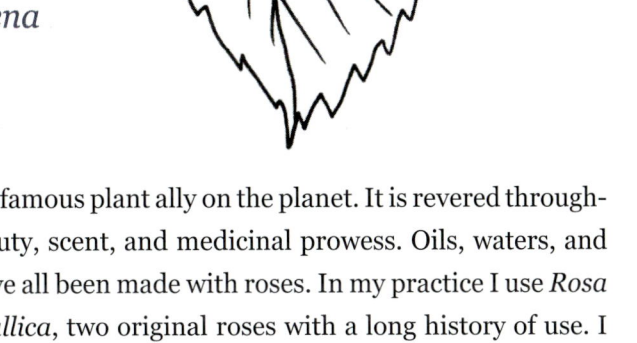

Rose is possibly the most famous plant ally on the planet. It is revered throughout the world for its beauty, scent, and medicinal prowess. Oils, waters, and food of the goddesses have all been made with roses. In my practice I use *Rosa damascena* and *Rosa gallica*, two original roses with a long history of use. I also love to use the flowers and hips of the wild dog roses that grow on the land around my home.

Rose is delicate petal, sweet intoxicating scent, nourishing hips, and wildly fierce thorns. It is a herb of boundaries and beauty. It uplifts and tends the spirit while cooling and calming us. It is a heart herb and along with hawthorn, lemon balm, and vervain may ease an aching heart. It is supportive in heart disease with hawthorn, lily of the valley, motherwort, and linden and brings down inflammation.

For women, rose can ease menstrual pain and menopausal hot flushes and it is helpful with urinary tract infections. It is packed with antioxidants and used in general infection, fever, and skin conditions. It can be taken by anyone internally and externally at any age.

I use rose a lot as a finishing herb to many blends. I see many patients with anxiety of some kind, and rose, as my teacher used to say, is love in a bottle.

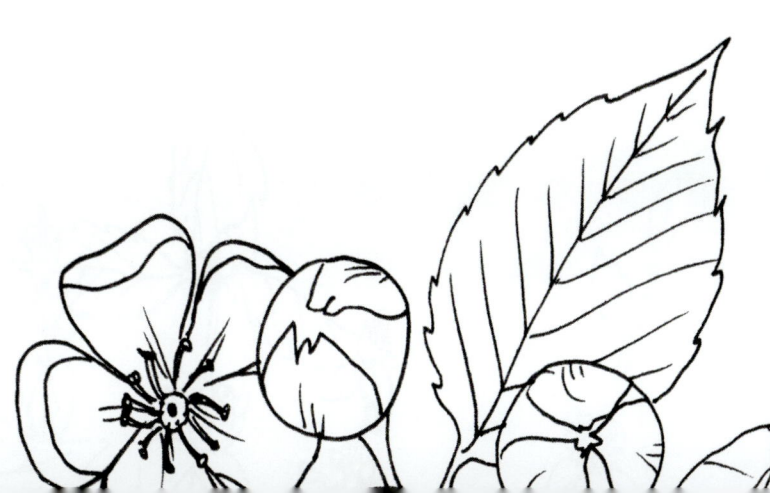

WILD HEART HEALING ELIXIR

Rose
Blackcurrant
Lemon balm
Vervain
Honey
Brandy

Macerate the herbs – you can use dried but I prefer fresh – in brandy (choose the ratio of each herb that you are drawn to and cover all with brandy). Leave to infuse over a full moon – starting on the maiden moon and straining on the crone moon. These herbs are all rich in volatile oils and don't take long to impart their wonder.

Strain. Add honey to taste and take a few drops daily to help strengthen the heart and release the ache.

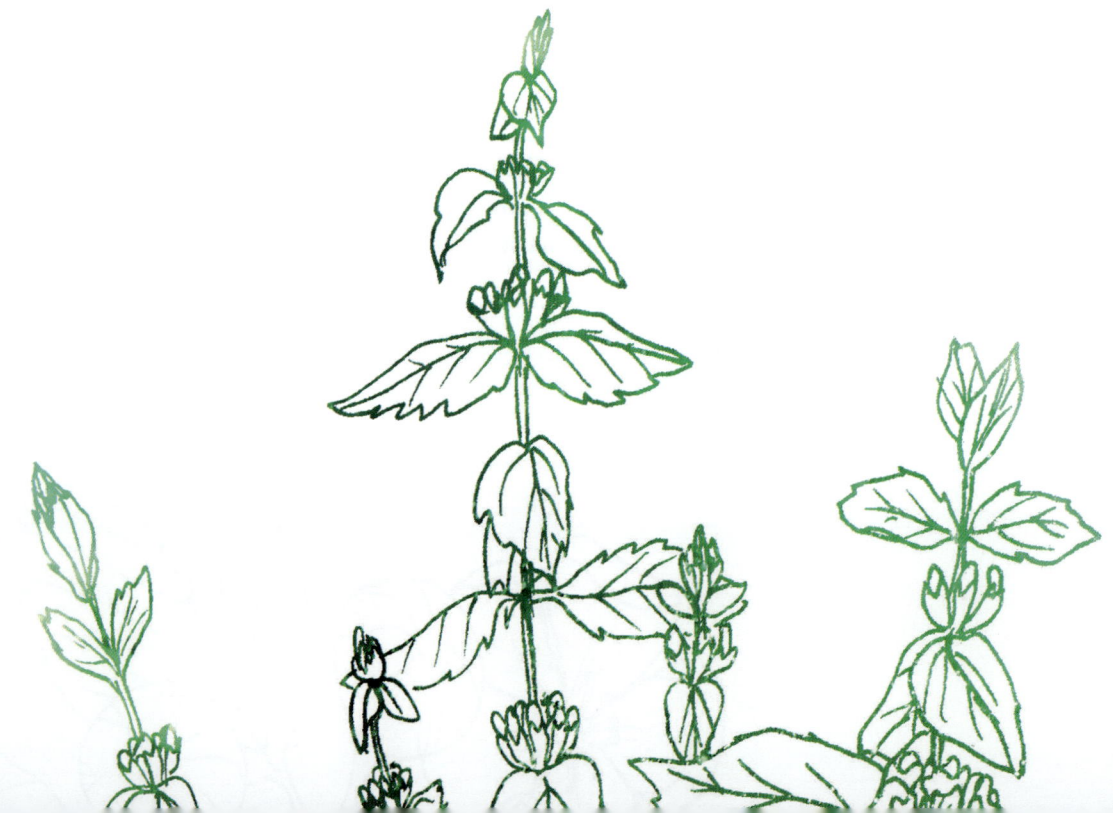

Lemon balm *Melissa officinalis*

Nature: temperate

Planet: Jupiter

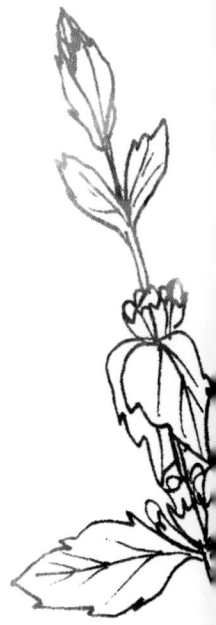

Where rose is a remedy of love in a bottle, lemon balm is a balm to our souls. This plant ally is deliciously uplifting and wonderfully refreshing. It carries an earthy lemon scent which is in itself enough to help you feel good. It is commonly and historically used as a specific for anxiety and low mood. If you are stuck in melancholy, this is the herb for you. If grief becomes too much to bear, this herb may shine the light and illuminate a path towards healing. Spend time with this herb if you are stuck in grief.

It is lovely with wood betony for those who worry and can't stop. For those who have built their walls high and have closed their hearts, lemon balm, or Melissa as I usually call her, will help you dismantle your walls and open up to love. If you have experienced trauma, especially sexual trauma, this little, sometimes straggly, sometimes lush herb will accompany you on your path to reconnecting with self.

This herb is also commonly used to ease physical ailments – skin conditions, digestive issues, viruses, headaches, respiratory conditions, and hyperthyroidism.

```
LEMON BALM BRANDY

Pick 100g lemon balm leaves and flowers - chop them
up a little

Pop into a small jar and cover with 200-300ml brandy

Seal and leave for 2 weeks

Strain and take a tipple of an evening when your heart is
sore or you need a little uplifting.
```

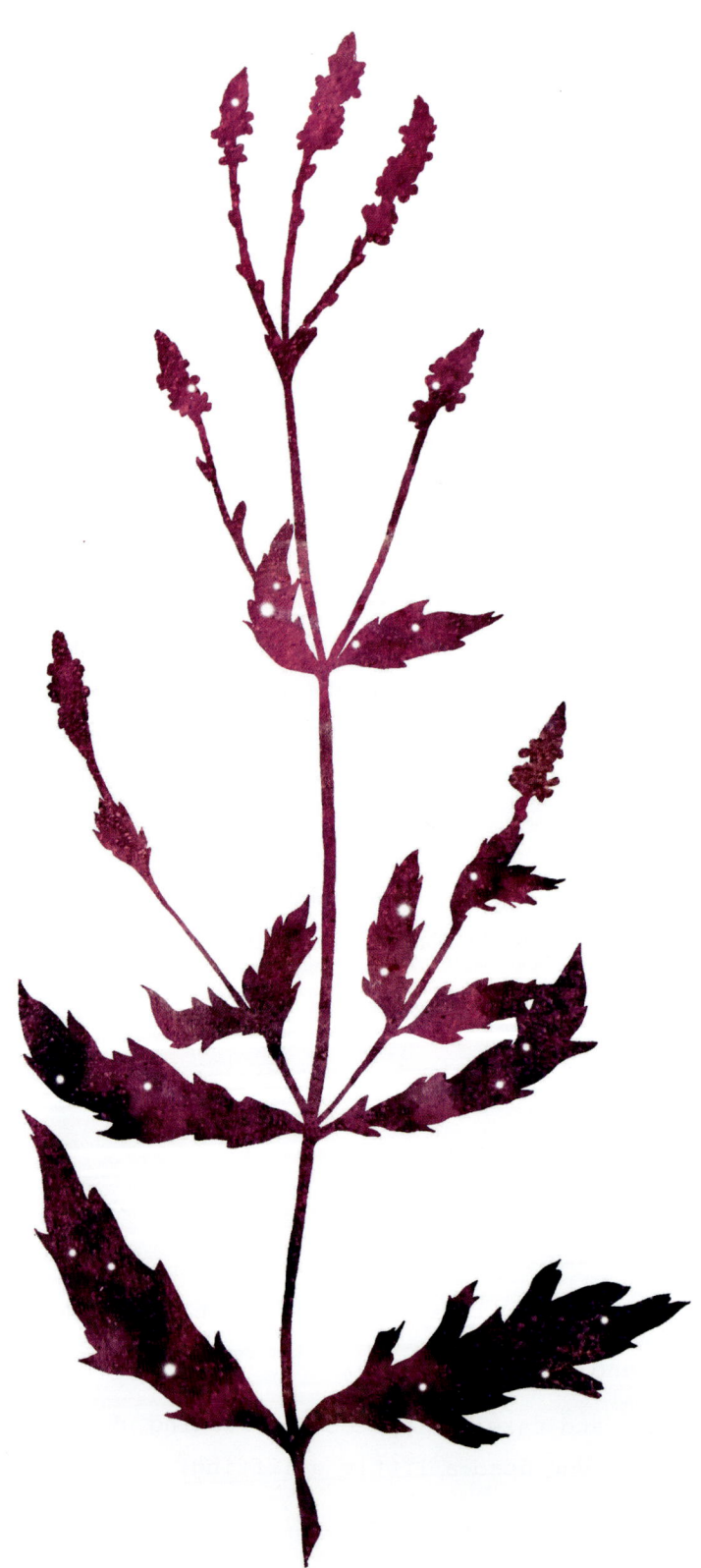

Vervain *Verbena officinalis*

Nature: hot/cold and dry

Planet: Venus

Vervain is a magical herb and long held in esteem. Its transformational magical powers were held in high regard by the druids, used in their lustral water and more. It is a plant greatly valued by herbalists. This herb is so easy to grow and is resilient and humble yet strong in its appearance.

Vervain is my go-to herb for grief. Being hot and cold (bitter) and dry it is transformative both in its physical effects, moving the blood and digestive juices, and acting as a liver tonic, and emotional effects. It gently encourages the self to let go while it supports us. It is tough and tender and reflects how we are when we grieve.

Vervain is predominantly used as a nervous system tonic and when we are grieving we all need this kind of support. Vervain is, however, a little pushy so if you're very tender just a little is enough. You might like to mix it with rose, as I often do in an elixir, which is comforting and nourishing while asking you to do the work.

Vervain can be used for fears, anxiety, low mood, sluggishness, fatigue, infection, stuck emotions, and much more. It is truly one of my most used herbs in the apothecary and where I go it seems to follow.

This is how people have described to me their experience of vervain and how they might use it or see it:

> For those emotionally blocked and frustrated whose spirits are not being watered.
>
> For stuckness in sexuality or relationships.
>
> For a woman who needs uplifting, some light energy (. . .) who needs warmth, energy, and releasing.

For those who are cold and clammy, they've no echo to their voice (. . .) timid and uncertain.

For people who are very bright, out there wanting to know.

For those who just live in their heads

For those who seek to move through what holds them back.

I have an interesting and close to my heart story of vervain.

I learned the plants that my teacher, Christopher Hedley, loved well. Vervain was one such plant. As I learned more, I longed to meet this plant ally.

I had never seen it before but had dreamed with it, grieved with it, and learned much from it.

In my first year as a baby herbalist I went to my childhood home and slept outside on the lawn I had grown up playing about on. After that night I asked my parents to let the grass grow long so that we might see a little wildness. And so they did.

When I returned a little while later, flourishing in the lawn were yarrow and vervain, just where I had been sleeping. It was as if magical seeds had sprouted, or more likely they had been there for decades and I had somehow been feeling their vibration for most of my life without knowing it.

Vervain is for grieving, for magic, dreams, and love to be attended to, and for our sorrow to be felt and gently let go of, bringing us a little further along the journey of self-love, connection, and wonder.

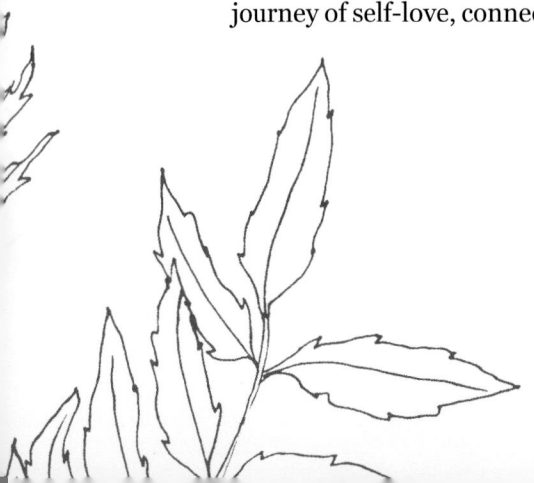

Vervain energetics

THE ROOTS: GRIEF

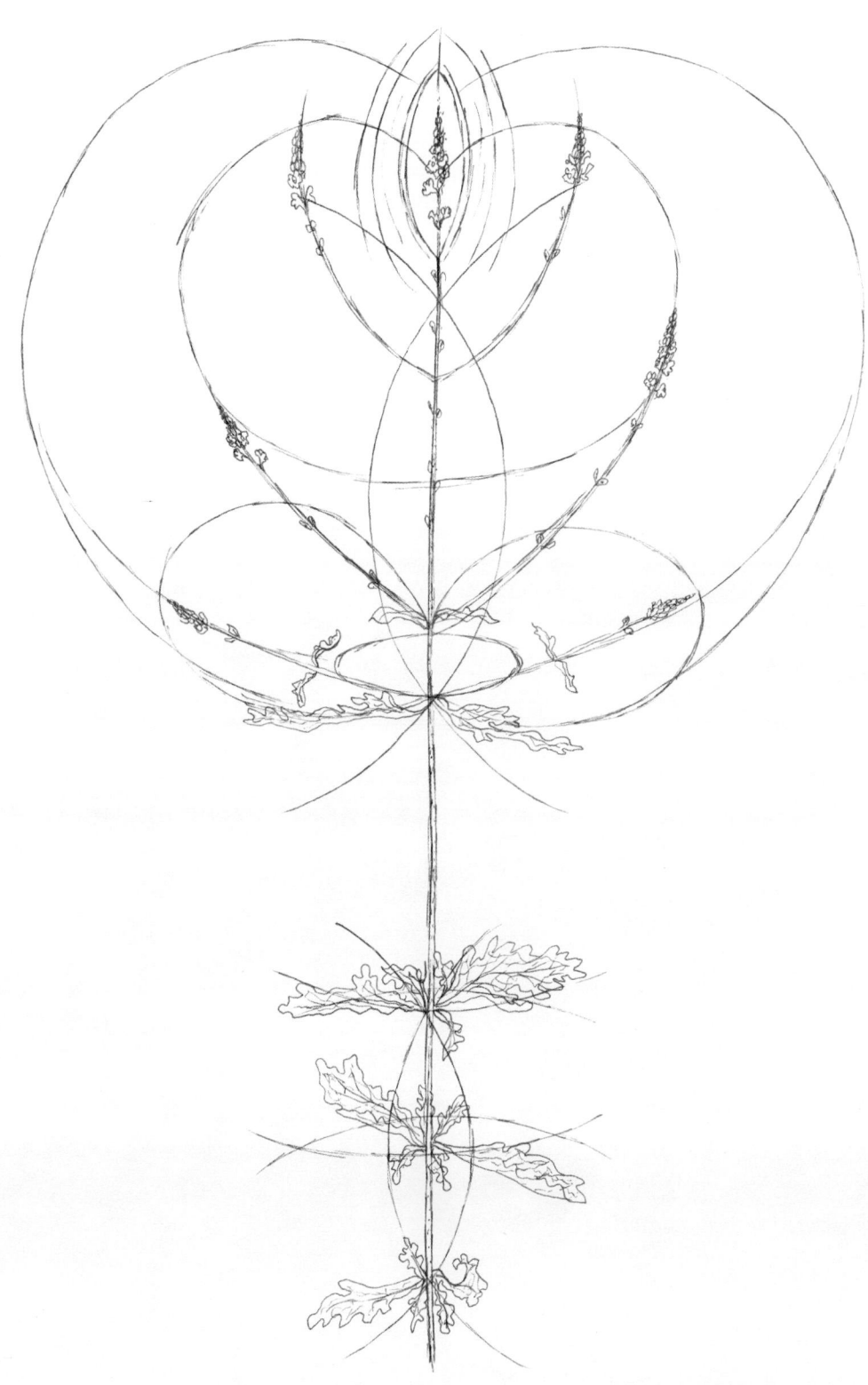

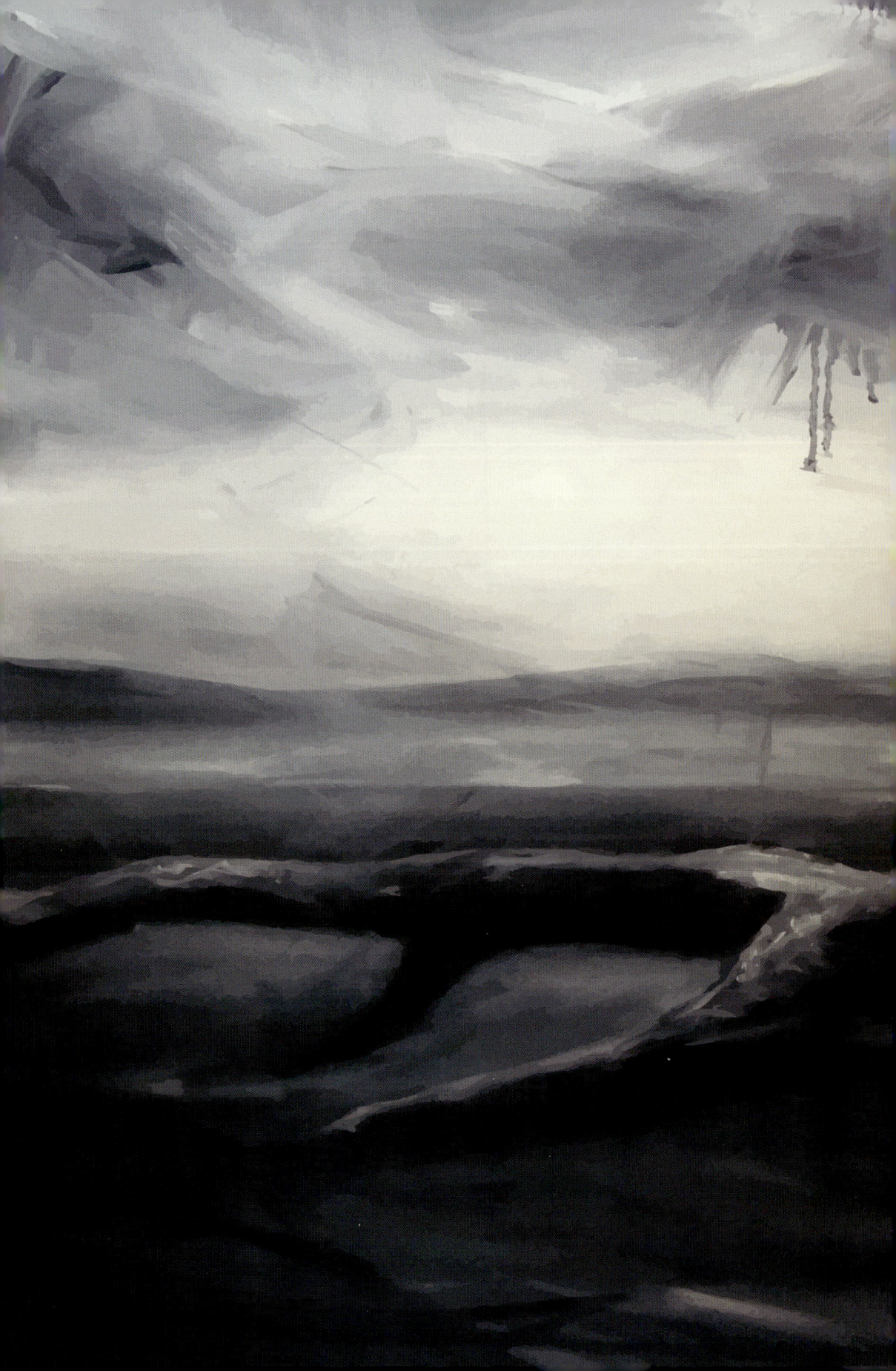

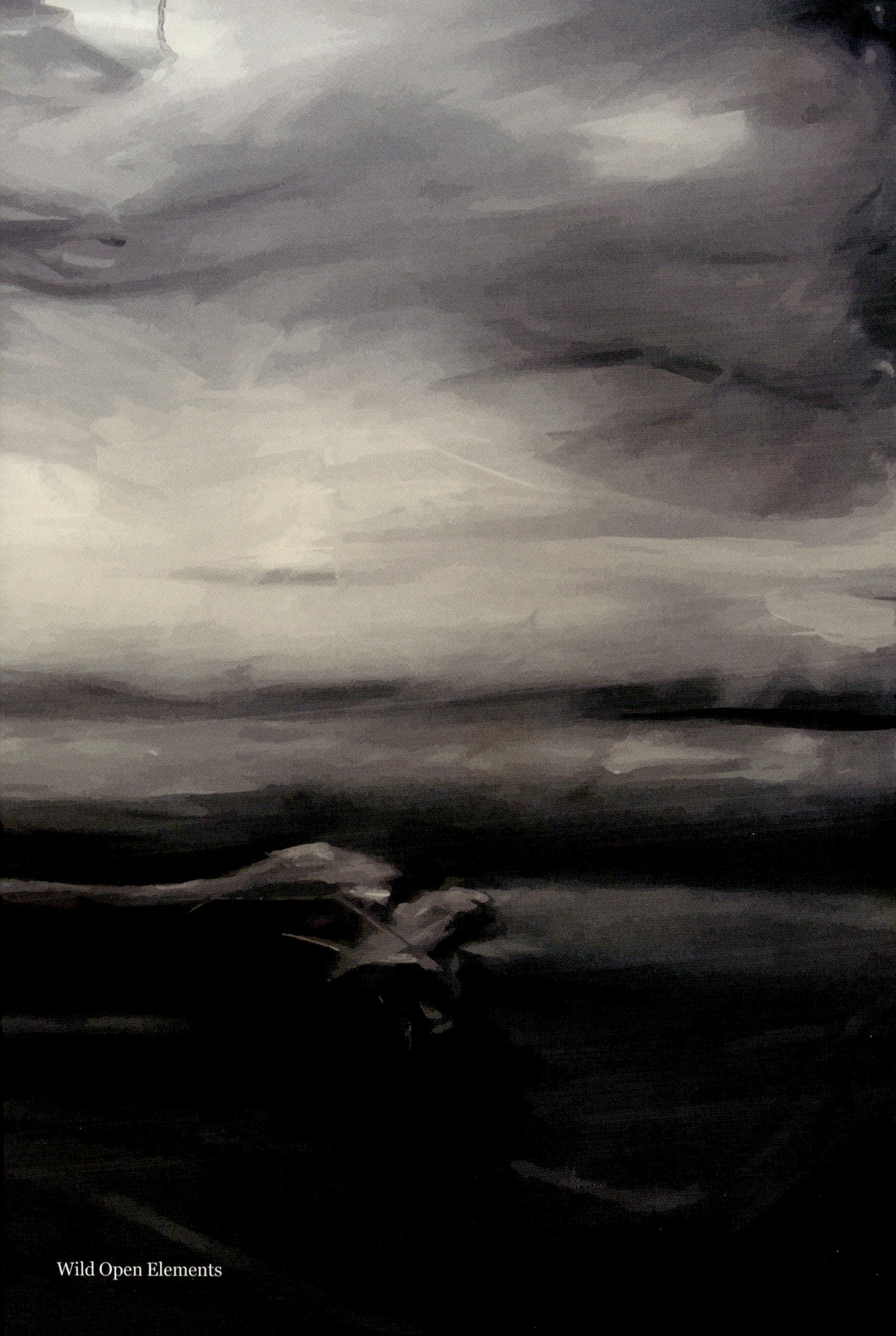
Wild Open Elements

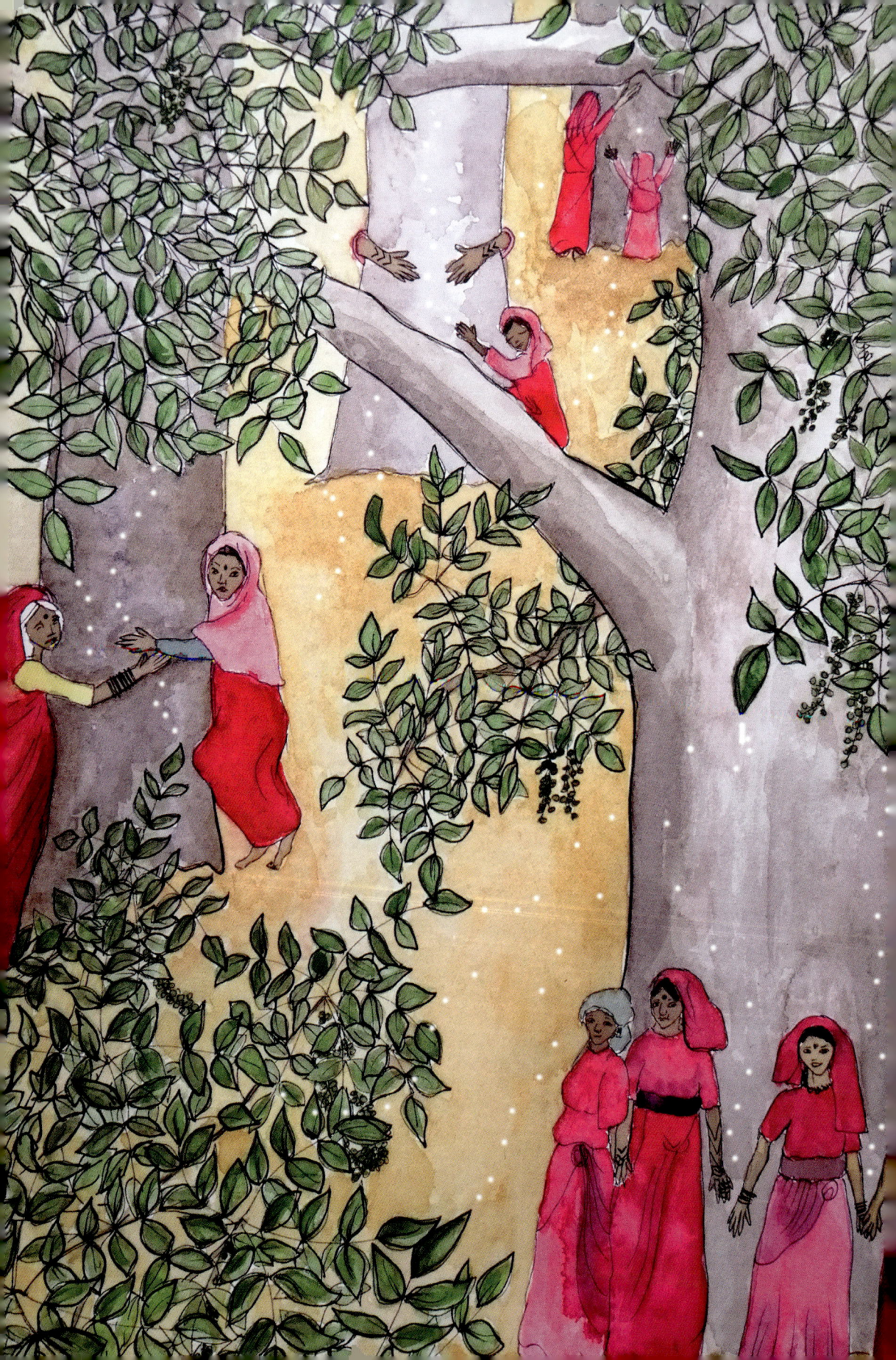

CHAPTER 11

RADICAL ROOTS: DECOLONIAL REFLECTIONS

By Claudia Manchanda, Radical Herbalist

Women defending ash trees as did the Chipko Tree Huggers in 1970s. The magenta pink in this illustration is to represent Gulabi Gang (Rose Gang) who formed in Uttar Pradesh to protect women, in response to the lack of police protection from domestic abuse.

Look at me
Get used to my face
My thick and slender frames
My weird and wild ways
Observe the many ways I display my femininity
Get used to what you see
Listen to what I have to say
Because whether you like it
And whether you do not,
I am here to stay
My bhindis, locs and traditional frocks
Mean more than a fashion statement,
More than appropriated symbols of identity
They are more than part-time adornments of the privileged
They survived because I did
As you have a history of theft
Taking from us, putting us on ships
Shackling our hearts and minds
Enslaving us for profit
Except I am free
It makes me smile to see that in your ignorance
In the wearing of my culture,
My heritage,
My colours and symbols,
My gifts and my curses
You are celebrating me
So copy, reinvent, try to obliterate who I am
But the truth is, and always will be that
I am here to stay
I have survived your famine
And now fill my belly with love
I have survived your wars
And replaced them with my peace
I have survived your poverty
And am rich in spirit

I have survived your technologies
And transformed your weapons
From the gun, into the sword, into the pen
With which I write these words
With which I will change the world
Because I was taught that
You were better than me
That God is white, that God is male
That this God was chosen to rule over us
Except I was born of a Woman
I grew in the womb
Was nurtured by breasts
And it was She that took my first breath
See, I am more than Kipling's "white man's burden"
I am more than the sum of my Ancestors' labour
I am my language,
I am my struggle
I am the glory of my heritage
Despite the crimes of colonialism
Capitalism and its father, neoliberalism
I am still the perfume of Arabia
I am still the silk of the Silk Route
I am still the comfort of cotton
I am the kohl Black that lines the eyes of the beautiful
I am the strength in the tin pots you mock
I am the pride of your Britain
Because I built this place
And now you protect your statutes, your histories
Yet these are my histories, of how I got here
And here I will remain
Occupying spaces you said I had no right to be in
I will fight despite your insults
I will be that thug and looter you claim I am
And you will insist that I get back, get back, get back to where you
once belonged!

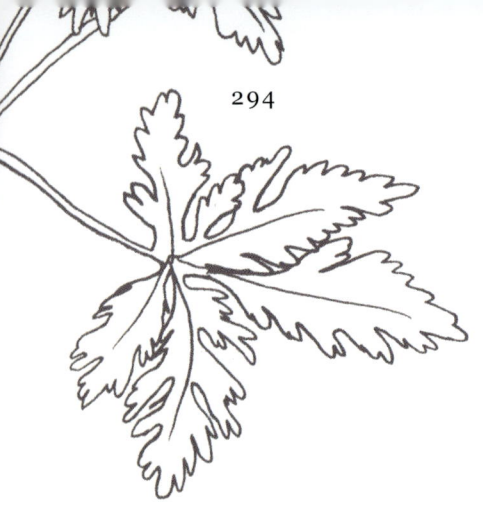

> But I am Here to Stay
> I am Here to Stay
> See my face
> Remember my name
> Because I have and always will
> Be here to stay.
>
> By RED MEDUSA, Mackayla Forde

I first met Amaia Dadachanji at the funeral of the esteemed British herbalist Christopher Hedley. Were it not for colonialism, we would not be writing in the coloniser's tongue, with our European/Indian names in the UK, the belly of the colonial beast. We are both "medical herbalists", that is, we have studied the BSc (Hons) in herbal medicine. Christopher Hedley had been a teacher to both of us at various stages of our training and was a non-conventional lecturer at Westminster University, London.

Christopher looked like an archetypical wizard. He was a tree-like, elegantly tall man, with wispy long white hair, shiny eyes, moving gently and with grace. Plant-centred, person-centred, and energetic traditional approaches were foundational to his herbal practice and teaching. He described modern herbal medicine as a "broad church", I think, referring to the welcoming of all traditions and systems with an open heart. Christopher once described a person with depression as the opposite of someone wearing rose-tinted glasses; he said that everything for them is grey, and the trick is to bring back the colour.

My own glasses are anti-colonial and anti-capitalist, and "the trick" in late stage capitalism is to learn and relearn the history, to reflect on "modernity". The political psychologist Ashis Nandy describes modernity as the liberal aspect of colonialism (and colonialism is the military wing of capitalism). It is impossible for colonialism to operate without modernity. Colonial modernity scuppered indigenous progress. To open and dig up the concrete, allowing the earth to breathe again and be watered is to rise up. To ensure self-sufficient food and medicine, to be able to access live, clean, non-chemicalised water, to return to Indigenous-led land protection and practices are the first steps to begin healing the ruins of imperial capitalism.

Once you've seen the world through decolonial glasses everything hurts continuously. However, reconnecting to nature and energetic medicine systems are fundamental to us, healing all.

The practice of holistic medicine is a culturally transformative act. Decolonising herbal medicine is the moral responsibility of contemporary herbalists. The year 2020 is a watershed moment. A global pandemic, appalling state negligence, erroneous lockdowns, a global public lynching have forced the gaze onto racist, socio-economic oppression and the failure of capitalism.

Enough is enough.

This generation has declared that they have come to finish what the ancestors started in terms of resisting oppression with radical activism, changing descriptors for identity, toppling statues of murderers; and throughout the so-called Commonwealth, votes are taking place to remove the British monarch as head of state. All with a consciousness for the need of health care, spirituality, and therapy and as forms of resistance.

The *Oxford English Dictionary* defines colonialism as "the policy or practice of acquiring full or partial political control over another country, occupying it with settlers, and exploiting it economically". This sanitised definition omits details of the genocidal exploitation and theft of our great-grandparents' lives, land, culture, identity, and herbs, resulting in intergenerational trauma and loss.

Britain alone colonised the lands known as Afghanistan, Antigua and Barbuda, Australia, the Bahamas, Bahrain, Barbados, Belize, Botswana, Brunei, Cameroon, Canada, Cyprus, Dominica, Egypt, Eswatini, Fiji, the Gambia, Ghana, Grenada, Guyana, India, Iraq, Ireland, Jamaica, Jordan, Kenya, Kiribati, Kuwait, Lesotho, Libya, Malawi, Malaysia, Maldives, Malta, Mauritius, Myanmar, Nauru, New Zealand, Nigeria, Pakistan, Palestine, Qatar, St Lucia and the Windward Islands, St Kitts and Nevis, Anguilla and the Leeward Islands, Saint Vincent and the Grenadines, Seychelles, Sierra Leone, Singapore, Solomon Islands, South Africa, Somaliland, Sri Lanka, Sudan, Tanzania, Tonga, Trinidad and Tobago, Tuvalu, Uganda, United Arab Emirates, United States, Vanuatu, Yemen, Zambia, and Zimbabwe.

The trauma of colonialism, post-colonial structures, and neo-colonialism is ever pervasive. What are the current conditions that people live in? Continued dispossession, water loss, land loss, bad health, loss of language and lineage. The lands named "Australasia", "Brazil", "Canada", "China", "India", "Indonesia", "New Zealand", "Pacifica" and "Palestine" are all sites of ongoing neo-colonialism, land appropriation, and resource extraction. The descriptions of uninhabited lands, *terra nullius* and "ripe for the picking" are always used to describe lands about to be invaded by colonisers, as happened in the Americas, Australia, Palestine, and even in outer space. These countries are known to us by their colonised names but traditional names are being reclaimed in international circles – Aotearoa, Turtle Island, and many more. Australia, for example, had no one name as its inhabitants are multilingual and name their own traditional lands rather than the whole land mass.

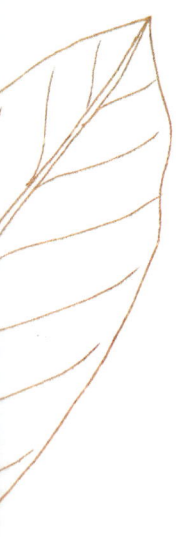

The word "West", as in Western herbal medicine, refers to the cultural assumption emanating from the "Western world", meaning Europe, European, White people in the colonised countries called America, Israel, Australia, New Zealand, and somewhat to colonisers in S. Africa. Identifying a herbal discipline that commonly incorporates global herbs, indigenous knowledge and naming it Western is problematic without reflection or acknowledgement. Using the herbs without the lore, empirical knowledge, and context is problematic at best. When I use the word "West", I am referring to colonial context and structure rather than geographical direction. When I use White, it is to describe relative privilege. When I use the term "BIPOC" (Black, Indigenous, People of Colour) it is to recognise a shared experience of colonised history that is capitalist-racism. However, the term "Indigenous" applies to where Indigenous peoples have had their ancestral land colonised.

Deconstructing language and considering the impact of language is an imperative process when decolonising thought and actions. The majority of the globe's population live in capitalist systems affected by empire, colonialism, white supremacy and classism. Every day, each one of us is engaging with the trajectory of nineteenth-century European invasion, where 75% of the globe had been colonised, stripping people of life, land, language, culture, belief, healing systems, resources, water, long hair, names, tattoos, clothes, music, and intimately intertwined herbal/spiritual practice. Colonial practices of deliberate genocide, banning of indigenous language, mass kidnap (enslavement), and ethnic divisions, child removal, and intergenerational trauma are still potent today.

Owning your ancestral name is a birthright not afforded to millions. Married women and often children are given men's names. Knowing your ancestral languages, customs, belief, and healing systems is a rarity. Even plants were stripped of their indigenous names, put into a classification system called taxonomy and given ludicrous names like *Rubus cockburnianus* which is a bramble named by the painter, Helmsley, to honour the Cockburn family. Bartholin's glands, which are pea-shaped secretory glands on each side of the vagina, are named after a White man! Imagine the glans of the penis being called "Boris Johnson"! That too would be ludicrous.

The language used by herbalists about our own practices can also be questioned. "Herbal Master Classes" are available – you can be a "master" of herbalism after a short online course. The idea that you can "master" herbalism implies that you are at the top of a knowledge hierarchy.

Western herbal medicine often describes itself as having an "essentially European heritage" without exploring how colonisers on Turtle Island appropriated Indigenous herbs. Where did Hippocrates, Galen, and Gerard receive their knowledge? Hippocrates studied in Alexandria, Egypt, Greece, and possibly Libya! It's important to note that rich complex Indigenous traditions existed and were repressed in Europe.

Western herbal medicine often uses the "medical model" as its foundation. It is colonial, racist, and sexist. Not holistic. Not person-centred. It doesn't assess/access the past, the environment, epigenetics, ancestry, poverty, oppression, energetics, the emotional and spiritual well-being of an individual/community. It does not celebrate puberty or the forty days post-partum as a rite of passage which require honour and guided support. Menopause and ageing are not regarded as a period of honour and respect where elders pass on learnings and reflection. It does not embrace and coexist with death. In fact, when we deviate from the White straight, athletic, mythical norms, we are subconsciously deemed deviant.

In the nineteenth century, plants were being reduced into constituents and ensuing pharmacological drugs, and borders of colonial lands were being imposed. White men were sectioning our bodies into bordered physiological systems, with subsequent separated disciplines presiding over them. The

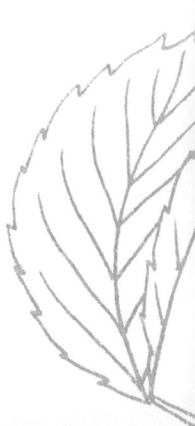

sciences of alchemy were reduced to chemistry, herbalism to pharmacology, astrology to astronomy, herbalists to heretics and witches.

Modern colonialism, late-stage capitalism, and hetero-patriarchal norms have all impinged on the way "we" relate to ourselves, our health, even our sense of beauty and true wealth. Our sense of peace and happiness is constantly being challenged.

CAROLUS LINNAEUS (1700s) AND THE NAMES OF PLANTS

"Should coconuts chance to come into my hands, it would be as if fried Birds of Paradise had flown into my mouth as I open my throat."

I used this Linnaeus quote as it evokes an image of gobbling up the exotic and the privilege of world domination and exploitation.

Linnaeus was a Swedish botanist who developed the system of categorisation called taxonomy. The largest category at the top is kingdom. At the bottom are species identified by two names: binomial nomenclature, denoting the genera and species, for example, *Homo sapiens* from the kingdom Mammalia. The word "kingdom" is male and imperial. The scientific formal name conforming to the international code of nomenclature for plants (and algae, fungi, etc.) is an internationally understood name for each plant, known as its botanical name.

Formal scientific names are italicised for generic, specific, and infraspecific botanical names and are European-dominated nomenclature. For example, daisy is *Bellis perennis*, the genus *Bellis* and epithet *perennis*. The epithets officinalis and officinale refer to medicinal plants such as dandelion (*Taraxacum officinale*). Binominal names, while often useful, are imposed and sometimes even bear the name of the coloniser. Common names reveal their properties and culture. For example daisy is also known as bruisewort, making its use obvious to all. I make an ointment from infused daisy oil for those having repeated cannulations for IV drips to prevent bruising and discomfort. When I learn plants, I like to know all of their names, as I do with people and places.

The legacy of nineteenth-century colonialism means that today's economic distribution of wealth is still reminiscent of the colonial era. However, in systematically ruined countries with climate "changed", the most profitable export is now people themselves, especially trained professionals and labourers who are forcibly exported to economically rich countries, due to lack of economic opportunity. In a quantified study of the diet of Brazilian sisal workers, the dire effect of world market capitalism on these agricultural labourers included malnutrition, increased morbidity, and abandoning traditional subsistence agriculture. Coupled with capitalism, this system is designed to make us reliant on exploitative production systems for sustenance: fast food, refined carbohydrates, synthetic sodium, rancid oils, synthetic clothes and shoes, aerial toxic particulates, flammable and toxic dwellings. All this renders our bodies chronically unwell with metabolic syndromes. We are stressed. We are post- and presently traumatised. We are at higher risk of metabolic disorders, Covid-19, cancer, mental illness, suicide, and death at the hands of the state.

When I was twenty-three, I had a baby and I decided I needed to pursue a formal education to support my child. I had worked as a chef and was interested in activism. I attended evening classes in astronomy, archaeology, pottery, and herbal medicine for one year. I went on community herbal walks. I was already becoming a budding herbalist.

On my first day of the herbal medicine degree course at Westminster University in 1999, we were taken into the dispensary in the Polyclinic and told that in three years we would be acquainted with all of the 200-plus tinctured herbs in brown bottles on the shelves, labelled in botanical binomial nomenclature. I looked at a bottle that said "*Elletaria cardamomum*". I figured it must be Elaichi, cardamom. I don't remember any context or introduction on the entire course as to how those herbs got in those bottles, who grew them, where, on what soils, what is their traditional use and folklore? How did these plants that are used in everyday life come to be there? On what land were they grown and by who?

How were they harvested and transported? Who packaged, labelled, and sold them? Who made the profit? How was the land treated? I couldn't picture any of the above. However, I was well acquainted with the resinous warming aromatic cardamom seeds from the pod used to give a depth and richness to my chai (tea), methai (Indian sweets), shrikand, kulfi, and keer. I vaguely remember an Indian love story from my childhood about the relationship between a clove and a cardamom pod. Elaichi is used as an aromatic digestive for indigestion, bowel spasm, loss of appetite, and general invigoration. It contributes rich aroma and indulgent depth to desserts, chai, coffee, and rice dishes.

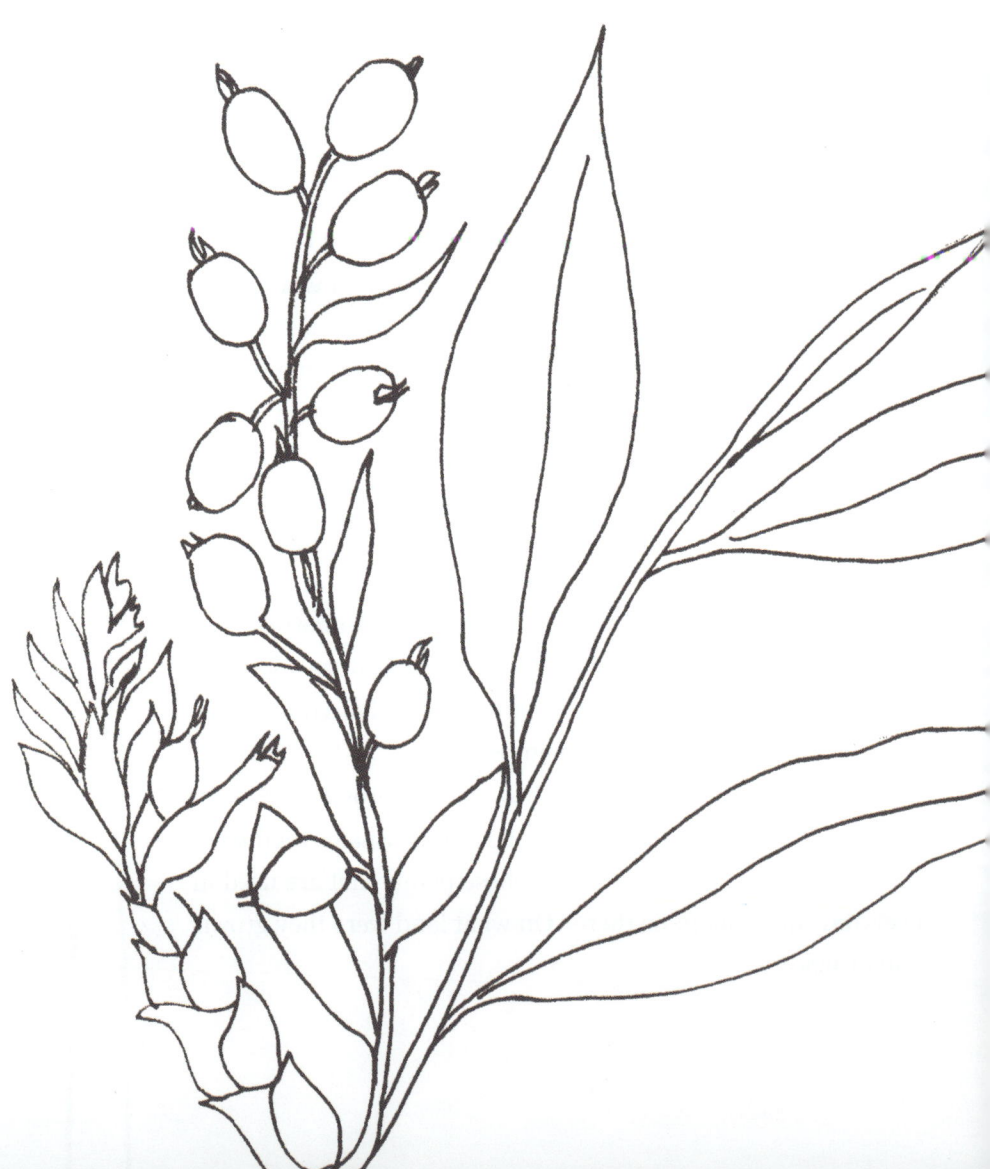

THE "ENGLISH" CUPPA: CAMELLIA SINENSIS. A METAPHOR FOR PLANT APPROPRIATION.

The epithet *sinensis* refers to a Chinese species. Tea may be considered as metaphor for plant food and plant relations available in the supermarkets. In the 1800s, tea was introduced to Europe as a herbal drug. It was exotic, exclusive, expensive, and unfamiliar. Within a century, it was a mass market commodity, consumed at least weekly by most people in the country. Did you know that if tea is called tea or té, it first arrived by clipper ship? If it's called chai, cha, or çhay, it came on land via the Silk Road. The origin of the word "tea" comes from its Chinese roots 茶 (chá in Mandarin and Cantonese).

In the Tang dynasty, through cultivation, it was developed into a tasty green tea beverage. Peasants were forced to grow "tribute tea" alongside their own food crops to pay the emperor, often sacrificing their own rice and provision crops, leading to famine. The tea-rich emperor was able to trade. Seventeenth-century tea houses and tea gardens became popular and black tea was made from fermenting green tea leaves. Tea was traded with Tibetans for war horses on the Tea Horse Road and was drunk with yaks' milk and yak butter. Buddhists moving along the Silk Road traded tea from Asia to the Middle East, from Burma in the south to Siberia in the north, from Korea to Japan and Turkey.

During the Ming dynasty, steeping loose tea became popularised through trading with Europeans for silver coinage. The Dutch bought a ship of tea in 1610. Europeans initially didn't like the cost of this expensive, bitter medicinal drink although they liked its ability to "vanquish heavy dreams, easeth the pain of heavy damps, and openeth obstructions in the bowel".

Catherine of Braganza, an avid tea addict, married King Charles II in 1661, influencing the popularity of tea among the upper classes. It sold for ten times the price of coffee. The demand for tea was high but it was only produced in China and so the clipper ship was designed for its capture. In 1848, the British East India Company, a state-run business, sent Robert Fortune on a mission of corporate cultural espionage to prohibited territories to steal horticultural and harvesting practices. At this time, the complex processing of tea had been established for 2,000 years. Fortune was responsible for appropriating cuttings in China for plant nurseries in India.

The British East India Company devised a heinous strategy to cause widespread opium dependence in China. By using opium poppies grown in India as payment for Chinese goods, they would buy tea as the Chinese would not trade for anything but silver. Rulers of the Qing dynasty were not impressed, initially destroying the 20,000 chests of opium (around 1,400m tonnes) and banishing British merchants but the Chinese were eventually forced to open up trade and Hong Kong was ceded to Britain. Then China paid reparations to the British for the cost of the war and opium became legalised. The Chinese nation had their livelihoods, possessions and silver forcibly taken. Whilst Opium was restricted in England, China became known as "the sick man of Asia" due to the drug addiction of twelve million people. The consequences included the Taiping Rebellion, a Christian-founded civil war killing 20–70 million. Death and drug addiction paid for British tea.

In 1827 and again in 1834 a prominent company botanist reported that India's Himalayan foothills would be suitable for tea growing. Under the auspices of the British East India Company the plant thief Robert Fortune brought 2,000 tea plants and 17,000 tea seeds to establish more than half a million acres. Impoverished peasants were recruited under contracts with harsh penal clauses in what was called "a new system of slavery" (Hugh Tinker, 1974). Plantations as such came late to the Asian colonies. The black tea now common in the UK is heavily oxidised, caffeinated, tanninised - the legacy of colonisation in India.

The lush western highlands of Kenya are currently one of the best tea growing regions in the world but in 1934, hundreds of thousands of Kipsigis and Talai people were violently driven out of their expansive homeland by White settlers for tea plantations supplying Unilever's Lipton's Tea and other well-known brands. The British Army used rape, arson, and murder and displaced the people from their homeland. The Kipsigi community and Talai clan are currently in the process of suing the British government for 2 trillion Kenyan shillings for crimes compared to genocide.

This is a synopsis of the tea story. However, there are similar histories to be found about coffee, cotton, cannabis, hemp, mahogany, sugar, pepper, Peruvian bark rubber, spices, and so on.

TRADITIONAL HERBAL MEDICINE AND SCIENCE

Traditional systems of medicine have used the same plants for millennia. Knowledge is contextual, refined, systematic, in tune with lineage, language, culture, times of day, seasons, rhythms, combinations of plants, planetary alignments, noting signs and instructions from nature. Connecting to someone's story is enough to ascertain their suffering and resulting stress. Additionally observing face shape, irises, the thickness of the skin and structures, body shape, personality, the pulse, tongue, the birth chart, provides constitutional cues allowing support for an individual make-up. Do we need a profit driven medical model to approve our medicine when we have observation, in addition to empathy, and compassion?

Today, the biomedical model for health care is the gold standard for legitimacy and prestige. Even the herbal medicine degree I attended was called Health Sciences: Herbal Medicine. Herbal medicine practices are disparaged as woo-woo and sayings like "old wives tales" are belittling to women's collective knowledge and generational empiricism. We may ask, what is science and what are energetics? Are they separate? Science is described as the intellectual and practical activity encompassing the systematic study of the structure and behaviour of the physical and natural world through observation and experiment. Surely this is energetic traditional herbal medicine? Today, science is

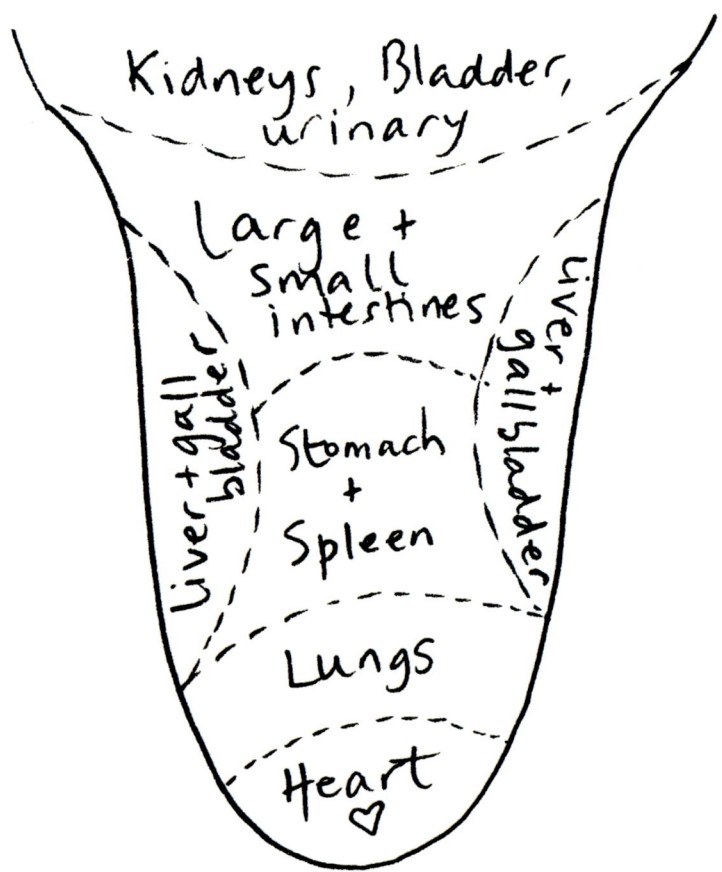

too often colonial and capitalist. White, male-led, sexist, racist, prejudiced, immoral, and unethical. Unscientific. Devoid of love. Devoid of compassion. Devoid of simply using common sense.

When I was first studying psychology, an experiment was described where baby rhesus monkeys were taken from their mothers then left alone or given a teddy to hug. Their response behaviours were observed. I felt very annoyed reading it. It hardly takes a genius to work out how babies torn from their mothers will respond. Another common experiment used to test herbal extracts is the burnt rat paw test. A rodent's paw is chemically injured and herbal extracts applied to see if they relieve it. These kinds of tests are accepted as a rational and moral aspect of science. Epigenetics, studying the mechanisms for turning genes on or off, is deemed as a legitimate science. However, herbalists have been identifying predispositions for thousands of years without ever having to draw blood or look at gene changes. It is common sense that abuse and loss is traumatic and consequential.

The scientific standard for testing herbal extracts for "legitimacy" starts with the separation of chemical extracts in vitro and evolves into the modern "gold standard" efficacy test – the double-blind placebo-controlled study, where people may be left to suffer without treatment while others may be extensively experimented on. As a student I found the ethics behind scientific experimentation often ghastly and unnecessary, such as the lethal dose test (LD50). Yet I marvelled at the wonders of scientific understanding when used with ethical foundation.

Understanding the science of plant medicine is necessary for herbalists, as is understanding the energetics of prescription drugs. Respectful integration is possible as exemplified by use of immune-modulating herbs alongside chemotherapy and radiotherapy in Chinese herbalism.

All traditional systems of medicine I have encountered regard the energetics and constitutions of humans and plants. Energetic medicines incorporate highly refined analyses to allow for individualised therapeutics in the context of real life. You may not want to give a hot person a heating medicine/plant, for example.

THE WHOLE IS GREATER THAN THE SUM OF ITS PARTS

There is a saying, "local herbs for local people". This refers to the mutual environment shared by plants and local life. Miraculously, but surely, plants we need for health appear in our local vicinity, producing varying constituents in different plant parts, places, and times. Even when our ancestors are not from the land we reside in, our bodies somehow know where we are in time and space, and the plants also know. Plants have their own microbiomes and exist symbiotically within nature; mycelium of fungi acts as inter-species communication. When we grow or harvest plants, we form a relationship with the plant and learn about its life. Interestingly, having an abundance of berries early on in the year and throughout the summer indicates a long, cold winter to follow, and during the beginning of this year's Covid-19 lockdown every single hawthorn in my street was both flowering and fruiting. I'd never seen this before but what we need, the plants provide; the leaves, flowers, and berries were needed for the heart and blood vessels during the pandemic.

Did you know that the bark protecting a tree commonly has protective chemicals like tannins and alkaloids which protect our barrier tissues? The red sun-tinged ends of lettuce leaves contain pigments which protect us from sunburn. The aromatic essential oils from the sexual organs of higher plants may bind to our sex hormone receptors. The roots of plants commonly have grounding properties.

Harvesting and preparing local plants provide an opportunity for relationship. Making herbal preparations can also be a meditative experience, infusing intentions of healing and care within the process. Herbalist colleagues are reclaiming the tradition of spagyric extractions where the solid part of the plants, that are generally discarded, are calcined and reunited into the liquid. This is truly honouring every part of the whole plant and produces a more potent medicine requiring lower doses. Holism also pertains to the environment and the social conditions a person is experiencing, now and intergenerationally, and colonial history is part of the whole story of herbal medicine in Britain.

KAVA KAVA

When I first began studying herbal medicine, there was a huge issue with the South Pacific root, kava kava, *Piper mythesticum*. Kava means bitter in Tongan and has been used for centuries by South Pacific people in a water-based extraction with neither drama nor adversity. I remember kava kava tincture being used in many prescriptions for overworked, stressed women in our training clinic.

In the Pacific islands the fresh root is chewed or ground, added to water and consumed fresh – chewing it fresh produces a stronger "euphoria". The herb was devoured in the West for its anxiolytic effects attributed to chemicals called kavalactones. The manufacture of standardised extracts soon ensued and were deemed as effective as pharmacological anxiolytic medications.

However, there was a stream of reports of liver damage (hepatotoxicity) associated with non-traditional tinctures and standardised extracts (with numerous postulations as to why, such as glutathione level variation, variances in flavokavains, cytochrome enzyme CYP2D6 deficiency). The extracts omitted protective elements of the herb (whole plant medicine) and the bottom line is that tradition was not respected.

Herbal medicine is an art that has been developed over millennia. Herbs given alone are called simples. In most traditions, herbs are given as balanced prescriptions complementing each other for the need of the recipient (human or animal). Some herbs may amplify the effects of another, some may behave as a vehicle to help to carry the medicine to where it's needed, some may nullify the toxicity of a plant, and so on. I once watched a BBC programme with a doctor explaining that the benefits of turmeric with fats and other spices had been "discovered". I sat and scratched my head thinking, isn't that how Indians eat their curries and Haldi has been consumed with milk for generations?

ITADORI

Itadori means "to remove pain". It is the traditional name for Japanese knotweed, indigenous to Japan, China, Korea, and Taiwan and apparently brought to the UK by Philipp von Siebold in the early 1800s. It has had numerous names but is known to botanists as *Polygonum cuspidatum*, in the buckwheat family. The cuttings from one female plant were shared among nurseries and popularised as an animal feed from 1840 and her progeny followed waterways so are now labelled as invasive, Japanese, foreign, and female. Demonised for affecting mortgage applications and the worth of properties, and declared a crime to make cuttings, of this plant the Telegraph newspaper went as far as to say, "The largest female on earth could strangle Britain."

A herbalist tends to look for deeper reasons for the presence/present of Itadori and can utilise the abundance of this plant nature has decided to bless us with. The fact she can grow through concrete and is tenacious

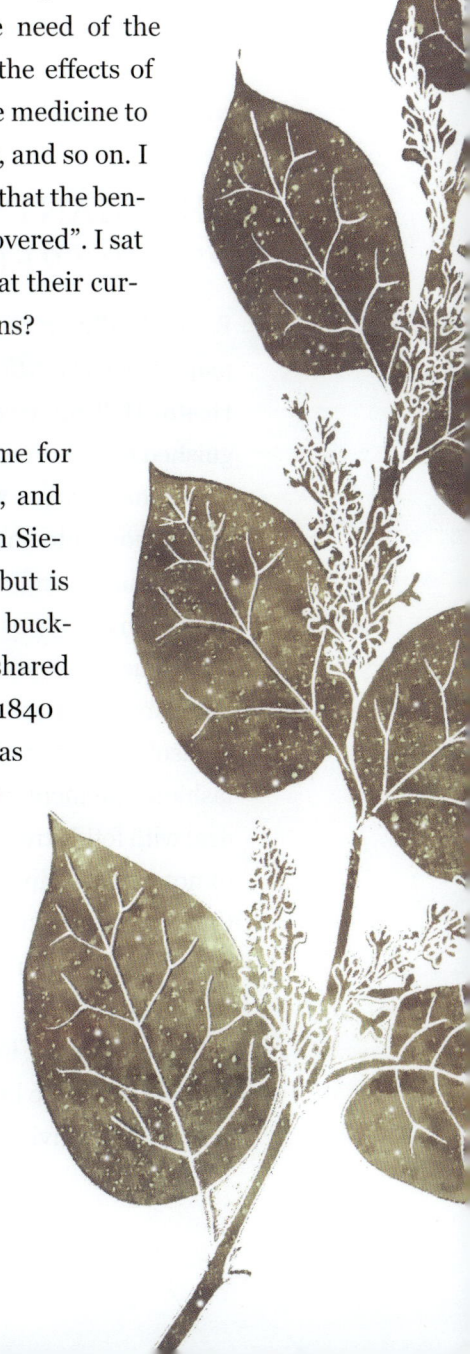

is mystically metaphorical and she provides food and medicine. Energetically, the plant is bitter and cold, especially the root, moves stagnation and invigorates Qi. It has affinity to the gall bladder, liver, lungs, and clears mucous. Traditionally useful in blood stagnation, haemorrhoids, bruising, inflammation, clotty periods, it is a rich source of red resveratrol and is a contemporary medicine for Lyme disease, even crossing the blood/brain barrier to calm intra-cranial inflammation. There have been investigations for its use in Covid-19. The young shoots can be used as a vegetable dish with a flavor reminiscent of asparagus/rhubarb. What is not to like? If we are to remove it because of damage to property, this should be done with reverence and not by contaminating the environment with mutagenic pesticides.

THE GIANTS OF LONDON, THE LONDON PLANE TREES

Before leading a recent radical herbal walk, I observed an avenue of London plane trees (*Plantinus x hispanicus*) leading to the entrance of Hampstead Heath. Half the trees in the city are London planes and they can be distinguished by flaky, camouflage-looking bark which is a marker of pollution. The closer the trees are to a busy road, the more frequent the turnover of bark and as you move into unpolluted areas, the bark becomes smooth and regular. They are not native and are a hybrid of the American sycamore and Oriental plane created in the 1600s.

Avenues of London plane trees line the Embankment on the Thames and I have images of aristocrats parading along the pavement with crinoline and parasols, showing off their stolen "exotic" wealth and plants as an upper-class fashion statement, displaying their pillaged wealth while the proletariat had to deal with fetid streams, open sewers, and back street butchery. (It is important to note that during this period there were only thirty physicians, whom only the rich could afford, permitted to practise for 400,000 Londoners. The poor had to rely on an underground army of illegal practitioners, in a time of witch hunts.)

London planes live for so long, require relatively small roots, and have adapted so well to living in the UK that few have died. They are a metaphor for resilience, surviving huge amputations (conventionally known as pollarding),

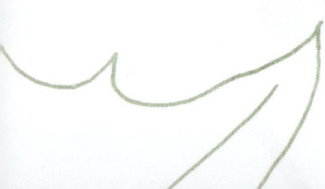

and represent strength after forced relocation and forced interbreeding and biological sex fluidity. Botanically, "perfect flowers" are bisexual or monoecious, having a male branch which pollinates in the spring and a female branch which fruits at the end of the summer. (Dioecious refers to separate male and female plants, for instance, stinging nettle and cannabis. I remember being a teenager and knowing that female ganja plants were a good thing.)

In Iran, the plane tree is called Barge Chenar. It has been used in folk medicine for dermatological (skin), gastrointestinal (gut), and rheumatic conditions. When I look up at them, I say "Barge Chenar, Barge Chenar", to honour their ancestors. I give them gifts of stones, seaweeds, or herbs to nourish their roots. I give them a hug. I appreciate how they protect us from environmental toxicity. The Hakims, Avicenna, and Momen mentioned the anti-inflammatory and analgesic properties (specifically for sore knees!) of the plant, later demonstrated by modern identification of flavonoids, pentacyclic triterpenoids, tannins, and caffeic acid. The leaves are cytotoxic, cytostatic, astringent, anti-microbial, and antiseptic. The leaf has also demonstrated anti-nociceptive properties.

The reason I use technical language is to show how modern science creates a language barrier which separates non-medics from the qualities of plants. If the tree was to be described energetically, it is drying. It would dry up the dripping water tears and snot from hay fever. An eye bath of the leaf tea might even soothe a red eye. If you tasted the tea of the leaves, it would be puckering to the mucous membranes lining your mouth and throat. This is very useful for inflamed gums, a mouth ulcer, a sore throat, or leaky gut. If the tree was in a polluted area I would not want to disturb it for medicine.

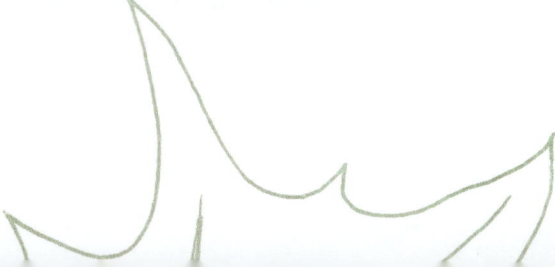

NICOLAS CULPEPER, RADICAL HERBALIST OF THE 1600s

Nicolas Culpeper was a learned, unlicensed radical apothecary, who wrote one of the best-selling books in English history. His father, the vicar of Oakley, died of typhoid when Culpeper was a child. He observed his mother's practice of using herbal medicine and roamed the countryside collecting for her. As a child he knew lady's mantle was for sagging breasts and honeysuckle ointment for sunburn. At sixteen he attended Cambridge University studying the "liberal arts" to equip him for Church life. He rebelled. He fell madly in love with a woman of gentry but she was tragically killed by a lightning strike while waiting for him under an oak tree. He was disowned by his family.

In 1634 Culpeper came to London, one of the most densely populated cities in Europe where life expectancy was just twenty-five years and disease was a viewed as a corruption of the air. Culpeper paid £50 to serve an eight-year apprenticeship, pledge not to marry, and learn how to compound, let blood, and brew herbs. As he had studied Latin (unlike common apothecaries), he could access the restricted applications withheld from the apothecaries who were specialists in collection and production of the medicines. Like me, Nicholas gathered herbs on Hampstead Heath, but also Greenwich and Putney.

He translated inaccessible Latin texts to English for commoners. He wrote political and radical pamphlets against the king, detailed astrological archetypes of plants, and believed no physician should be without astrology in the application of herbal remedies. He dedicated his service to the poor people of London and set up illegally in Spitalfields in 1644. In 1653 he wrote The English Physician, against which the Royal College of Physicians protested and he was accused of witchcraft. Culpeper regarded the body as a whole, that each organ has a humour, a voice, and a spirit.

PERSECUTION

In 1592 Parliament had passed the Witchcraft Act which defined witchcraft as a crime, punishable by death.

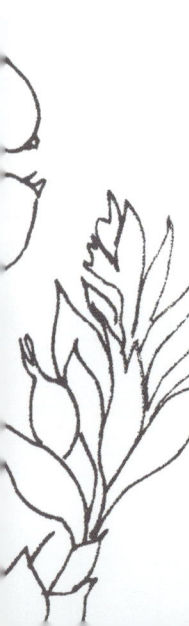

In Western Europe from 1484 until around 1750 some 200,000 witches, and by that I mean poor people, those possessing the "evil eye", non-conformists, someone with a freckle, a hairy upper lip, queers, someone with a flea bite perhaps, were tortured and tested for witchcraft, burnt or hanged. In 1590, Agnes Simpson of Keith was burned at the stake for using herbs to alleviate the pains of childbirth. In Puritanical fervour, the "pilnie-winks" (thumb screws) and iron "caspie-claws" (a form of leg irons heated over a brazier) forced confessions from the accused witches. Matthew Hopkins, the Witchfinder General, would use a three-inch-long jabbing needle to see if the person was insensitive to pain. There are tales of women thrown into deep water with their thumbs tied to the opposite big toes, if they drown they are innocent, if they float then they must be killed.

BOTANIC GARDENS

Imperial botanic gardens were centres for colonial expansion. They were, and still are, repositories of colonial ("economic") botany with the superficial allure of paradise masking lies, history, and espionage.

Today's Millennium Seed Bank at Kew, with its mission of saving indigenous species, was created without acknowledgement that the very systems on which Kew was founded were responsible for biodiversity destruction. Kew has a building named after Sir Joseph Banks. Once you find out about his history, you may decide his statue is worthy of throwing in the Thames.

The modern European botanic garden has its roots in the *Hortus Medicus* attached to medical schools of the Renaissance universities. In the eighteenth and early nineteenth centuries a surgeon-naturalist customarily sailed on each of the many worldwide voyages of exploration sponsored by learned societies or national governments.

In 1770, Captain James Cook and his mercenary compadres arrived off the east coast of Australia in Ka-May, renaming it Botany Bay while claiming Australia for Britain in one voyage (1768–1771). Some of the plants they looted were placed in Kew Gardens. Banks and his colleague Solander, two White men and students of Linnaeus, appropriated plant specimens and gave them new names. They described land which had been inhabited for at least 65,000 years as *terra nullius* – blank and unknown. Banks was responsible for designating New South Wales a penal colony where convicts provided free muscle power or faced hanging.

Hugely wealthy and Eton-educated, Banks paid for his own passage, and for the scientists, equipment, and wages on the Endeavour. On arrival, Banks saw space between trees ripe for cultivation, oblivious to Aboriginal bush-burning practices and land maintenance as they "were too ignorant in the art of cultivations and wandered from place to place". Aboriginal resistance was met with murder and pillage including the shooting of the Gweagal warrior, Cooman. His shield and spears are stolen trophies still sitting in the British Museum. The Gweagal people want their ancestors' belongings back.

Banks later hatched a scheme for exploitation in the plantations of the then-named "West Indies". He decided that the non-native but cheap and nutritious food source, breadfruit, could feed the suffering, kidnapped, African "slaves" so they would be fit to work in large-scale cotton cultivation which drove Lancashire's mills and increased UK exports to Asia. He had no regard for African humanity but rather a heart for profits. The breadfruit was brought from the central Pacific on HMS Bounty, finally arriving in 1793 and planted in the St Vincent botanic garden. Plantation owners then obtained cuttings to start growing it and feeding it to their workforce.

Kew's first official director (1841 to 1865), William Jackson Hooker, a former protegé of Banks and professor of botany, was the founder of the Hooker dynasty at Kew. The Palm House was built in 1845 and drew thousands of visitors every year within Kew's acres of plantings and labelled specimens. Its greenhouses and museum collections were essential for the new expanding science of taxonomy and a laboratory was built in 1878 for plant study, publishing, drawing, and information storage and retrieval, with a library and herbarium, all from Hooker's private collection. Today it holds seven million dried and mounted plant specimens, the world's largest herbarium. A training programme was formalised in 1878, which sent hundreds of students to all the colonial gardens, to the universities, and to "the great" commercial nurseries.

Kew Gardens and its colonial affiliates emerge as a vital capital asset, transforming knowledge into profit and power for Great Britain. The Gardeners' Chronicle stated that "it was not originally designed as a pleasure ground" and "most of the visitors are incapable of enjoying the higher branches of horticulture, much less botanical science, and they could not be expected to take more than a languid and vague interest in supply of plants to the colonies". Kew opened at 1pm, any earlier and it would have been regarded as a park (imagine!) One afternoon in 1877, 58,000 people visited Kew and it was noted by John Tyndall that: "Kew has been made so beautiful that there is a danger that its scientific importance is being overlooked" (Endersby, 2019). Kew was never primarily for the joy of common people.

At this time, when developments in shipbuilding, navigation, and weaponry meant the acquisition of plants/herbs (and resources) bypassed land trade routes, new medicinal wonders were arriving at the docks. Plants were and are a source of imperial wealth. Economic botanical acquisition consisted largely of tea, coffee, and cocoa. Archers reported that vegetable commerce comprised three-quarters of economic wealth. At Chelsea Physic Garden (est. 1653) there is still a gate with access to the River Thames where plant products would have been delivered. By 1900, European countries had control of 75% of the world with "the scramble for Africa" from 1870.

ELITISM

Day 1, Westminster Polyclinic: We were directed how to dress in clinic for future reference. This included: always wear a clean white coat, "smart clothes", specific shoes, no perfume, no nail varnish, hair back. A photo of Prince Charles in royal regalia was on the wall. We were to assume the role of clinician in allopathic apparel. For my departing honours dissertation in 2001, I requested to write about the colonisation of herbal medicine and was refused. Naïve, inexperienced, and seeking a high grade, I complied. By the end of the full-time, four-year degree, I left as a theoretical polymath with first class honours, scientific curiosity, and rigour, but it was just the beginning of my journey to becoming a herbalist and I am still decolonising this path. Becoming a qualified medical herbalist is an expensive and exclusive affair. Once I had finished, I was heavily in debt and never had the funds to pay for a dispensary, practising space, insurance, or accreditation. Accrediting bodies do not represent me or my radical essence. I call myself a radical herbalist, not a medical herbalist.

A colleague recently used the term "Pale, male and stale" to describe herbal medicine institutions. When you look at herbal medicine textbooks, "Michaels" and "Christophers" feature often, they are not all stale – however, they hold a gravitas and confidence not afforded, on the whole, to "BIPOC" women. Still, in 2021, the UK's National Institute of Medical Herbalists – of which many herbalists are members – has a tradition of

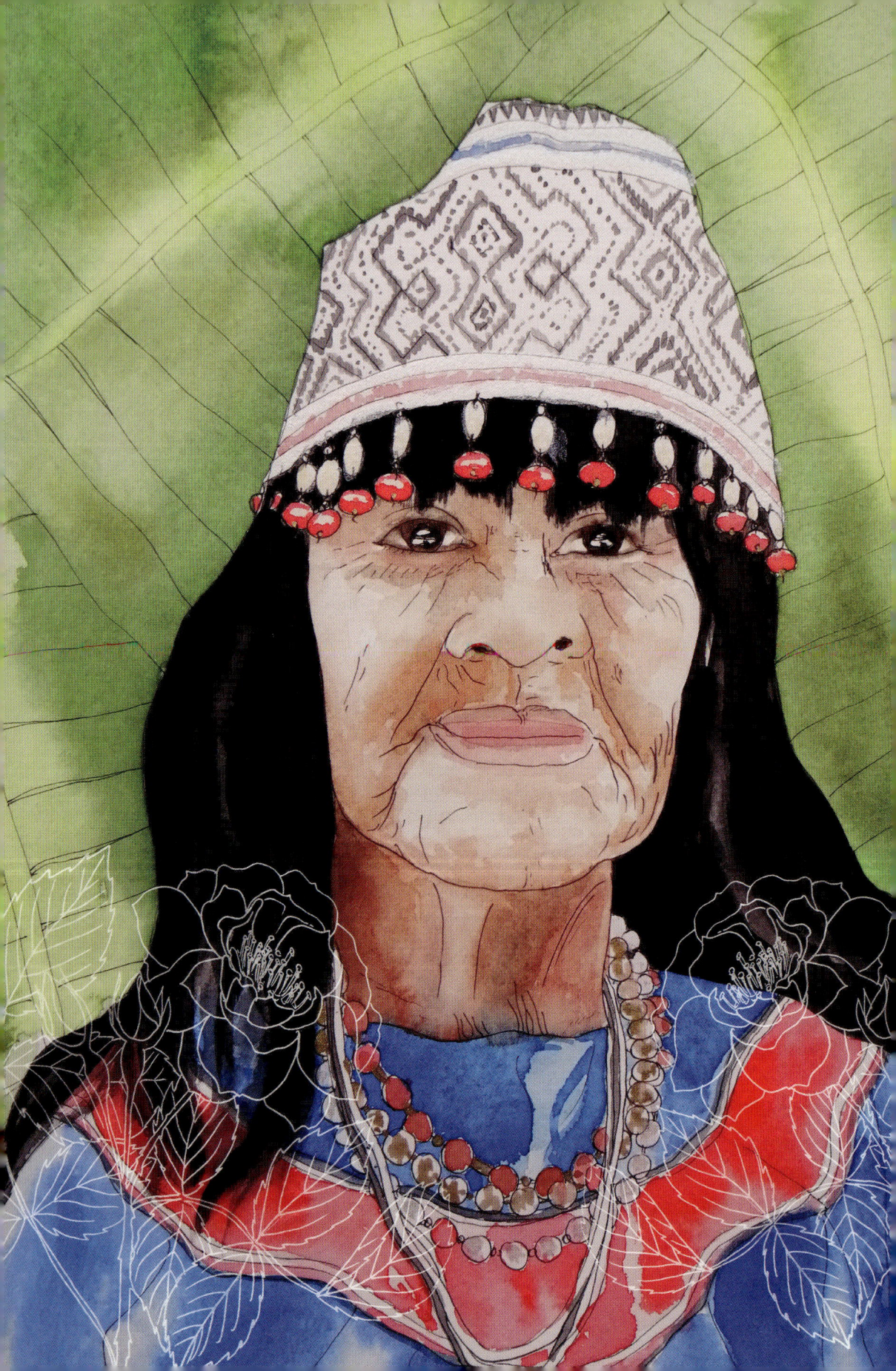

sending "loyal greetings" to Queen Elizabeth, the Head of Empire, at its annual conference. As Benjamin Zephaniah said when rejecting the OBE: "'Empire' reminds me of slavery, thousands of years of brutality, it reminds me how my foremothers were brutalised . . ."

APPROPRIATION AND AYAHUASCA: PERU, UCAYALI, 19TH APRIL 2018

Olivia Arevalo, RIEP, an eighty-one-year-old Shipibo-Conibo curandera (healer) and human rights and environmental activist, was shot twice in her chest on her doorstep by a foreign visitor, a White man, Sebastian Woodroffe. Her body was left bleeding on the ground for everyone to see.

She was a custodian of traditional ways and her murder a painful act of aggression to the Shipibo-Conibo community. A local curandero Walter Lopez said that "Because the authorities did not condemn her killing, people had to take matters into their own hands. Indigenous people are clearly not their priority. One of our curanderas was murdered in her own community, it fills you with hatred, pain, rage and sadness. All of the riches in our community and villages, foreigners took everything. Their only goal is to extract and absorb everything we have. Now they also want to take our spirituality or wisdom, using ayahuasca incorrectly. The main problem with Westerners is their mind. Their minds carry a great deal of anxiety and stress. These problems become piling up in the body making it sick."

Taking ayahuasca, a sacred herb, is not a frivolous experience and the cost is concerning and destructive. Every year 20,000 Westerners go to Iquitos, Peru, seeking aya as it's known. Ayahuasca has become big business. Dissatisfied Westerners who don't find relief in the Western medical system go searching for a quick fix to help themselves, to heal deep psychic wounds, for an epiphany or curiosity.

Traditionally, ayahuasca is the mother of all medicinal plants and part of a complex indigenous medical system. To prepare the brew takes hours and you need two plants, chacruna and ayuhuasca vine. Each person has their own way of cooking. In Amazonia, if a person gets sick they may go to their "shaman" who drinks ayahuasca to commune with the Spirit allies. The sick person does NOT take the ayahuasca. The curandero or curandera will channel a particular

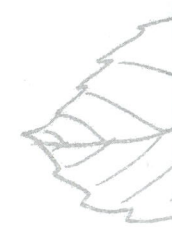

Olivia Arévalo, Indigenous Shipibo medicine woman, murdered in 2018

song to the "patient" called ikaros. These songs are the medicine. Westerners do not want to pay two thousand dollars for a song. For them, everything revolves around the consumption – they want to experience the entheogenic effects and locals give them what they want, "whenever westerners get what they want, they take over and take it for them, transform it . . . it's happened with ayahuasca". Like other psychedelics, ayahuasca can shift intractable depression, post-trauma, and addiction but at what cost? This is not what Christopher Hedley was referring to when discussing removing the depressive lenses.

It is probable that the word "shaman" comes from šamán, the Evenki word for "one who knows", and it relates to communicating with the spirit world through altered states, such as a healing trance. The fact it is applied to other indigenous spiritual traditions and is so readily appropriated as a term is a product of colonialism. Traditionally, a shaman inherits the practice or is trained for many years in the art, often including local healing plants, preparations, and rituals. This practice has existed in every continent. The term shamanism in "Western society" is often coupled with the appropriation of varied ancestral cultural practices which are not theirs.

I have attended festivals and seen first-hand the exploitation of white sage smudge sticks, Tibetan bowls, Djembe drums, African dance without African people, essential oils for internal consumption, yoga, Tai chi, Indian clothes, Afghani jewelry, selling Dhal and Buddha bowls.

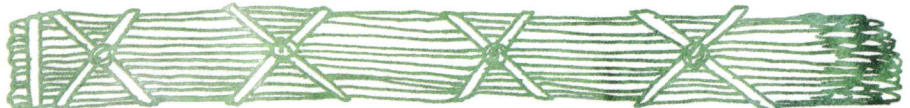

When I was growing up, although non-religious, I took part in havan poojas, where herbal offerings of saamagri (Bhimseni Kapoor-camphor, rose petals, sandalwood powder, lobaan, ghee, agarbatti, chandan, and turmeric) were consecrated in fire in a special havan. This practice connected me to ritual and my Indian heritage after the death of my father. I would collect dry twigs from the garden or neighbourhood to put in the havan pot. An elder, Kamala would recite the mantra:

दीन दयाल विरद सम्भारी
हरहु नाथ मम संकट भारी

"Deen dayal Viradh Sambhari
Harahu Nath Mamah Sankat Bhari"

(Lord you are the protector of the weak and destroy the great obstacles. Please take away the great danger which has been befallen on me! You take away all pains as Vedas say it.)

She recited the mantra 108 times using her mala as a guide. Upon saying "Sva ha" at the end of the mantra, my Aunty Leena would spoon ghee on the fire with saamagri. The herbs would spit and hiss in the pot. The ceremony would evoke an auspicious and peaceful atmosphere. It would connect me to my Indian culture and a sense of peace.

The word incense comes from the Latin *incendere* – to burn. Smoke and incense are used for cleansing, ritual, spirituality, and health. From Chinese joss sticks, bamboo core, dhoop, frankincense, copal, palo santo, champa with sandalwood and frangipani, feathers, nests, to dragons blood, burning of a plant product creates nano-particles and particulates which can clean the air and enter the body.

The manufacture of incense is important. Many believe burning incense may be spiritually uplifting but are unaware that the combusted chemicals in many modern mass manufactured incense sticks releases noxious gases creating a risk to respiratory health and possible mutagenesis in enclosed spaces.

Smudging is a cultural practice pertaining to some indigenous nations in Turtle Island and the practice is regional. Herbs burnt are aromatic and may include white sage, sweet grass, and red cedar for specific reasons. Until 1978 it was illegal for the Indigenous people of Turtle Island to use their own traditions and currently smudging has been prohibited in university campuses and hospitals. The popular misappropriating, particularly by New Agers and Neopagans widely using white sage smudge sticks, has caused brutal over-harvesting. Smudge sticks are available in spiritual sets with crystals, a feather, palo santo, and a pāua shell to burn them in. Palo santo, frankincense, copal are other unnecessary sources for smoke in the West. Mugwort and local aromatics

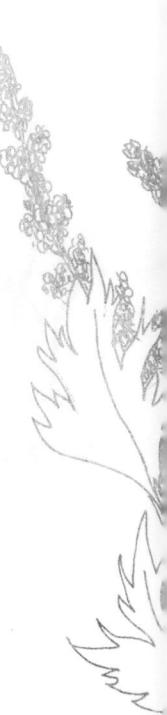

including other salvia species may be used for burning in the UK. There is really no need to appropriate species from abroad when we have an abundance of aromatic slow burning plants locally. This year I experimented with pineapple weed sticks with great success.

TREES AS MEDICINE, EXPLOITED

Wild tree resins generate billions of dollars in revenue annually but many species face extinction. The endangered lansan tree (*Protium attenuatum*) is native to the Windward Islands and to Dominica, Guadeloupe, Martinique, St Lucia, and St Vincent in the Eastern Caribbean. A member of the "incense tree" family (Burseraceae), it exudes a highly aromatic oleoresin. Some 60% of St Lucians use lansan resin for shrines, churches, and international trade. Over-slashing and tapping of the trees mean it is now granted conservation status and new methods of applying diluted sulphuric acid to the injury sites are being adopted.

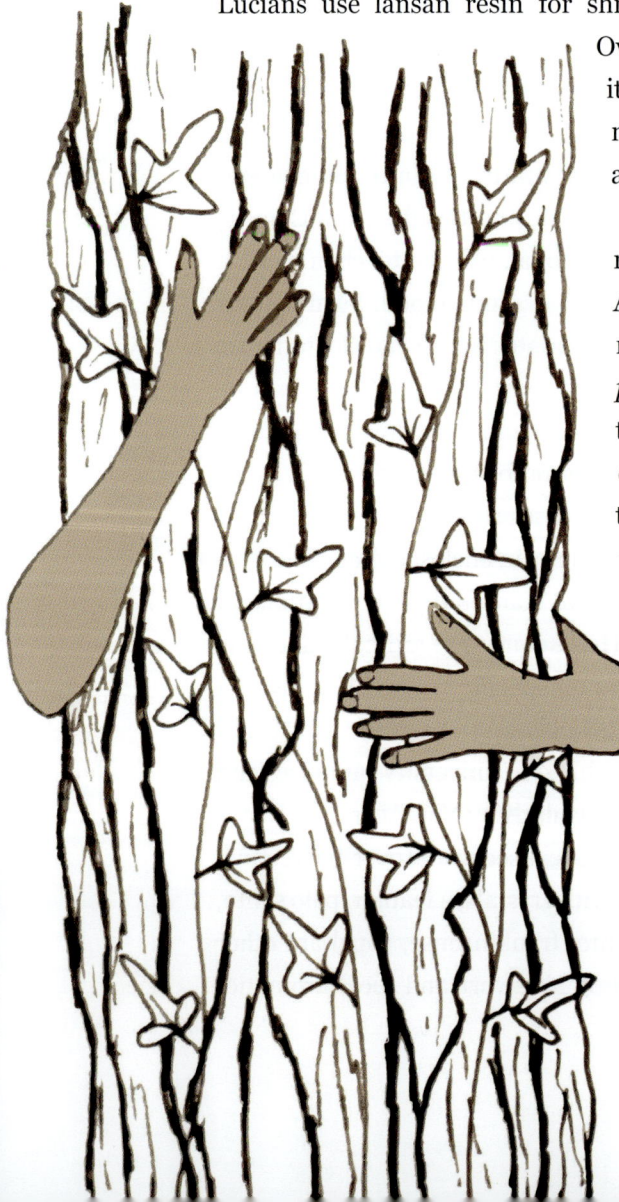

Frankincense is native to the ravines and rocky slopes of north-east Africa and the Arabian peninsula. The scientific binomial names for Frankincense are *Boswellia papyifera*, *carterii*, and *sacra*. It was mentioned in the Bible. The ancient Egyptians described the resinous sap as the sweat of the gods condensing on earth and used it for smoke and to embalm its revered. The phoenix rises from the ashes of burnt frankincense. Its resin is extracted by injuring the plants to produce a protective sap which is then harvested for imparting protection on to humans. Thousands of tonnes are harvested each year.

The abuse of this sacred tree is a metaphor for the destruction of natural habitats, super exploitation of people and land, climate change, and the desperate measures Indigenous people are forced to take to veer away from their preferred ways of living. Sustainable tapping techniques have been disregarded due to poverty and demand by the economically rich. The more a tree is injured the more opportunity for insects to take over. Climate "change" has caused saplings to die and fires to wipe them out.

As a plant is on earth, so it is in the body. The sap from the above-mentioned *Boswellia sp.* protects the tree from disease and parasites. It is a powerful sacred protector of the human body. The resinous constituents, specifically the boswellic acids consumed with fats, cross the blood-brain-barrier and inhibit inflammation of the brain inside the skull in critical situations. This is the only time I use this herb. The oil from *Boswellia carterii* induces tumour cell specific cytotoxicity – it selectively kills cancer cells. Its use is heavily in demand by people desperate with cancer.

ANTI-BLACKNESS

The legal prohibition of traditional healing and autonomy occurred in all colonial structures. The Obeah Act 1898 is an active yet archaic law which prohibits African people kidnapped to the Caribbean from access to spiritual healing and ancestral power.

Black people are marginalised in herbal medicine institutions and textbooks. When studying there was not one mention of African traditions at all, yet Africa is the dawn of all civilisation. There was repeated reference to Ayurvedic, Chinese, and Indigenous Turtle Island medicine. Terms like doshas, five elements, qi, prana, and herbs like echinacea are familiar to herbalists in the West.

I figured *Pygeum africans* and Kola nut were from Africa when looking at bottles in the dispensary. When studying psychopharmacology to lecture, I learned about the alkaloids of iboga and khat and taught myself their indigenous use. But I wondered why the medicine of Africa, South "America", Australasia and Pacifica were absent?

Medical papyri from Ancient Egypt that are held in vaults across Europe were given European names. These include the twenty metre long so-called Ebers Papyrus (1500 BC) written in Hieratic, containing magic and folk medicine. It describes contraception with paste of dates, honey, acacia on wool. It has over 700 remedies for dementia to diabetes. It has the Book of Hearts which describes depression. The Kahun Papyrus (1800 BC) is the oldest Egyptian medical text, inscribed on flattened clay. It describes gynaecological disease, fertility, contraception, pregnancy. It is kept in premises of University College London. There are many more papyri all with the names of European men.

The saying "As above, so below. As within, so without" originates from Hermetic texts found in Nag Hammadi in 1945, describing Ancient Egyptian concepts. Today this term is used in astrology, alchemy, astro-herbalism, and Tarot acknowledging that the microcosm and macrocosm are intertwined.

The West African Dogon people, I learned from herbalist Kandaké, are famous for their rich traditions of mask dancing, sublime sandstone architecture, and astronomical knowledge. The Dogon understand what is not seen in the material world and the essence of African traditional medicine. Dogon teachings are through oral ancestral lineage and the medicine is extremely localised from village to village.

Divination, amulets, prayer, dance, particular body movements, personal and communal elevation are aspects of healing. Igbo'gi (yorubá medicine) is West African herbal medicine, also practised in the Caribbean, and has long recognised microscopic pathogens (kororo). Bitter herbs are used for parasitic infection, although symbiosis with microbes has a place. There is emphasis on herbal baths, deep inner reflection, and herbal remedies. There are ceremonies for each occasion. Initiates into Egbo'gi protect their customs from colonial theft. Oral traditions carry these sacred practices circumventing white cultural appropriation.

Water purification and herbal baths still form a major part of traditional medical practices of the Maroon descendants, escaped from slavery, who fought for their freedom and settled in the tropical rainforest of Suriname. Baths used are baby strength, adult strength, skin disorders, respiratory ailments, spiritual ailments, and genital steams. It is common to have a mixture of leaves in water standing in a plastic tub or a big earthenware or wooden dish in front of the house for days, to be used many times by one or more family members by adding new water to it before pouring the mixture over the head and/or body with a calabash (Crescentia cujete). Aromatic plant species, such as *Campomanesia aromatica* and *Lantana camara* are often added to baths. Winti wasi (Aucan) spiritual baths are used to cleanse metaphysical toxicity and danger, for an individual or the whole family, and for genital steams.

Black women are more likely to die in childbirth, of chronic disease, and are commonly dehumanised. The super-exploitation of Black women occurs when racism, classism, sexism, misogyny and even freedom of expression is intersected. Black women work harder for less pay than men and White women. Recently the mayor of Islington, a London borough, resigned after eight years because she was battling a system that allows "white men to have what they want when they want". Historically there has been a conscious omission of Black knowledge and healing traditions. Sade Musa describes reclaiming herbal traditions and body autonomy as a key to anti-colonial struggle: "When we give people the skills to heal themselves it is an act of resistance and self-determination, they get the confidence to push back against the running narrative." Musa goes on to say that people who want pharmaceuticals should have access to them, but they should also have access to alternative modes of healing should they so choose.

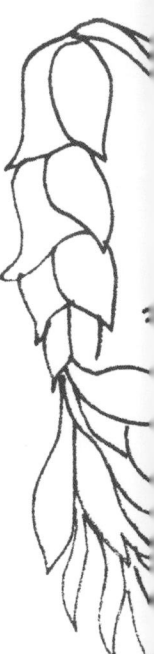

Colonial ideology deemed non-Christians and Indigenous people as uncivilised cannibals with no moral code, animalistic, with no fixed homes, and considered it was a duty to civilise "them". This notion is perpetuated in many guises today and is used to justify the murder of Black and poor people routinely on British soil. Illustrations from colonial voyages depicted Indigenous people as hideous savages and plants as beautiful specimens.

Studies have demonstrated the healing nature of forest bathing and being immersed in nature. In 2019, Harvard scientists demonstrated that just twenty minutes spent interacting with nature reduced blood markers of stress such as cortisol.

"BIPOC" in the UK spend less time in nature than White people. Only 1.9% of Black people and 2.6% of Asian people live in the countryside. The English countryside is the bastion of Empire reflected in studies demonstrating inaccessibility

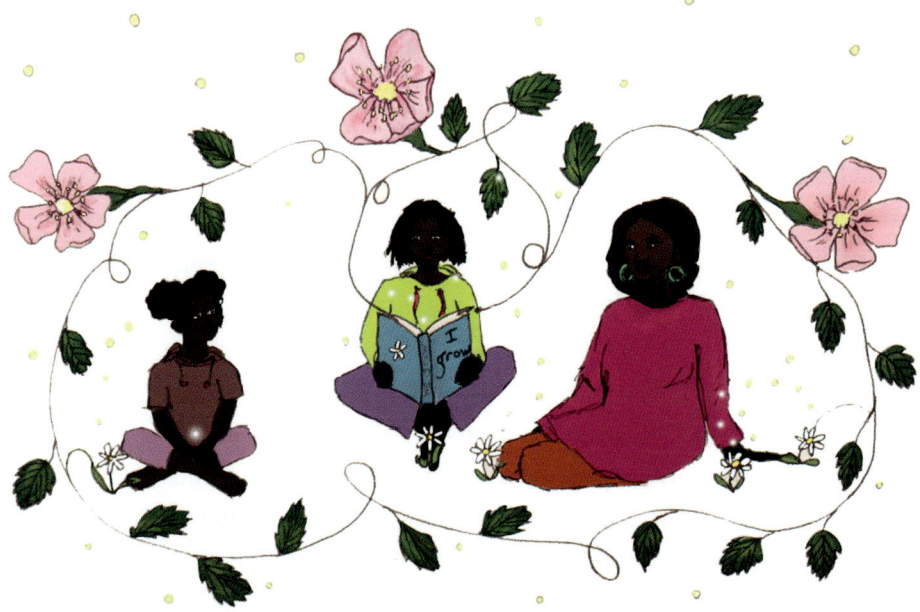

and inhospitality from White people exemplified by name calling, physical violence, and exclusion. Louisa Adjoa Parker is mapping the experience of Black and Brown people in rural landscapes and racism is a huge part of why "BIPOC" are less present in nature, countering the whole notion of attaining peace and creating a barrier to simple enjoyment and healing.

In The Ecologist, Beth Collier explored the ongoing colonial narrative that White people regard themselves as "true" custodians of nature. She describes nature as a support for spiritual, physical, and emotional uplift and the connection to nature is present in our heritage countries. Black men have described the pressure of being treated with suspicion and having to modify their behaviour to prove they are not a threat, whereas it is perfectly respectable for a White man to be walking his dog. Collier also describes how "BIPOC" may be disconnected from rural England as their parents were dealing with survival issues, and coupled with racism a chain of disconnect may occur. Translocation means our elders may not have a connection with British nature and thus cannot pass on knowledge from ancestral locations.

Other experiences described include the historical trauma and abuse in the fields that leads to the abandonment of nature and, once in the city, the value codes mutate into material consumerism, screen-based lifestyles, and mud is seen as dirty. Collier goes on to describe how Gina Yashere and Romesh

Ranganathan incorporate material into their comedy that mocks closeness to nature.

The National Trust is a legacy of Octavia Hill (1838–1912) who campaigned for access to nature for the "urban poor", enabling those who did not own a country residence to have access to fresh air and purification. The Trust is Britain's largest landowner and has run for 125 years. It has six million members, 65,000 volunteers, and 28 million visits per year. A report published in its September 2020 report showed that at least one third of its properties have links to the slave trade and colonialism.

The £200,000 lost due to the pandemic means that the proposed scrapping of self-led school visits will hit "worst off children" (Guardian newspaper, 29th Aug. 2020).

At least one quarter of the school visitors are from Black, Brown, and UK "minority" and working-class children, who would lose the opportunity to visit the vast openness, greenery, woodland, mountains, and streams and to inspire naturalists of the future.

RADICAL HERBALISM AND THE RADICAL HERBAL NETWORK

Radical herbalism exists to address what is lacking from medical herbalism.

Colonialism continues worldwide through corporate damage to and theft of Indigenous peoples' lands and medicines, and it is the role of radical herbalists to raise consciousness of this violence.

"Rad" derives from Latin, meaning root. *Taraxacum officinale* radix refers to the root of dandelion for example. The radical herbalist network acknowledges that health is inextricably linked to the health of ecosystems, that health care is a right and should be accessible to all people regardless of their ethnicity, culture, nationality, economic class, sexual identity, gender, age, or abilities.

Radical herbalism is committed to dismantling barriers that stand in the way of this access.

Radical herbalism is founded on supporting health with minimal harm and meeting community needs, while staying committed to long-term social change, considering models of land use that nourish our communities rather than harm them; Indigenous precedents of conscious cultivation incorporating ethical wildcrafting and sustainable harvesting; the need for sustainable freedom from our dependence on systems, institutions, and individuals that exploit, neglect, and degrade us physically, emotionally, socially, and financially. This means recognising the harm caused by states and capitalism and the need for creative and radical alternatives. Part of this holistic approach requires the necessity of self-care, mutual aid, and community responsibility for cultivating our well-being.

Radical health practitioners strive to end discrimination, oppression, poverty, and other forms of social injustice through herbal practice and community organising. Herbalists Without Borders (HWB) is an international group run

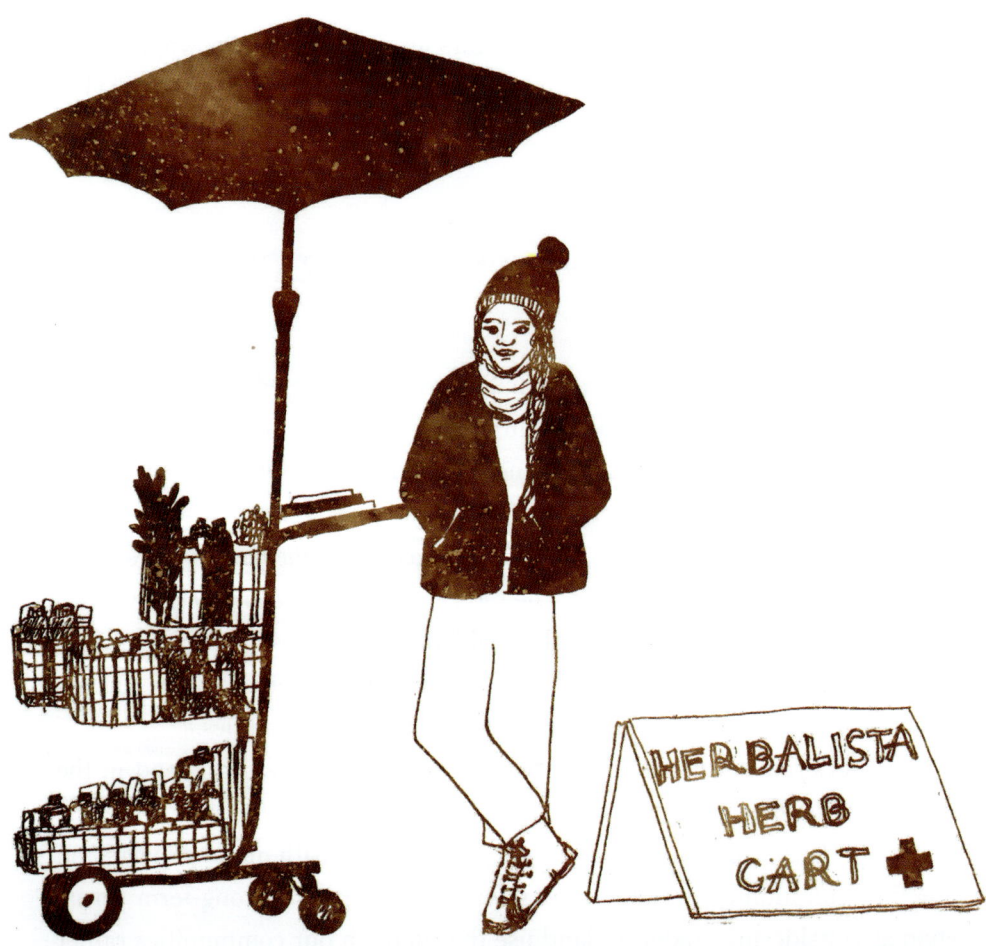

by radical herbalists promoting herbal support through the making of medicines by the community and the provision of them to those in immediate need of support. They provide:

Community growing spaces and community apothecaries.

Free people's clinics trauma trainings.

Accessible herbal education, and advocacy technical assistance

Community gatherings.

Herbal First Aid at events such as protests (nursing eyes burnt by pepper spray for example).

HWB also promotes nourishing community gardens, medicinal seed swapping, seed banks/libraries, healthy food in food deserts, herbal education and advocacy, and social justice related to herbalism and herbal health access. In the past year HBW has travelled to Calais and Dunkirk working with displaced people providing cough syrups, chest ointments, bruise ointments, antimicrobial vinegars, bespoke creams, and has helped people to clean and dress wounds where appropriate.

There are diverse traditions and practices of plant medicine globally. They all should be honoured. The Prisoner's Herbal by Nicole Rose, from Solidarity Apothecary, details plants which grow through the cracks of concrete in prison yards and are a metaphor for those of us living in incarceration and urban confines. The omission of African, European indigenous, Mexican, and other almighty traditions were obvious to me at university.

Auto-destruction of European sacred culture means that people who are robbed of a healing tradition have to search in the past or look to other systems of medicine still intact, especially when allopathic systems fail them. Today we see more Chinese medical clinics on the high streets and expensive health food shops in gentrified areas. We see popularity for particular herbs such as moringa and frankincense when we have nettles, herb Robert, feverfew, rosebay willow, and marsh pennywort in our localities.

In 2020 there has been a boom in community growing projects. The impact of the pandemic highlighted the fragility of food supplies: food banks don't provide fresh green vegetables; a precarious government allied with Trump, with talks of chlorinated chickens and abandoning EU safety regulations.

Community gardens and growing spaces utilise land for collective growing, they provide an aesthetically pleasing space for cultivation, physical, mental, social well-being, and space for intergenerational and cultural exchange. Medicinal and culinary herbs, fruit, and vegetables can be grown. Beehives and bug houses can be installed. Herbal medicine based community projects exist throughout the country.

> "Where is imperialism? Look at your plates when you eat . . ."
>
> Thomas Sankara Faso, 1987. Assassinated 1987

As above, so below. Everything is interconnected. Of course we need entire system change and there is no quick fix. Historical entitled privileged behaviour makes it possible to use medicines from around the world and call it "Western" herbal medicine, without honouring any single one of the traditions the herbs come from, even the indigenous ones. Much of what I've read historically is from the White male gaze, primarily because that is what I have had access to.

This is why everything has to be continually unpicked and questioned. How did the plants and herbs you use in everyday life come to be here? When I look in my cupboard of teas and spices, I question: what land did they grow on? Who cultivated it? Who tended to the plants? Harvested? Packaged? Labelled? Sold? Made a profit? Did the tea, té, or chai in the jar on my counter arrive by clipper ship or land? Sadly, many brands of tea use polypropylene plastic to form the tea bag. This takes hundreds of years to biodegrade and contributes towards plastic contamination in compost. Studies have demonstrated these heat resistant plastics cause a stress response in cells and interfere with androgen metabolism.

There are a myriad of questions we need to ask for the health of the earth and ourselves.

Recent news reports show matters of real concern: the mass burning of heather (releasing carbon) and goshawks allegedly being murdered so the aristocracy can hunt grouse. The phosphate, nitrogen, and ammonia run-off from intensive factory farming of "livestock" is causing toxic algae blooms, poisoning our rivers, and killing the fish. Companies invested in "fracking" have been

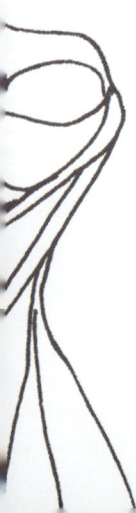

Illustration inspired by Farmers March (2020-21) where 300,000+ agricultural workers congregated in Delhi to protest 3 Acts laws to erode autonomy of what to grow, who to sell to and regulation.

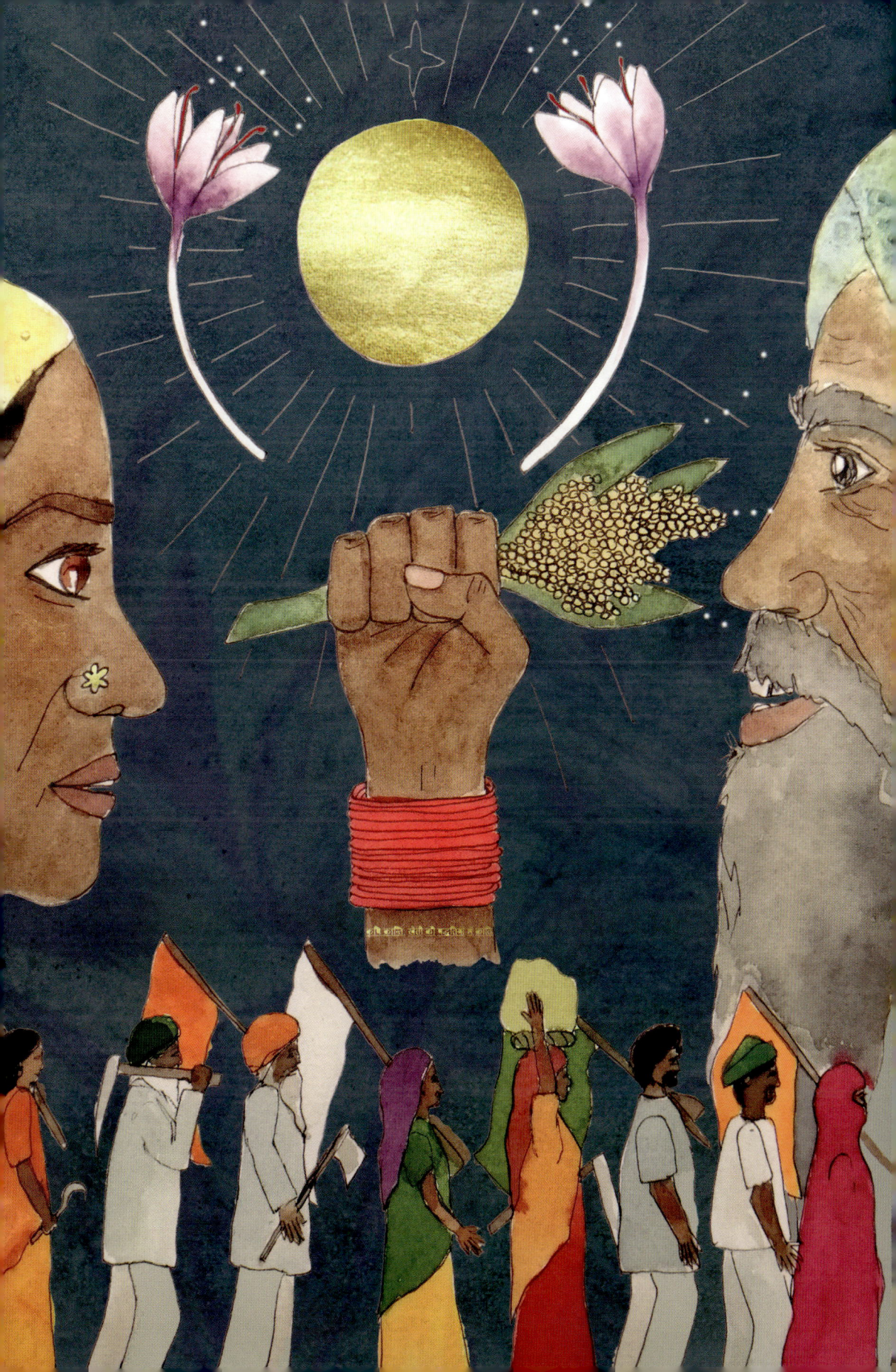

bailed out by government Covid schemes. Wind and solar farms in Kent are to produce energy to be sold abroad, destroying the local ecosystems with industrial-scale battery storage systems. The chopping down of the 300-year old oak tree at Cubbington Woods to make way for the HS2 railway that will save thirty minutes of journey time. The pain of deaths in custody. Frontline workers exposed to high viral loads of Covid-19 while people complain that wearing masks is muzzled tyranny. The pain of knowing Belly Mujinga was spat in the face in a racist assault resulting in her death from Covid-19.

Even with this as a backdrop, the wonder of nature and beauty of natural resistance is ever present and constant.

Plant medicine, self-care, and sourcing it may not feature as a priority or even be immediately accessible, yet it is a powerful holistic tool to connect us back to the unified source of the natural world, the astral world, our ancestral heritage, and to connect to ultimate healing. The art of herbalism is

The three finger sign has been used as a sign of resistance to oppression in Myanmar and Thailand. The Flower Strike lays flowers at the sites of killed activists during the coup in Myanmar.

founded on the art of justice. Being a radical herbalist connects us to our ancestors, our relations, kindred spirits, health, and existence. I hope this book facilitates a deeper connection to the plant beings because they know we are here and connect with us. I hope we protect them as they protect us. As above, so below, as without, so within.

References

A New System of Slavery: The Export of Indian Labour Overseas 1830-1920 by Hugh Tinker, 1974

Gardens of Empire: Kew and The Colonies by Professor Jim Endersby, 2019

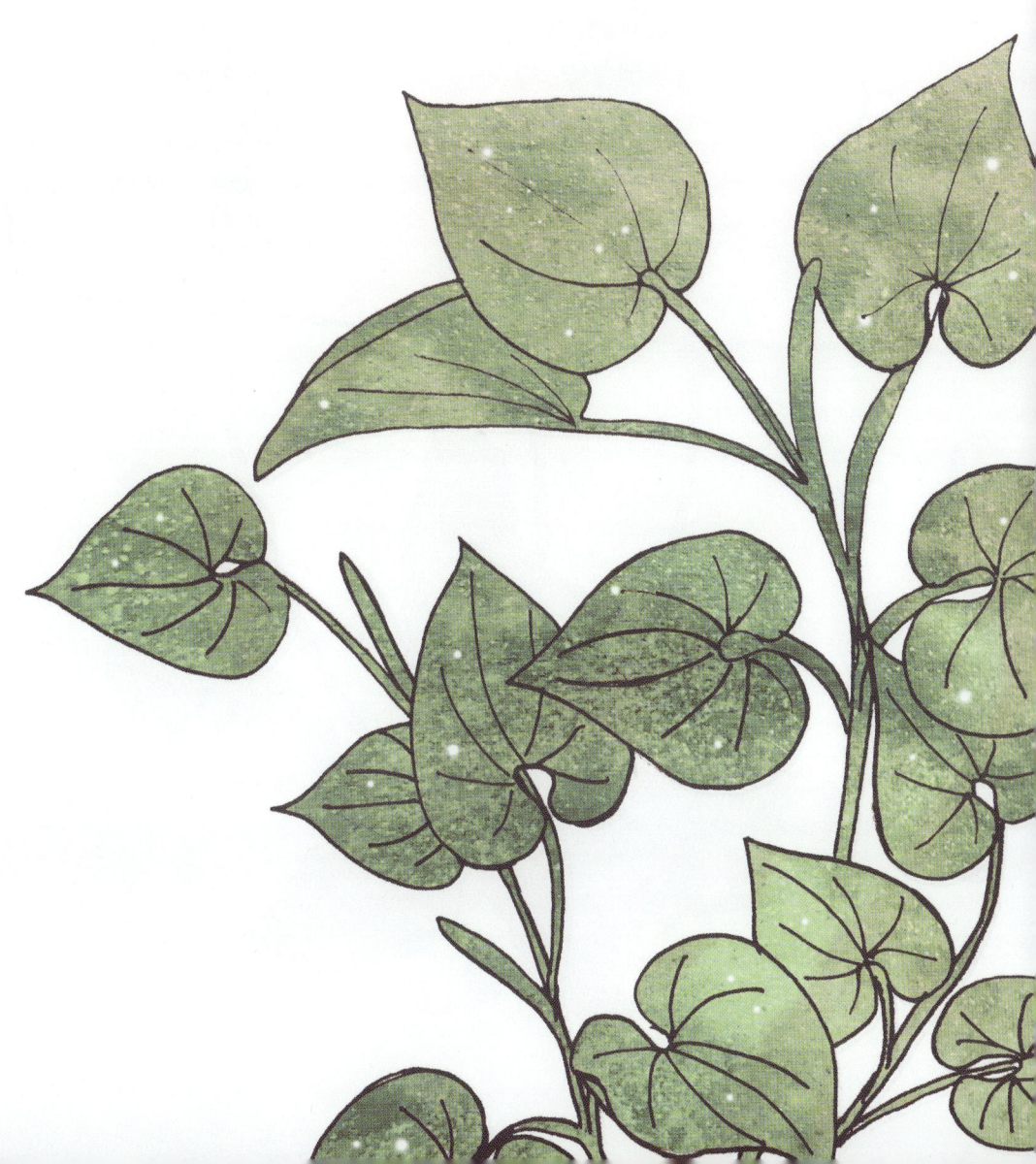

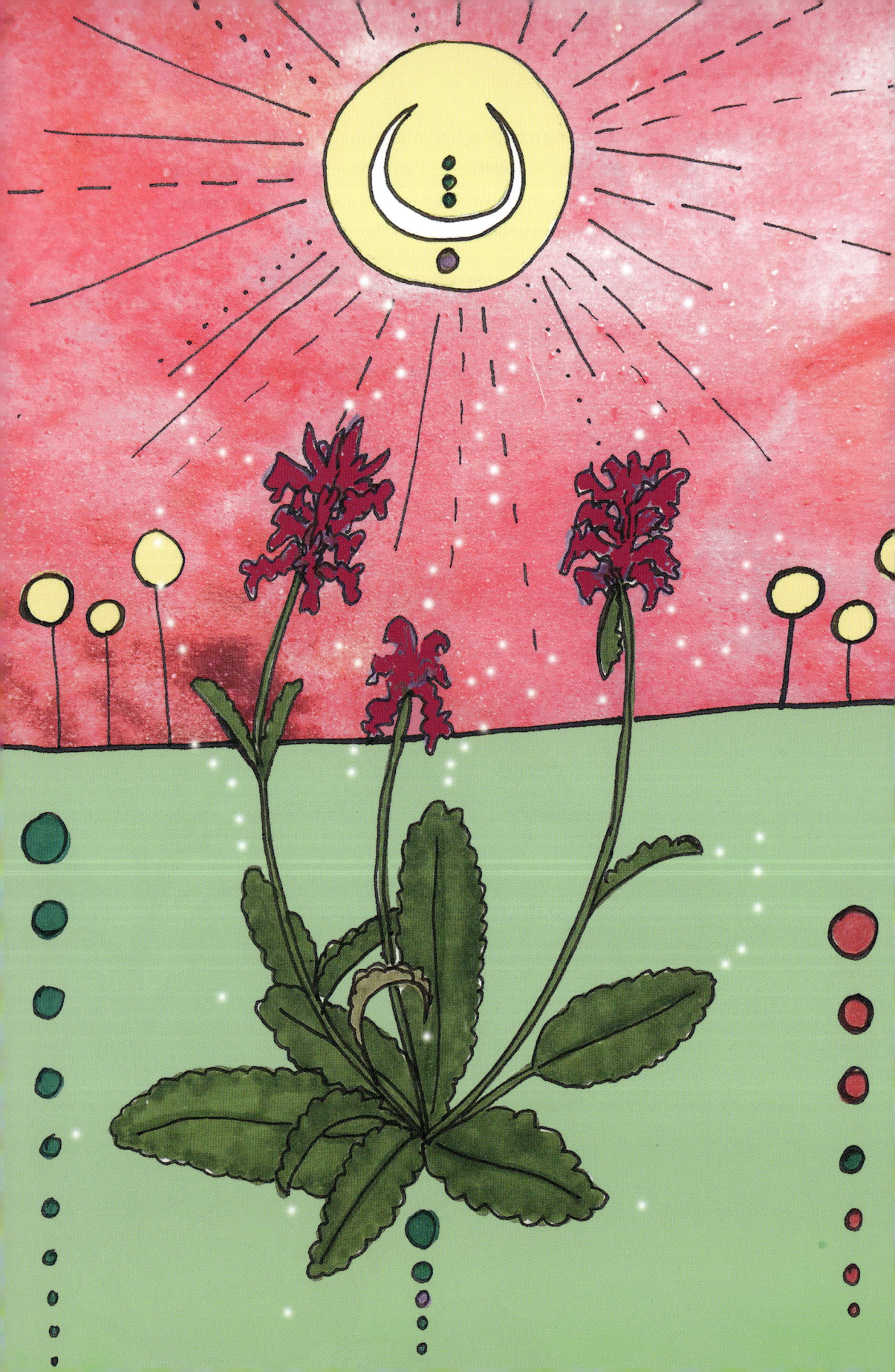

THE WILD JOURNEY AHEAD

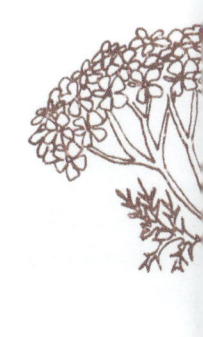

Could you allow
For just a while
Your feet to take you
forward
Your eyes to relax
Your skin to feel?

Just for a while.
Breathing in.
Feeling in.

And hear that birdsong
In your heart,
Where tenderness and
Yarrow reside.

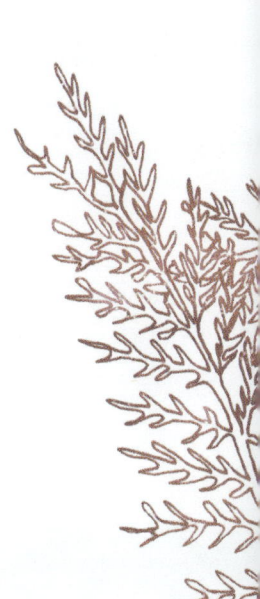

Betony for the wild journey ahead

Thank you for reading these words. For many of you this will be the beginning of a fruitful journey with plant allies and deep connection with nature and self. We are all one, remember; we can learn, share, and care, make reparation. The journey that history has brought upon us is one of self-care, community care, and global care. To make better than we have done, or have had done to us, to use the power of now to heal the wounds of the past, even if we can only do so by understanding our past; it is a step forward. If we can learn to give, share, embody wisdom with ethical care then we begin to walk the path to reparation. It will be a difficult path. Which glasses do you have on now?

If you can journal, practise rewilding, breathe fresh air, make medicines, and spend time with plants you will be shown gifts that you too can pass on, creating a huge mycelium-like network of folk knowledge and plant medicine within our communities.

Find your wildness, find your plant allies, find yourselves. This is your moment, these are your moments; let's cherish mama earth with our respect, love, and care and let's find ways to nourish each other with knowledge, acceptance, rebellion, or wisdom.

Let us find the most nourishing path for all and reclaim the ways we have lost through elitism, capitalism, patriarchy, and colonialism.

May your cupboards be filled with wild medicines and your hearts be merry with the laughter of plant magic.

But . . . how to make that next step? How to become the herbalist, do the work, relearn, rewild? How do we take all that is on offer for us to learn in balance – that is, give back? How do we even recognise our colonialist or capitalist tendencies and conditioning? How do we reclaim the knowledge that has been ripped away from us by patriarchy? It is not easy. We cannot even see colonial traits in many respects – be you Black, Brown, White, or Yellow. Here are some ways to connect in and move forward:

COMMUNITY

Learning our communities – for many of us, we have to somehow find our communities; it isn't always easy to blend, to make friends, to align with our neighbours. However, if we strive to find those who nourish us and can help us, we can reciprocate. Sometimes this is too painful and tending our wounds is needed. Community can bring the most support you have ever felt, despite the worst having occurred. True community takes the ego away from just me and allows me to spread my wings and be involved.

COMMUNICATION

Asking for help. Do you do it? It is hard. Learning how to communicate well is a skill long lost for many of us with conditioning and patterned behaviour that do not serve us well. Let us learn to communicate with each other so that we might help, receive, and find ourselves and each other.

LISTENING

Just as communication is hard, so too is listening. Often we are only hearing ourselves mirrored in the words of the other, or if you're like me you might always be trying to fix things when all that is wanted is someone to hear, someone to listen with no judgement and no fixing. Listening is a skill many of us need much practice in. Some refer to deep listening as listening has become a superficial affair but if we take responsibility and tune in to the needs of others, we can begin to listen well.

PLANTS

Oh! Plants! How much wisdom, joy, and healing they hold. We all have our favourites, we all have some plants we notice and some we just don't. There is a tree on the common near me that I have noticed and been drawn to for years but only today did I really look at its leaves and see it was a hornbeam. An old beautiful hornbeam. Gifting wisdom to many if they stay for a while and listen. Plants are our peers, our mentors, our allies, our benefactors, our beauty; we exist only with them and yet many of us don't know them and all too often, destroy them or take them for granted. Let's big up the plants and find a better way.

LEARNING

We never stop learning. Every day we learn. Let's come together to share our learning, to weave each other's stories into wisdom we can embody. Through plant medicine, tending and remaining open to learning, we start to break down the structures that tame us, dull us, oppress us. We open up connection and understanding that we may have lost. We become the wild apothecary many of us dream of.

Get outside and use all your senses to begin to feel your landscape and the magic that is all around.

With love, Amaia

Wild Apothecary, Gloucestershire, 2021

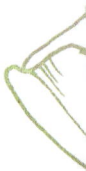

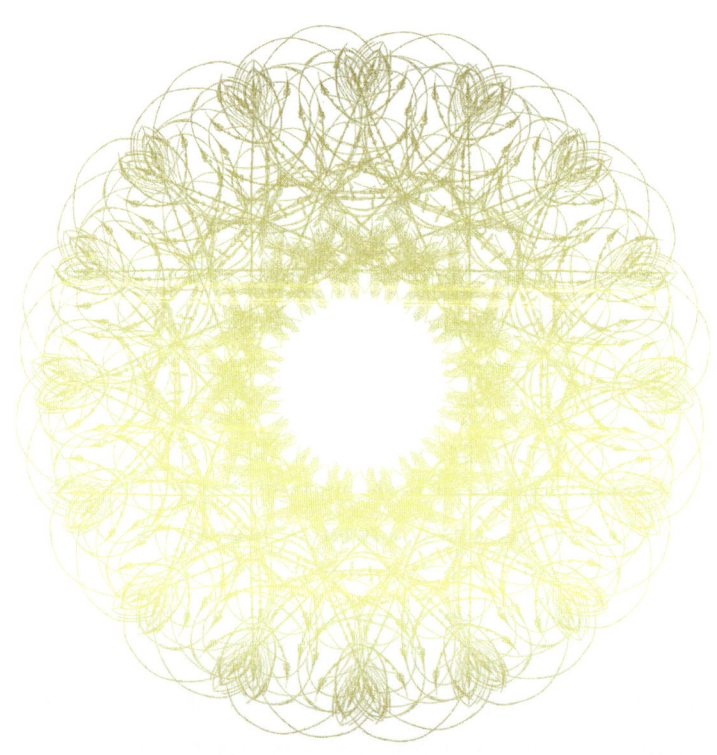

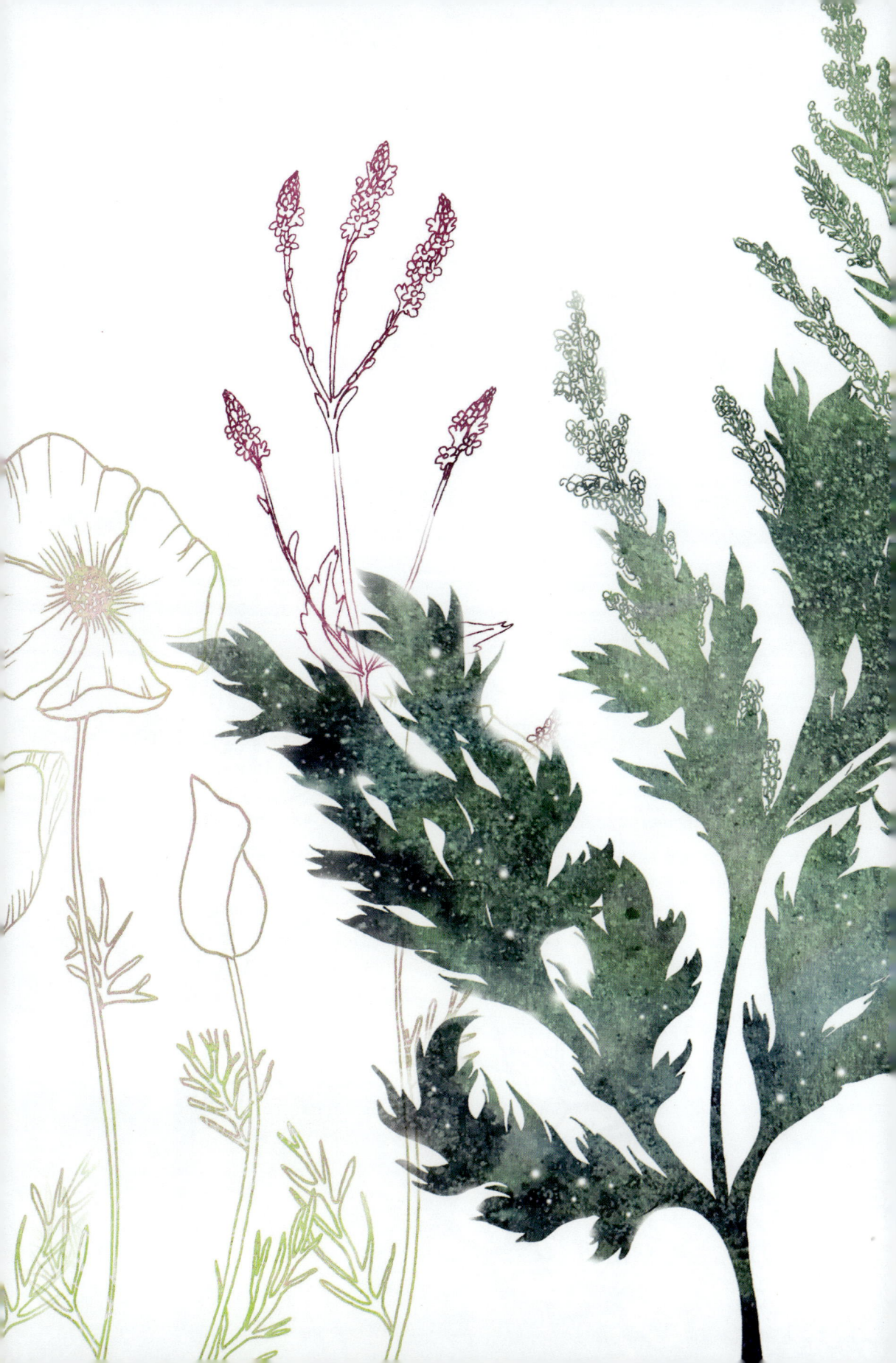

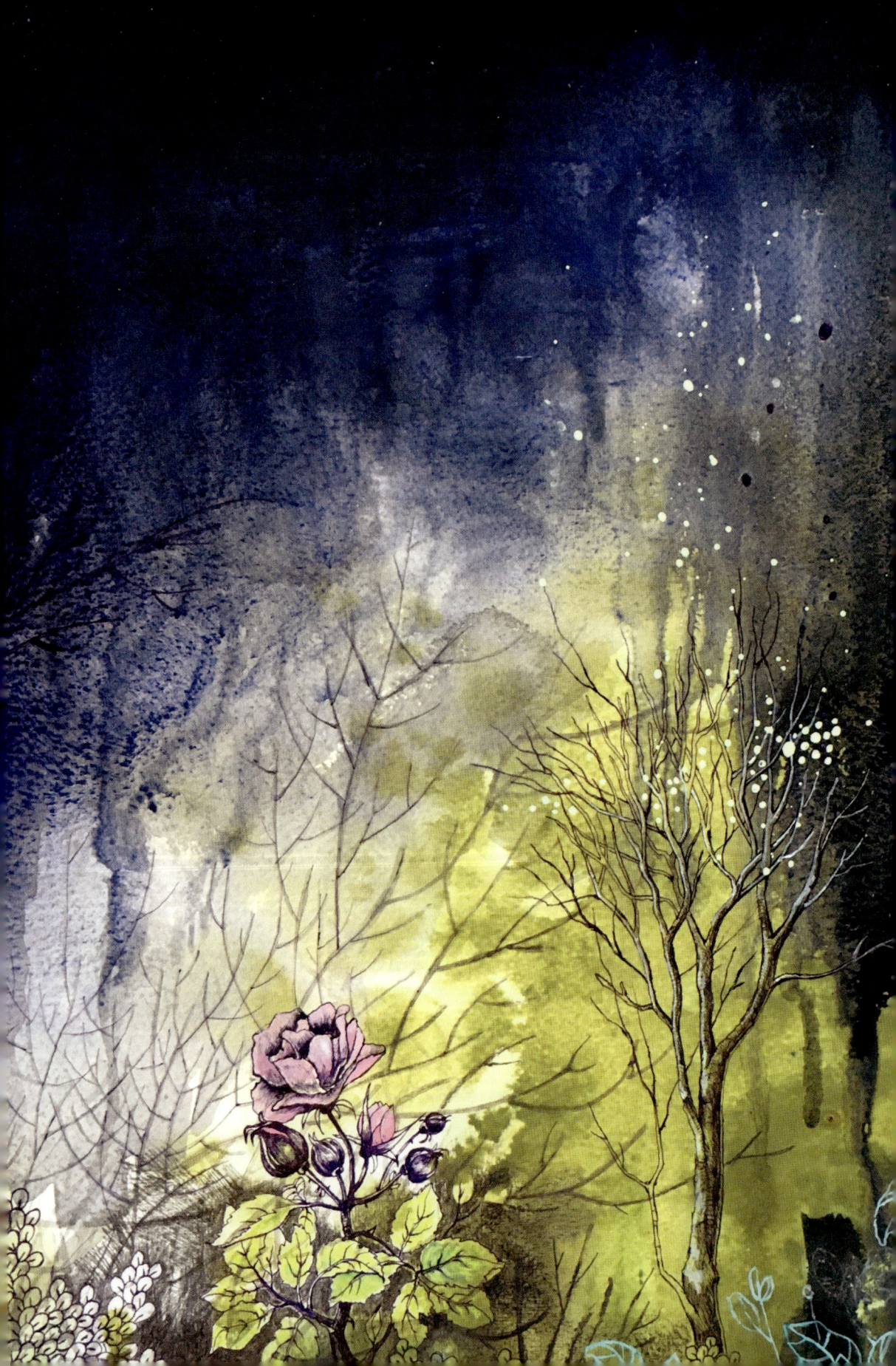

A FEW RESOURCES

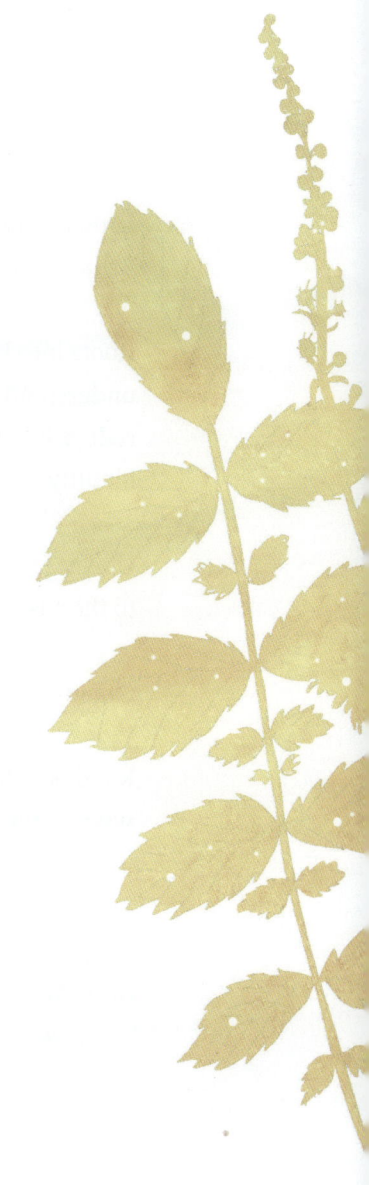

Rose and nellikai by Chitra Merchant

There are hundreds more amazing folk I could think of and thousands more I don't know but here are some for your own interest.

HERBALISM

Amaia Dadachanji MNIMH. Wild Apothecary: herbal medicine clinic, teaching, botanicals. **amaia@wildapothecary.com, wildapothecary.com**

Land Is She. Women's health, women's empowerment through land based connections, connection, rewilding, healing, intuiting, tending, landing, ceremony, plant allies, sisterhood. **landisshe.earth**

Claudia Manchanda. **claudiamanchanda@yahoo.co.uk**

Land in Our Names (LION). Reconnecting Black communities with Land in Britain, Climate Justice, Racial Justice.

Rootz into Food Growing Project. The project aims to more clearly identify, understand, plan and implement a series of interventions which subsequently reduce barriers to entry into the social enterprise growing system and begin to identify appropriate land for commercial food growing purposes.

Ubele. The Ubele Initiative is a social enterprise with a mission to contribute to the sustainability of the African Diaspora community.

Organic Lea. Workers Co-op growing food in Lea Valley London.

Kandake Makonnen, Medical herbalist, holistic consultant. **www.instrumentahealth.co.uk**

Julie James, **greenpathherbschool.com**

Anne McIntyre, **https://annemcintyre.com**

A FEW RESOURCES

Favourite books

Christopher Hedley and Non Shaw, *The Herbal Book of Making and Taking*. I still check in with the little gem when I need to!

Robin Wall Kimmerer, *Braiding Sweetgrass*. A gem of a read.

Leslie Feinberg, *Transgender Warriors: Making History from Joan of Arc to Dennis Rodman*.

Hokkanen, Markku, Kananoja, Kalle (eds.) *Healers and Empires in Global History: Healing as Hybrid and Contested Knowledge*.

Hugh Tinker, *A New System of Slavery: The Export of Indian Labour Overseas 1830–1920*, 1974.

Online

The Herbarium, **https://theherbarium.wordpress.com/**
Excellent site by different herbalists with lots of information on medicine making.

The Plant Medicine School, **www.theplantmedicineschool.com**
Nikki Darrell is a herbalist in Ireland running this school with grace and beauty.

Alice Nugent, **www.hippopot.co.uk**. Herbalist in Buckinghamshire, mixing traditional medicine from Mozambique, Mali, and Zimbabwe with Western medicine.

Rasheeqa Ahmad, **www.hedgeherbs.co.uk**. Community herbalist in London, community apothecary.

Rocio Alarcon, **www.iamoe.org**. Centre in the Ecuadorian rainforest.

Elisabeth Brooke, **www.elisabethbrooke.com**. Magical herbalism and astrology.

Rosemary Gladstar, **www.sagemountain.com**

Rebecca Altman, **www.wonderbotanica.com**

Herbalists Without Borders, **www.hwbglobal.org**. HWB local to me is in Bristol, for example: **www.bristolhwb.org** – there are others too near you (hopefully).

Radical herbalism, **www.radicalherbalism.org.uk**

Melissa Ronaldson, **www.herbalbarge.co.uk**. Community herbalist providing loads of help in the refugee camps in Calais.

Solidarity Apothecary, **www.solidarityapothecary.org**. Herbal medicine as mutual aid.

Hackney Herbal, **www.hackneyherbal.com**. Social enterprise promoting health.

Kara Sigler, San Francisco Herbalist. Information for anyone transitioning and would like to know more about herbs. Kara has made an audio recording which (at time of writing) you can access here: **http://sfherbalist.com/articles**

Queering Herbalism – free offering online resource by Toi Scott **www.static1.squarespace.com**

Queering Herbalism BIPOC group, **https://facebook.com/groups/1208833482527978**

BIPOC herbalists, **https://facebook.com/groups/2585604575085942**

Kathie Bishop, **www.intothewylde.com**. Clean, toxin free, vulva loving care – lubricant with herbs.

A FEW RESOURCES

Henriette Kress, **www.henriettes-herbal.com**. A huge site with loads of great information.

7Song, **www.7Song.com**. Lots of free articles and classes, 7Song also works in a free clinic in Ithaca, New York.

Dylan Warren Davis, **www.myddfaiherbs.co.uk**. Works in Myddfai where the Physicians of Myddfai practised and works with some of their very plants (descendants!)

Entheogens and mushroom cultivation, **https://darrenlebaron.com**

Grass Roots Remedies (Edinburgh), **www.grassrootsremedies.co.uk** Worker's co-operative with accessible herbalism.

Herbal Unity Clinic, **www.radicalherbalscotland.co.uk**

Herbalista Network (Dublin and USA), **www.herbalista.org** Mutual aid and lots of free resources.

Aviva Romm, **www.avivaromm.com** herbalist, midwife, doctor.

Kandake Makonnen, medical herbalist, holistic consultant, **www.instrumentalhealth.co.uk**

There are also many excellent books written by herbalists and plant nerds.

Herb nurseries

www.poyntzfieldherbs.co.uk, excellent herb nursery in Scotland.

https://herbsforhealing.net/ tiny herb nursery and beautiful products – run by the daughters of the late amazing Davina Wynne Jones.

WILD APOTHECARY

INSPIRATIONS

Caroline Criado Perez, **www.carolinecriadoperez.com**. Writer, speaker, campaigner – her book *Invisible Women* is a shocking account of patriarchy and how it affects women.

Hannah Gadsby, **www.hannahgadsby.com.au** Hannah's show Nanette was mind-blowingly funny and devastating.

Journeyman, **www.journeyman.co.uk**. Supporting boys in their journey to manhood.

Red School, **www.redschool.net**. Alexandra Pope and Sjarnie Hugo Wurlitzer – women's leadership, creativity, and spiritual life based on a uniquely feminine way – the menstrual cycle.

www.criposium.wordpress.com

Jennie Martin, **jenniemartin.co.uk**. 'Dirt-time'.

GRIEF AND EARTH MENTORSHIP AND PRACTICE

Azul Valerie Thome, **www.souland.org**

Sobonfu and Malidoma Somé, **www.malidoma.com**. Sobonfu was a Burkinabe teacher – her teaching in African spirituality and grief reached far and wide, **www.sobonfu.com**. Malidoma still teaches spirituality and healing.

Francis Weller, **https://francisweller.net/** Soul work, mentoring, and community building.

A FEW RESOURCES

DIVERSITY

Land In Our Names, **www.landinournames.community**. Reconnecting Black communities with land.

Ancestral Voices, **https://ancestralvoices.co.uk**

POC IN NATURE

Black Outside, **www.blackoutside.org**

Black2Nature, **www.birdgirluk.com**. Visible Minority Ethnic (VME) led campaign for equal access to nature for all VME communities.

Black Girls Hike, **www.facebook.com/bghmcr/**

Brown People Camping, **www.brownpeoplecamping.com**. Promoting greater diversity of people on public lands.

wildwise.co.uk

May Project Garden, **www.mayproject.org**. Reconnecting with nature for personal, social, and economic transformation, includes the Hip Hop garden.

ARTISTS

Chitra Parvathy Merchant, **www.chitra.co.uk**. Amazing plants and landscapes.

Lucinda Warner, **www.whisperingearth.co.uk**. Herbalist and artist, writing excellent blogs.

MUSIC

Rising Appalachia, **www.risingappalachia.com**

POETS

Indigo Mudbhary, Brown Girl. Winner Top 15 Foyle Young Poets of the Year Award 2020.

Kat Francois, **www.katfrancois.com**

RED MEDUSA, **www.poetrybyredmedusa.squarespace.com**
Mackayla Forde, RED MEDUSA is a poet, academic, and activist hailing from South-East London.

OF ADDITIONAL INTEREST

MOBS, "mothers offering breastfeeding support", **https://gbsn.org.uk/groups/mobs-stroud/** This is in my home town – see what is in yours, a great source of support.

Sprout Distro, **https://www.sproutdistro.com/catalog/zines/**

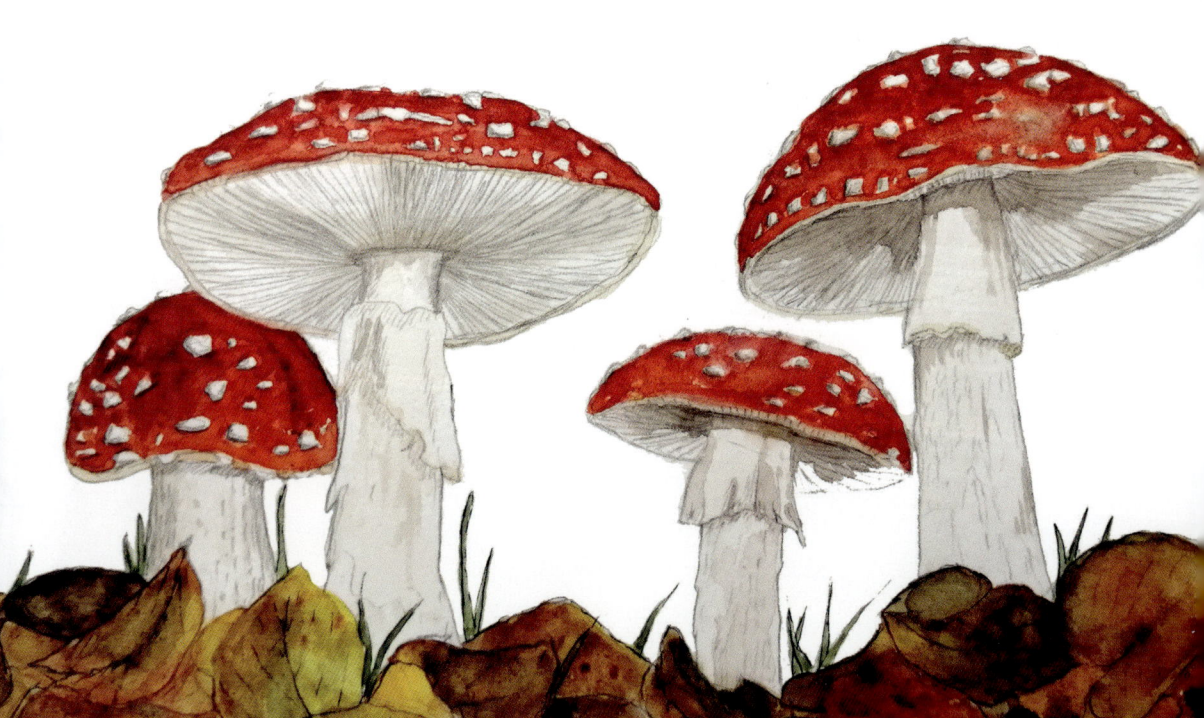

INDEX

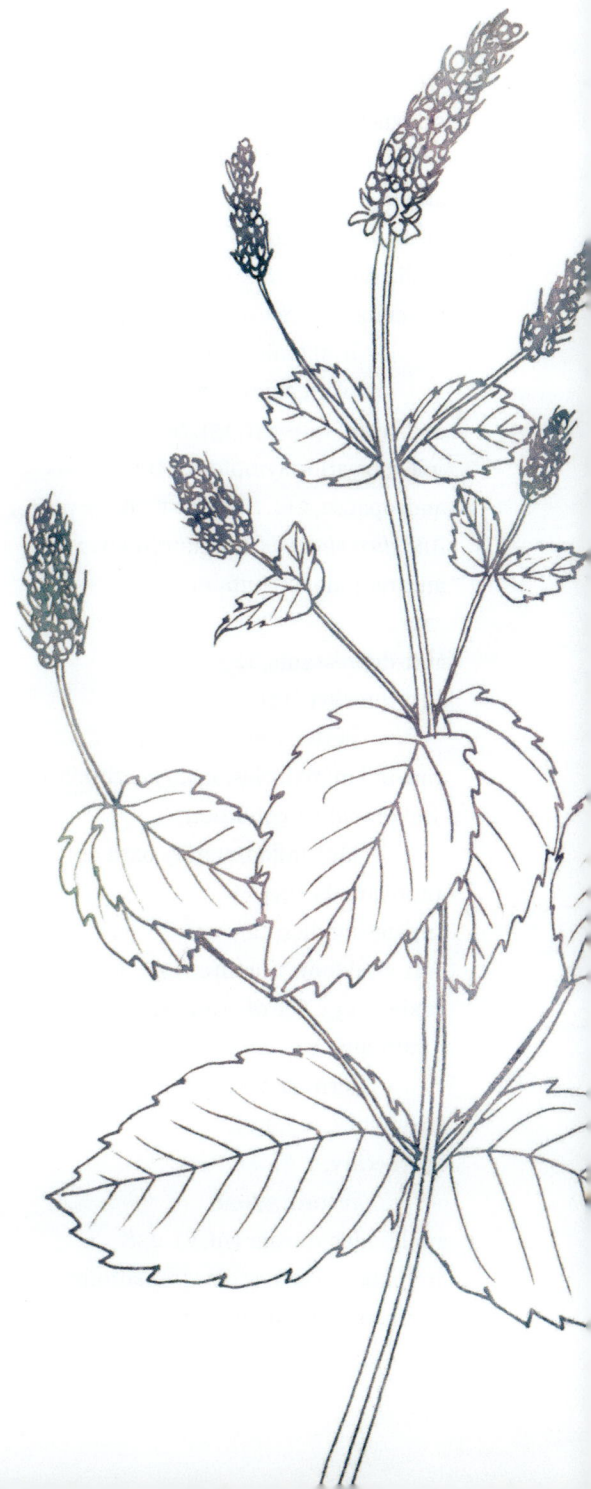

Achillea millefolium. See yarrow
acne, 130–131. *See also* menstruation symptoms
ACV. *See* apple cider vinegar
adaptogens, 127, 131, 135, 152, 223
air (sanguine), 66. *See also* energetics of wild medicine
Albizia julibrissin. See Mimosa
Alchemilla vulgaris. See lady's mantle
alfalfa, 196
alterative, 131, 240
Alzheimer, 253. *See also* dementia
anaemia, 176. *See also* pregnancy
    iron tonic, 176, 177
    plant allies, 176
androgen, 130–131, 151. *See also* menstruation symptoms; transitions
andropause, 214. *See also* men
Angelica sinensis. See dong quai
anthraquinone-containing bitters, 257
anti-depressants, 127
anti-infective, 131
    herbs, 102
anti-inflammatories, 131, 172, 240. *See also* inflammatory conditions
    anti-inflammatory bath, 239
antioxidants, 254
antispasmodics, 125, 240
anti-viral tonic tincture, 99
anxiety, 133. *See also* menstruation symptoms
    formula tincture, 135
anxiolytics, 127, 135
apothecary, x
    record, 57–58
apple cider vinegar (ACV), 258
aromatase, 151. *See also* transitions
aromatase inhibitors, 151

aromatic
    plant species, 321
    waters, 48
arthritis, 238, 240. *See also* inflammatory conditions
arthropathy, 238
ashwagandha, 221
asthma, 101. *See also* babies and children
    bronchease tea for kids, 102
astringent herbs, 92
ayahuasca, 315–318
Ayurveda, 63, 64. *See also* energetics of wild medicine

babies and children, 73
    asthma, 101–102
    bed-wetting, 96–97
    betony, 109–110
    chamomile, 105–108
    chickenpox, 98–99
    colic, 78–79
    conditions affecting, 77
    coughs and colds, 89–91
    diarrhoea, 81–82
    differences in baby's weight, 80–81
    eczema, 103–104
    energetics and elements, 74–77
    eye wash, 100
    factors affecting immunity, 89–90
    fever, 85–89
    insomnia and night terrors, 92–96
    journaling, 114
    marigold, 110–112
    measles, 100
    nappy rash, 82–83
    nourishing and caring, 75
    plant allies for children, 105–113
    rewilding exercises, 76–77
    sanguine temperament, 74

INDEX

teething, 84
tonsillitis, 91–92
yarrow, 113
baby's weight, 80–81. *See also* babies and children
Barge Chenar, 309
bedtime calm balm, 95
bed-wetting, 96–97. *See also* babies and children
beetroot, 258–259
benign prostastic hyperplasia (BPH), 214. *See also* men
    plant allies, 215–216
    prostate, 214
    stages of, 214
    tonic tincture, 216
betony (*Stachys betonica*), 109. *See also* plant allies
    calming kiddie drops, 110
binomial nomenclature, 298
"BIPOC" (Black, Indigenous, People of Colour), 296
bitters, 125, 152, 257
blackberry vinegar, 46. *See also* vinegars
black haw, 173
Black, Indigenous, People of Colour. *See* "BIPOC"
blood pressure, 247. *See also* hypertension
bones, healthy, 195–196. *See also* menopause
boney vinegar, 195. *See also* osteoporosis
Boswellia sp. See Frankincense
botanic gardens, 311–313
botany, 13–14
    understanding botanical language, 15–16
BPH. *See* benign prostastic hyperplasia
breastfeeding, 179. *See also* pregnancy
    low milk flow, 180

    mastitis, 181
    sore nipples, 181–182
breast tenderness, 129–130. *See also* menstruation symptoms
bronchease tea, 102
bronchitis, 245. *See also* lung conditions
brown bottle herbalist, 2
bulk laxatives, 257
burnt rat paw test, 304

calendar, 59
Calendula officinalis. See marigold
California poppy, 95–96
calm and nourish tonic, 127. *See also* menstruation symptoms
Capsicum annuum. See cayenne
cardiotonics and vascular tonics, 251. *See also* hypertension
carminative herbs, 78, 79
cayenne (*Capsicum annuum*), 263–264
celery family, 17–18
cerebral circulatory stimulants, 254
ceremony, 26–27, 28. *See also* natural cycles
chamomile (*Matricaria recutita*), 81, 105–108. *See also* plant allies
    German, 86
    hydrosol, 83
    and yarrow bath, 88
chasteberry (*Vitex agnus castus*), 173, 184, 203–204. *See also* plant allies
chest rubs, 91
chickenpox, 98–99. *See also* babies and children
    anti-viral tonic tincture, 99
    cooling gel, 99
Chinese angelica, 205
choleric. *See* fire
choleric humour, 117

Christopher's calendula (marigold) cream, 54. *See also* creams
chronic obstructive pulmonary disorder (COPD), 245
circulatory stimulants, 240
circumcision, 218. *See also* men
    plant allies, 219
    rewilding visualization, 219–220
cleavers (*Galium aparine*), 137. *See also* plant allies
cold. *See also* hot flush
    sage tea, 192
    vegetables, 84
colic, 78. *See also* babies and children
    tummy love tea, 79
colonialism, 294, 295. *See also* radical roots and decolonial reflections
    Britain colonies, 295
    colonial ideology, 321
    impact of, 296
    legacy of nineteenth-century, 298–299
comfrey
    infused oil, 51–52
    leaf, 241
    ointment, 53
compresses, 57. *See also* external remedies
constipation, 257. *See also* elders
    daily beetroot, 258–259
    plant allies, 257–259
cool and calm tea, 192. *See also* hot flush
cooling. *See also* hot flush
    gel, 99
    insomnia mix, 192
COPD. *See* chronic obstructive pulmonary disorder
coughs and colds, 89–90, 91. *See also* babies and children
COX 2 enzyme, 186
crampbark, 173
creams, 53. *See also* external remedies
    marigold cream, 54
crone goddess drops, 194. *See also* depression and anxiety
Culpeper, N., 310
cultivation of herbs, 11. *See also* herbalism
    botany, 13–14
    drawing, 20
    herbarium, 19
    herb sovereignty, 20–22
    nomenclature, 18
    own herbs, 11–13
    plant families, 16–18
    plant initiation, 22–23
    rewilding exercise, 14, 19, 20
    tastings, 23–25
    understanding botanical language, 15–16
Curcuma longa. *See* turmeric

D&C. *See* dilation and curettage
daisy family, 17
damiana (*Turnera diffusa*), 173, 197, 221, 227–228. *See also* plant allies
decoctions, 43. *See also* wild apothecary
    reduced, 43–44
deep breathe tea, 247. *See also* lung conditions
dementia, 253. *See also* elders
    dusk and, 254
    memory, 254
    memory boosting smoothie, 255
    plant allies, 254–255
depression and anxiety, 192–193. *See also* menopause
    crone goddess drops, 194
    no more anxietea, 193
    plant allies, 193–194
DHT. *See* dihydrotestosterone
diarrhoea, 81–82. *See also* babies

INDEX

and children
dihydrotestosterone (DHT), 213
dilation and curettage (D&C), 187
dioecious, 309
dirt time, 8, 11
disease, 63
diuretic herbs, 256
dong quai (*Angelica sinensis*), 173, 186, 199, 205. *See also* plant allies
doshas, 64. *See also* energetics of wild medicine
drawing, 20
dried herbs, 33. *See also* wild apothecary

ear infection oil, 100
earth (melancholic), 66. *See also* energetics of wild medicine; women
    temperament, 167
Ebers Papyrus, 319
eczema, 103. *See also* babies and children
    skin-calm balm, 104
    skin-ease cream, 104
    triggers, 103
elder and echinacea tincture, 88
elderberry syrup, 44–45. *See also* syrups
elders, 233
    arthritis, 238
    bronchitis, 245
    cayenne, 263–264
    conditions affecting, 238
    constipation, 257–259
    dementia, 253–255
    energetics and elements, 235
    hypertension, 247–252
    incontinence, 255–257
    inflammatory conditions, 238–244
    journaling, 273
    lung conditions, 244–247
    medicinal mushrooms, 271–272
    metaphor for body, 235
    nettle, 269–270
    osteoarthritis, 238
    phlegmatic time of life, 235
    plant allies for, 259–260
    pneumonia, 244
    rewilding exercise, 235–237
    rosemary, 265–266
    sage, 261–262
    turmeric, 267–268
    ulcers, 252–253
    useful herbs for, 261–272
elemental elixirs, 154. *See also* transitions
elitism, 313, 315. *See also* radical roots and decolonial reflections
endogenous hormones, 150. *See also* transitions
endometriosis, 185–187. *See also* gynaecological conditions
energetics of wild medicine, 61
    air (sanguine), 66
    earth (melancholic), 66
    elements affecting temperaments, 66–68
    energetics and elements, 62–66
    fire (choleric), 66
    flavours affecting our body, 67
    gender specific herbalism, 62
    herbs for particular actions, 68–69
    humours of body, 63
    modern herbalists, 65
    system of philosophy based healing, 62
    tastes and feelings, 67
    temperature of herbs, 68
    virtues of herbs, 66
    water (phlegmatic), 67–68
Epigenetics, 304–305
erectile dysfunction, 220. *See also* men

    plant allies, 221–222
    sexual stimulation, 221
expectoration, 44
external remedies, 51. *See also*
 wild apothecary
    compresses, 57
    creams, 53–54
    infused oils, 51–52
    liniments, 55–56
    lotions, 56
    ointments, 52–53
    poultices, 57
eye wash, 100. *See also* babies and children

fatigue, 135–136. *See also* menstruation symptoms
feminising herbs, 151. *See also* transitions
fennel (*Foeniculum vulgare*), 157–158
fertility, 169–171, 222.
 See also men; women
    fertilitea, 174
    plant allies, 172–174, 222–223
    tonic for men, 223
    yoga, 174
fever, 85–88. *See also* babies and children
feverfew, 128, 186
fibroids, 185. *See also* gynaecological conditions
fire (choleric), 66. *See also* energetics of wild medicine
fleeceflower, 223
flower remedies, 50–51. *See also* wild apothecary
Foeniculum vulgare. See fennel
follicle stimulating hormone (FSH), 150
foraging, 2, 3
forms of body, 64. *See also* energetics of wild medicine
Frankincense (*Boswellia sp.*), 318
FSH. *See* follicle stimulating hormone

GAD. *See* generalised anxiety disorder
galactogogues, 180
Galen, 65
Galium aparine. See cleavers
Ganoderma lucidum. See Reishi
Gardeners' Chronicle, 312
gargles, 44. *See also* wild apothecary
gender dysphoria, 145. *See also* transitions
genderisation, 144. *See also* transitions
genders, 144
generalised anxiety disorder (GAD), 133
gentle bitters, 257
German chamomile, 86.
 See also chamomile
ginger, 128, 176, 186
ginkgo, 102, 221–222
ginseng ren shen (*Panax ginseng*), 222, 229. *See also* plant allies
glycerine, 44
Glycyrrhiza glabra. See liquorice
gotu kola, 186
grief, 275
    energetics, 276
    five gates of grief, 278
    lemon balm brandy, 283
    lemon balm, 283–284
    plant allies, 281–286
    rewilding exercise, 279
    rose, 281–282
    vervain, 285–286
    wild heart healing elixir, 282
gynaecological conditions, 182.
 See also women
    endometriosis, 185–187
    fibroids, 185
    pelvic inflammatory disease, 189
    polycystic ovarian syndrome, 182–184

INDEX

harvesting, 3, 8–11. *See also* wild crafting
    and preparing local plants, 305–306
hawthorn, 250
    heart brandy, 252
headaches /migraines, 127–128. *See also* menstruation symptoms
    drops for premenstrual, 129
healing based on philosophy, 62
healthcare system in Britain, xvii
heartease tea, 250. *See also* hypertension
heart protect chai, 252. *See also* hypertension
hepatics (liver herbs), 127, 131, 152
herb. *See also* cultivation of herbs; wild apothecary
    androgenic, 151
    anti-infective, 102
    antispasmodic, 125, 240
    for arthritis and rheumatism, 240
    feminising, 151
    fennel, 157–158
    for fevers, 86–87
    for particular actions, 68–69
    important, 34–37
    liquorice, 159–160
    liver, 223
    progesteronic, 151
    red clover, 161
    sourcing, 33
    sovereignty, 20–22
    temperature of herbs, 68
    virtues of, 66
herbal
    antibiotics, 187
    medicine, 307
    roots, 87
herbalism, 2
    approaching the plant, 4–6
    astrology in, xviii
    "BIPOC" health and, xvii–xviii
    botany, 13–14
    ceremony, 26–27, 28
    cultivation of herbs, 11
    dirt time, 8, 11
    drawing, 20
    ethical wild crafting of herbs, 3–4
    ethics of intention, 4
    foraging, 2
    gathering medicine, 6–8
    growing own herbs, 11–13
    harvesting, 3, 8–11
    herbarium, 19
    herb/plant sovereignty, 20–22
    journaling /sketching, 6
    kinds of medicines, 38
    labeling herbs, 2
    natural cycles, 25
    nature literacy, 7
    nature's gems, 27–29
    nomenclature, 18
    patch, 8
    plant families, 16–18
    plant initiation, 22–23
    rewilding exercise, 5–6, 14, 19, 20, 26, 29
    tastings, 23–25
    understanding botanical language, 15–16
herbalist, becoming, 331
    communication, 333
    community, 333
    learning, 334
    listening, 333
    plants, 333
Herbalists Without Borders (HWB), 324, 325

herbalist toolkit, 40. *See also* wild apothecary
    general materials, 41
    tools, 40
herbal medicine and science, 303–305
Herbal Rebellion: Stroud Community Medicine Garden, 21
herbal teas, 41. *See also* wild apothecary
    for babies, 79
    bronchease tea, 102
    cold infusions, 43
    fever tea, 88
    guide to make, 42
    teething tea, 84
    tummy love tea, 79
    wild woman tea blend, 42
herbarium, 19
Hericium erinaceus. *See* Lion's mane
Hippocrates, 62–63, 64
hirsutism, 183
holism, 306
holistic medicine, 295. *See also* radical roots and decolonial reflections
hops, 196
hormone
    modulation, 127, 131
    regulation/fertility tonic, 172
hormone replacement therapy (HRT), 189
horny goat weed, 222
hot comfrey balm, 242. *See also* inflammatory conditions
hot flush, 191. *See also* menopause
    cold sage tea, 192
    cool and calm tea, 192
    cooling insomnia mix, 192
    plant allies, 191–192
    tonic, 191
HPA. *See* hypothalamus pituitary adrenal
HRT. *See* hormone replacement therapy

humour, 166. *See also* energetics of wild medicine
    of body, 63
    melancholic, 166
HWB. *See* Herbalists Without Borders
hydrosols, 48–49. *See also* wild apothecary
hydrotherapy, 124
hyperemesis gravidarum, 175–176. *See also* pregnancy
hypertension, 247. *See also* elders
    blood pressure, 247
    cardiotonics and vascular tonics, 251
    diet and life style, 248
    galactic heart and plant allies, 251
    hawthorn heart brandy, 252
    heartease tea, 250
    heart protect chai, 252
    plant allies, 250–252
    rewilding exercise, 248
hypogonadism, 222
hypothalamus pituitary adrenal (HPA), 126

Igbo'gi (yorubá medicine), 320
Imhotep, 62–63
immunity. *See also* babies and children
    factors affecting, 89–90
    modulators, 216
    support, 172
incense, 317
incontinence, 255. *See also* elders
    lifestyle, 256
    overflow, 256
    plant allies, 256–257
    stress, 256
    total, 256
    urge, 256
indigenous, 296
infertility, 171. *See also* fertility

inflammatory conditions, 238.
  See also elders
    anti-inflammatory bath, 239
    arthritis, 238
    diet and life style, 239
    herbs for arthritis and
      rheumatism, 240
    hot comfrey balm, 242
    nettle stings, 244
    osteoarthritis, 238
    recipes, 241–243
    rheuma tea, 241
    wild heat bath salts, 243
inflammatory foods, 182
infused oils, 51. See also external
  remedies
    comfrey, 51–52
infusions. See herbal teas
insomnia and night terrors, 92–93. See also
  babies and children
    bedtime calm balm, 95
    exercise, 93–94
    night ease drops, 96
    rewilding exercise, 93
iron tonic, 176, 177
irritant purgatives, 257
itadori (*Polygonum cuspidatum*),
  307–308

journaling, 58–59, 206, 230. See also
  wild crafting
    aspects of, 230
    about childhood, 114
    feel in winter, 273
    menstrual cycle and fertility, 206
    moon cycle, 141
    sketching, 6
    transitions, 162
jujube, 199

Kahun Papyrus, 320
kava kava (*Piper mythesticum*), 306–307
kidney tonics, 152

labeling herbs, 2
lady's mantle (*Alchemilla vulgaris*), 173,
  201–202. See also plant allies
Land in Our Names (LION), 338
lavender, 196–197
LD 50. See lethal dose test
lemon balm (*Melissa officinalis*), 283–284.
  See also tinctures
    brandy, 283
    specific tincture, 47–48
lethal dose test (LD 50), 305
LH. See luteinising hormone
Ling zhi. See Reishi
liniments, 55. See also external remedies
    cooling, 56
    heating, 55
Linnaeus, C., 298–300
LION. See Land in Our Names
Lion's mane (*Hericium erinaceus*), 271.
  See also medicinal mushrooms
liquorice (*Glycyrrhiza glabra*), 159–160,
  184, 213
liver
    herbs, 223. See hepatics
    support, 172
London plane trees, 308–309
loose stools, 125–126. See also menstruation symptoms
lotions, 56. See also external remedies
lung conditions, 244. See also elders
    bronchitis, 245
    deep breathe tea, 247
    galactic lungs and plant allies, 245
    plant allies, 246–247
    pneumonia, 244
    rewilding exercise, 246

luteinising hormone (LH), 150
lymphatics, 127, 131

male pattern baldness, 213. *See also* men
marigold (*Calendula officinalis*), 179, 182, 196, 110–112, 253. *See also* plant allies
    Christopher's calendula (marigold) cream, 54
mastitis, 181. *See also* breastfeeding
Matricaria recutita. *See* chamomile
measles, 100. *See also* babies and children
medical papyri, 319
medicinal mushrooms, 271
    Lion's mane, 271
    Reishi, 271
    Turkey tail, 272
medicine making, 38–39. *See also* wild apothecary
melancholic. *See* earth
melancholic humour, 166
melancholic work, 166
Melissa officinalis. *See* lemon balm
memory boosting smoothie, 255. *See also* dementia
men, 209
    andropause, 214
    benign prostastic hyperplasia, 214–216
    circumcision, 218–220
    conditions affecting, 213
    energetics and elements, 210–211
    erectile dysfunction, 220–222
    fertility, 222–223
    journaling, 230
    male pattern baldness, 213
    orchitis, 216
    patriarchy, 210
    plant allies for all men, 225–229
    rewilding exercises, 211–212
    toxic masculinity, 211

menarche, 120. *See also* periods
menopause, 167, 189. *See also* women
    depression and anxiety in, 192–194
    healthy bones, 195–196
    hot flushes, 191–192
    HRT and mainstream treatment of, 189
    osteoporosis, 194–195
    phytoestrogens in, 199–200
    stages of, 189
    vaginal dryness, 196–198
menstrual cramps, 124. *See also* menstruation symptoms
    no cramps tincture, 125
menstruation symptoms, 124
    acne, 130–131
    acne infusion, 131
    androgens, 130–131
    anxiety, 133
    anxiety formula tincture, 135
    breast tenderness, 129
    calm and nourish tonic, 127
    constipation or loose stools, 125–126
    fatigue, 135–136
    headaches, 127–128
    menstrual cramps, 124
    moods, 126–127, 132–133
    no cramps tincture, 125
    nourish tea, 136
    plant allies, 125, 127, 128–129, 131, 135, 136
    premenstrual headache drops, 129
    tea for anger, 132
    tea for scared, emotional youth, 133
    tender breast tea, 130

INDEX

migraine. *See* headaches/migraines
Millennium Seed Bank at Kew, 311
Mimosa, 193
mint family, 16–17
mittelschmerz, 187
MOBS. *See* mothers offering breastfeeding support
modern
    herbalists, 65
    herbal medicine, 294
modernity, 294. *See also* radical roots and decolonial reflections
monoecious, 309
mood, 132–133. *See also* menstruation symptoms
    changes, 126–127
moon pain mix, 189. *See also* pelvic inflammatory disease
mothers offering breastfeeding support (MOBS), 78
motherwort, 250
mugwort, 126
myrrh, 253
    tincture, 83

nappy rash, 82–83. *See also* babies and children
National Trust, 323
natural cycles, 25. *See also* herbalism
    ceremony, 26–27, 28
    living in city, 29
    nature's gems, 27–29
    rewilding exercise, 26, 29
nature literacy, 7
nature's gems, 27–29. *See also* natural cycles
nausea, 175–176. *See also* pregnancy
nervine, 131, 135, 146
    cooling, 132

nerviness, 94, 97, 152
    betony, 109–110
nettle (*Urtica dioica*), xviii, 176, 269–270. *See also* inflammatory conditions
    beer, 269
    root, 215
    stings, 244
night ease drops, 96
nocturnal enuresis, 96
nomenclature, 18
no more anxietea, 193. *See also* depression and anxiety
nourishing juice, 153. *See also* transitions
nourish tea, 136. *See also* menstruation symptoms

oat sock, 99
Obeah Act 1898, 319. *See also* radical roots and decolonial reflections
oestrogen blockers, 151. *See also* transitions
ointments, 52–53. *See also* external remedies
old wives' tales, 21
opium dependence in China, 302
orchitis, 216. *See also* men
osteoarthritis, 238. *See also* inflammatory conditions
osteoporosis, 194. *See also* menopause
    boney vinegar, 195
    plant allies, 194–195
oxymel, 47. *See also* vinegars

padsicles, 178
Panax ginseng. *See* ginseng ren shen
Passiflora incarnata. *See* passionflower
passionflower (*Passiflora incarnata*), 138. *See also* plant allies
    and skullcap, 94
patch, 8
patriarchy, 166, 210. *See also* men

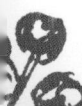

PCOS. *See* polycystic ovarian syndrome
pelvic inflammatory disease (PID), 187.
  See also gynaecological conditions
    moon pain mix, 189
    plant allies, 187–189
peony, 184
peppermint oil, 128
perfect flowers, 309
periods, 120
    menarche, 120
    rewilding exercise, 121–123
    vagina, 122
Persian silk tree. *See* Mimosa
phlegmatic. *See* water
phytoandrogens, 150
phytoestrogens, 150, 151, 194
    dong quai, 199
    jujube, 199
    in menopause, 199–200
    red clover, 199
    sage, 199
    shatavari, 199
    wild yam, 199
phytoprogesterones, 150
phytotestosterones, 150
PID. *See* pelvic inflammatory disease
Piper mythesticum. See kava kava
plant. *See also* radical roots and decolonial reflections
    appropriation, 301–303, 315–318
    initiation, 22–23
    matter, 32
plant allies, 184
    betony, 109–110
    chamomile, 105–108
    chasteberry, 203–204
    for children, 105. *See also* babies and children
    cleavers, 137
    damiana, 227–228
    dong quai, 205
    ginseng ren shen, 229
    lady's mantle, 201–202
    marigold, 110–112
    for men, 225. *See also* men
    passionflower, 138
    saw palmetto, 225–227
    skullcap, 139
    transitions, 149, 150–156
    violets, 140
    for women, 201
    yarrow, 113
    for youth, 137
pneumonia, 244. *See also* lung conditions
pollarding, 308
polycystic ovarian syndrome (PCOS), 182.
  See also gynaecological conditions
    galactic womb and plant allies, 183
    plant allies, 184
    symptoms, 183
    tincture blend, 184
Polygonum cuspidatum. See itadori
post-partum care, 178. *See also* pregnancy
poultices, 57. *See also* external remedies
pregnancy, 174–175. *See also* women
    anaemia in, 176–177
    bloom tea, 174, 175
    breastfeeding and associated conditions, 179
    conditions affecting woman in, 175
    low milk flow, 180
    mastitis, 181
    nausea and hyperemesis graidarum, 175–176
    post-partum care, 178
    sore nipples, 181–182
    varicose veins in, 177–178
progesteronic herbs, 151. *See also* transitions

pruritic urticarial papules and plaques of pregnancy (PUPPP), 178
PUPPP. *See* pruritic urticarial papules and plaques of pregnancy

radical
    health practitioners, 324
    herbalism, 323–329
    herbal network, 323–329
radical roots and decolonial reflections, 291
    anti-blackness, 319–323
    appropriation and ayahuasca, 315–318
    binomial nomenclature, 298
    botanic gardens, 311–313
    Britain colonies, 295
    burnt rat paw test, 304
    Carolus linnaeus, 298–300
    colonial ideology, 321
    colonialism, 294, 295
    impact of colonialism, 296
    elitism, 313, 315
    exploitation of Black women, 321
    Frankincense, 318
    Gardeners' Chronicle, 312
    harvesting and preparing local plants, 305–306
    HBW, 324, 325
    herbal extract testing standard, 305
    herbal medicine and science, 303–305
    holism, 306
    incense, 317
    itadori, 307–308
    kava kava, 306–307
    legacy of nineteenth-century colonialism, 298–299
    London plane trees, 308–309
    Millennium Seed Bank at Kew, 311
    modernity, 294
    Nicolas Culpeper, 310
    Obeah Act 1898, 319
    opium dependence in China, 302
    perfect flowers, 309
    persecution, 310–311
    plant appropriation, 301–303
    practice of holistic medicine, 295
    radical health practitioners, 324
    radical herbalism and network, 323–329
    shaman, 316
    shamanism, 316
    simples, 307
    smudging, 317
    taxonomy, 298
    tea, 301–302
    tea plantation, 302
    trees as medicine, 318–319
    West African herbal medicine, 320
    Witchcraft Act, 310
raspberry leaf, 173
red clover (*Trifolium pretense*), 161, 199
rehmannia, 187
Reishi (*Ganoderma lucidum*), 271. *See also* medicinal mushrooms
resources, 337–344
rewilding, xx–xxii
rheum, 238
rheuma tea, 241. *See also* inflammatory conditions
rooting tea, 155. *See also* transitions
Rosa damascene. *See* rose
rose (*Rosa damascene*), 281–282
    family, 16
rosemary (*Salvia rosmarinus*), 213, 265–266

saamagri, 316
sage (*Salvia officinalis*), 199, 261–262

Salvia officinalis. See sage
Salvia rosmarinus. *See* rosemary
sanguine. *See* air
sanguine temperament, 74
saw palmetto (*Serenoa repens*), 213, 215, 223, 225–227. *See also* plant allies
science, 303
Scutellaria lateriflora. *See* skullcap
sedatives, 135
self-love elixir, 153. *See* also transitions
Serenoa repens. See saw palmetto
sex determination, 149. *See also* transitions
sexual identity, 144. *See also* transitions
shaman, 316
shamanism, 64, 316
shatavari, 173, 197, 199
simples, 307
skin-calm balm, 104
skullcap (*Scutellaria lateriflora*), 139. *See also* plant allies
slippery elm, 81
slow-releasing carbohydrates, 125
smudging, 317
soothing herbs, 256
specific tincture (ST), 48
ST. *See* specific tincture
Stachys betonica. *See* betony
steroidal saponins, 150
St John's wort, 39
stress relief, 172
syrups, 33. *See also* wild apothecary
    elderberry syrup, 44–45

Taraxacum officinale radix, 323
tastings, 23
    and feelings, 25
    tea, 24
taxonomy, 298
tea, 301
    for anger, 132
    plantation, 302
    for scared, emotional youth, 133
    tender breast tea, 130
teething, 84. *See also* babies and children
testosterone. *See also* transitions
    hormonal replacement therapy, 152
    production blockers, 151
throat spray, 91
tinctures, 33. *See also* wild apothecary
    lemon balm, 47–48
tonsillitis, 91–92. *See also* babies and children
toxic masculinity, 211. *See also* men
Trametes versicolor. *See* Turkey tail
transitions, 143
    androgenic herbs, 151
    androgen receptor blockers, 151
    aromatase inhibitors, 151
    elemental elixirs, 154
    endogenous hormones, 150
    energetics, 146
    feminising herbs, 151
    fennel, 157–158
    gender dysphoria, 145
    genderisation, 144
    journaling, 162
    liquorice, 159–160
    nourishing juice, 153
    oestrogen blockers, 151
    and plant allies, 149, 150–156
    progesteronic herbs, 151
    red clover, 161
    rewilding exercise, 147–148
    rooting tea, 155
    self-love elixir, 153
    sex determination, 149
    sexual identity, 144
    social constructions of gender

INDEX

    binary, 144–145
    testosterone production blockers, 151
trees as medicine, 318–319
Trifolium pretense. See red clover
Turkey tail (*Trametes versicolor*), 272. *See also* medicinal mushrooms
turmeric (*Curcuma longa*), 267–268
Turnera diffusa. See damiana

ulcers, 252, 253. *See also* elders
urticaria, xviii

vagina, 122. *See also* periods
vaginal dryness, 196. *See also* menopause
    galactic vulva, 197
    plant allies, 196–198
    vaginal pessaries for dryness, 198
Varicella zoster virus, 98
varicose. *See also* ulcers
    ulcers, 253
    veins, 177–178
Verbena officinalis. See vervain
vervain (*Verbena officinalis*), 186, 285–286
vinegars, 46. *See also* wild apothecary
    blackberry, 46
    oxymel, 47
Viola odorata. See violets
violets (*Viola odorata*), 140. *See also* plant allies
vitamins, 90
Vitex agnus castus. See chasteberry

water (phlegmatic), 67–68. *See also* energetics of wild medicine
West African Dogon people, 320
West African herbal medicine, 320. *See also* radical roots and decolonial reflections
Western herbal medicine, 296, 297
white peony, 187

wild, x. *See also* inflammatory conditions
    bath salts, 243
    heart healing elixir, 282
    tree resins, 318
    woman tea blend, 42. *See also* herbal teas
    yam, 199
wild apothecary, x, 31
    calendar, 59
    choice of herb sourcing, 33
    compresses, 57
    creams, 53–54
    creating, 38–41
    decoctions, 43–44
    dried herbs, 33
    external remedies, 51–57
    flower remedies, 50–51
    gargles, 44
    herbalist toolkit, 40–41
    herbal teas, 41–44
    hydrosols, 48–49
    important herbs, 34–37
    infused oils, 51–52
    journaling, 58–59
    liniments, 55–56
    lotions, 56
    medicines, 41
    ointments, 52–53
    poultices, 57
    record, 57–58
    syrups, 33, 44–45
    tinctures, 33, 47–48
    vinegars, 46–47
    ways to connect with plants, 32
wild crafting, 3–4. *See also* herbalism
    approaching plant, 4–6
    ethics of intention, 4
    gathering medicine, 6–8
    harvesting, 8–11
    journaling, 6

rewilding exercise, 5–6
Witchcraft Act, 310. *See also* radical roots and decolonial reflections
women, 165
    anaemia in pregnancy, 176–177
    breastfeeding and associated conditions, 179
    chasteberry, 203–204
    conditions affecting pregnant woman, 175–182
    dong quai, 205
    earth temperament, 167
    endometriosis, 185–187
    energetics and elements, 166
    fertility, 169–174
    fibroids, 185
    gynaecological conditions, 182–189
    infertility, 171
    journaling, 206
    lady's mantle, 201–202
    low flow breast milk, 180
    mastitis, 181
    melancholic humour, 166
    melancholic work, 166
    menopause, 167, 189
    nausea and hyperemesis graidarum, 175–176
    pelvic inflammatory disease, 187–189
    plant allies for, 201
    polycystic ovarian syndrome, 182–184
    post-partum care, 178
    pregnancy, 174–175
    rewilding exercises, 167–168
    sore nipples, 181–182
    varicose veins in pregnancy, 177–178
wood betony, 95

yarrow (*Achillea millefolium*), 113. *See also* plant allies
    bath, 88
Yin elements, 167
yorubá medicine. *See* Igbo'gi
youth, 117
    acne, 130–131
    anxiety, 133–135
    breast tenderness, 129–130
    choleric humour, 117
    cleavers, 137
    conditions affecting, 120
    constipation or loose stools, 125–126
    energetics and elements, 118–119
    fatigue, 135–136
    headaches or migraines, 127–129
    journaling, 141
    menstrual cramps, 124
    mood changes, 126–127
    moods, 132–133
    passionflower, 138
    periods, 120–124
    plant allies for, 137–140
    rewilding exercise, 118–119
    skullcap, 139
    symptoms accompanying menstruation, 124
    violets, 140